Public Health: Emerging Issues and Innovative Solutions

Public Health: Emerging Issues and Innovative Solutions

Edited by Joshua Grayson

hayle
medical

New York

Hayle Medical,
750 Third Avenue, 9th Floor,
New York, NY 10017, USA

Visit us on the World Wide Web at:
www.haylemedical.com

ISBN: 978-1-63241-748-0

Cataloging-in-Publication Data

Public health : emerging issues and innovative solutions / edited by Joshua Grayson.
    p. cm.
Includes bibliographical references and index.
ISBN 978-1-63241-748-0
1. Public health. 2. Medical care. 3. Health care reform. I. Grayson, Joshua.
RA425 .P83 2019
613--dc23

Table of Contents

Permissions

List of Contributors

Index

Preface

This book was inspired by the evolution of our times; to answer the curiosity of inquisitive minds. Many developments have occurred across the globe in the recent past which has transformed the progress in the field.

Public health is concerned with the prevention of diseases and the promotion of human health through organized efforts of society, organizations, communities and individuals. Some of the common sub-branches of public health include environmental health, sexual and reproductive health, gender issues in health, community health, and mental health and occupational safety. Distribution of condoms, delivery of vaccinations and promotion of breastfeeding are some important preventive public health measures. The personnel involved in promoting public health mainly consist of public health nurses, epidemiologists, midwives, medical assistants and environmental health officers. This book is a compilation of chapters that discuss the most vital concepts and emerging trends in the field of public health. It explores all the important aspects of public health in the present day scenario. For all readers who are interested in this discipline, the case studies included in this book will serve as an excellent guide to develop a comprehensive understanding.

This book was developed from a mere concept to drafts to chapters and finally compiled together as a complete text to benefit the readers across all nations. To ensure the quality of the content we instilled two significant steps in our procedure. The first was to appoint an editorial team that would verify the data and statistics provided in the book and also select the most appropriate and valuable contributions from the plentiful contributions we received from authors worldwide. The next step was to appoint an expert of the topic as the Editor-in-Chief, who would head the project and finally make the necessary amendments and modifications to make the text reader-friendly. I was then commissioned to examine all the material to present the topics in the most comprehensible and productive format.

I would like to take this opportunity to thank all the contributing authors who were supportive enough to contribute their time and knowledge to this project. I also wish to convey my regards to my family who have been extremely supportive during the entire project.

Editor

1

Using the Theory of Planned Behavior to Explain Expecting Couples Birth Preparedness Intentions in a Rural Setting: A Cross-Sectional Study from Rukwa, Southern Tanzania

Fabiola V. Moshi ⓘ,[1] **Stephen M. Kibusi** ⓘ,[1] **and Flora Fabian**[2]

[1]School of Nursing and Public Health, The University of Dodoma, P.O. Box 259, Dodoma, Tanzania
[2]School of Medicine and Dentistry, The University of Dodoma, P.O. Box 259, Dodoma, Tanzania

Correspondence should be addressed to Fabiola V. Moshi; fabiola.moshi@gmail.com

Academic Editor: Carol J. Burns

Background. According to the Theory of Planned Behavior, an intention to carry out a certain behavior facilitates action. In the context of planning for birth, certain preparations and planning may better ensure maternal and neonatal survival. Little is known on the predictors of birth preparedness intention among expecting couples. The aim of this study was to determine the predictors of birth preparedness intentions among expecting couples. *Methods.* A community based cross-sectional study targeting pregnant women and their partners was performed from June until October 2017. A three-stage probability sampling technique was employed to obtain a sample of 546 couples A structured questionnaire based upon the *Theory of Planned Behavior* was used. The questionnaire explored three main domains of birth preparedness intentions. These three domains included (1) attitudes towards birth preparedness, (2) perceived subjective norms towards birth preparedness, and (3) perceived behavior control towards birth preparedness. *Results.* The vast majority of study participants had birth preparedness intentions. This included 521 (95.4%) pregnant women and 543 (99.5%) of their male partners. After adjusting for the confounders, the predictors of birth preparedness intentions among pregnant women were attitude (AOR=70.134, 95% CI=12.536-392.360, p<0.001) and perceived behavior control (AOR=7.327, 95% CI=1.545-34.761, p<0.05) which were significant. Among male partners, only attitudes (AOR=31.315, 95% CI=1.497-655.149, p<0.05) influenced the birth preparedness intention. *Conclusion.* Birth preparedness intention among male partners was higher compared to their female partners. The reason for the difference could be the concern each group puts on the issue of birth preparedness. Among the three domains of intention, attitude and perceived behavior control were statistically significant predictors of birth preparedness intention among pregnant women. Attitude was the only domain which influenced birth preparedness intention among male partners. Therefore, interventional studies are recommended targeting attitudes and perceived behavior control in order to boost birth preparedness intention.

1. Introduction

Globally, maternal mortality has declined by 45% per year since 1990 [1]. The estimated number of maternal mortality was 289,000 in 2013 worldwide [1]. Sub-Saharan Africa accommodated the largest share of the maternal mortality as 179,000 maternal deaths occurred in this region in 2013 [1].

Tanzania is among the countries in Sub-Saharan region committed to reduce maternal mortalities by increasing the use of facility deliveries and quality of childbirth care [2] but maternal mortality remains unacceptably high. According to 2010 and 2015 Demographic and Health Survey, maternal mortality was 454 [3] and 556 [4] per 100,000 live births, respectively.

Despite the fact that improving access to skilled attendants during child birth and emergency obstetric care are vital strategies towards reduction of maternal and neonatal mortalities, the use of skilled attendants during childbirth is unacceptably low in developing countries [5]. Forty million births in this region were not attended by skilled health personnel, but by traditional birth attendants or relatives in 2012, and over 32 million of those births occurred in rural areas [5]. Despite the fact that the use of skilled birth attendants in developing countries was 68% in 2012, the use of

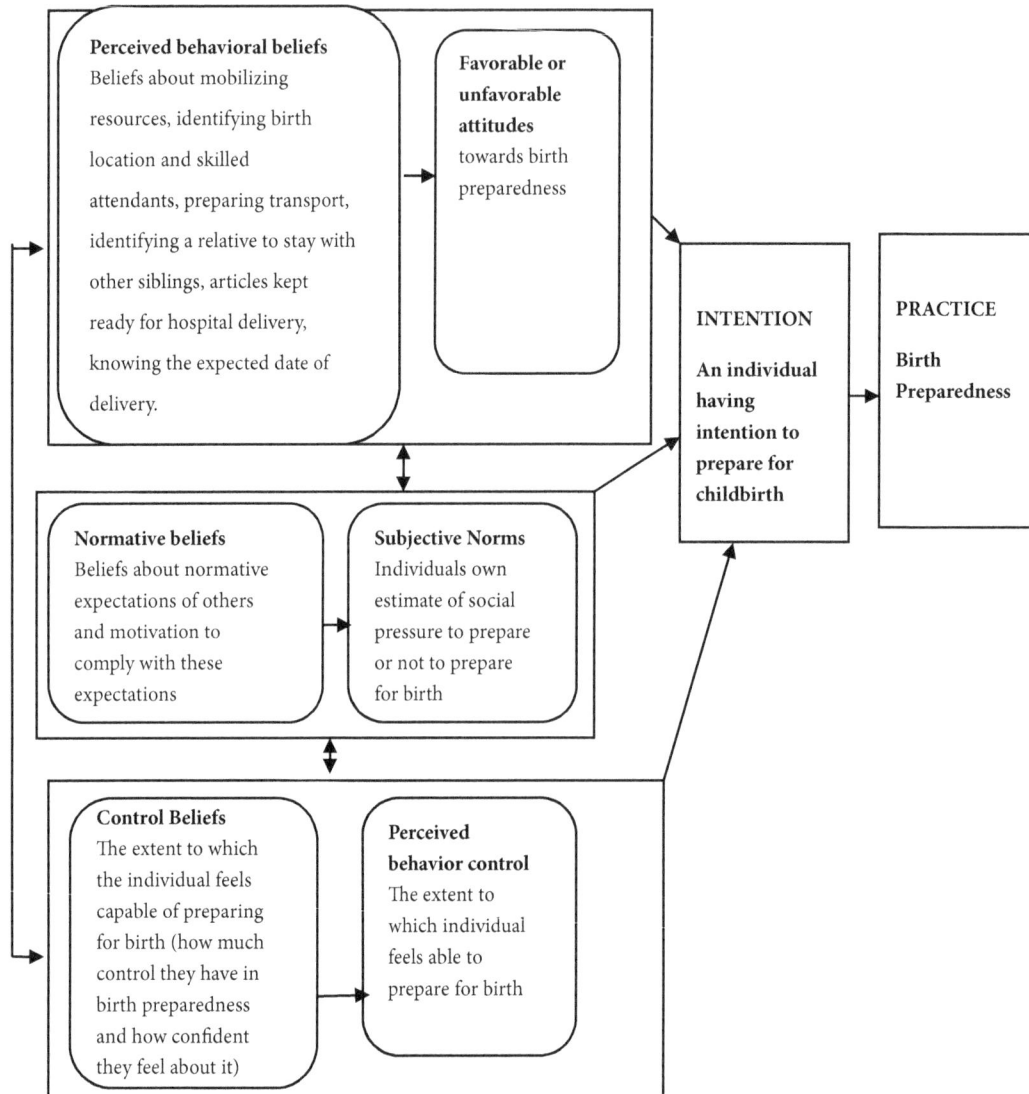

FIGURE 1: Theoretical framework of birth preparedness based on the Theory of Planned Behavior.

skilled birth attendants in Sub-Saharan Africa was only 53% [5] while only 51% used skilled birth attendants in Tanzania [3].

As previously demonstrated in the literature, a main cause of low utilization of maternal health services is low levels of birth preparedness [6]. Birth preparedness has a potential to reduce all three phases of delays to access maternal services. These delays include delay in decision-making to seek healthcare, delay in reaching a health facility, and delay in obtaining appropriate care upon reaching a health facility [7].

Studies have reported low-birth preparedness in developing countries, especially in South Asia and Sub-Saharan Africa [6, 8–11]. A study conducted in Tanzania reported that only 0.8% of expecting mothers identified skilled birth attendants, 10.2% identified transport, and 47.2% saved money for emergency [12]. Similar studies conducted in Nigeria and Uganda also reported low levels of birth preparedness [10, 11].

According to the *Theory of Planned Behavior*, an individual will have the intention to perform a behavior when they evaluate it positively, believe that the important others think they should perform it, and perceive it to be within their own control [13]. The intention to prepare for childbirth is influenced by the way an individual evaluates birth preparedness. If they evaluate it positively, believing that important others think it is something worth doing and perceive they can do it then they will have the intention to prepare.

An attitude toward a behavior refers to the degree to which a person has positive or negative feelings of the behavior of interest. It entails a consideration of the outcomes of performing the behavior [13]. A subjective norm refers to the belief about whether important others think he or she will perform the behavior. It relates to a person's perception of the social environment surrounding the behavior [13]. Perceived behavior control refers to the individual's perception of the extent to which performance of the behavior is easy or difficult [13] (see Figure 1).

There is a close link between preparation for childbirth and use of health facilities for childbirth [14]. Previous studies have reported several factors which influence birth preparedness. A few key factors include maternal level of education, male involvement in birth preparedness, living in either an urban or rural setting, and walking distance to the health facility [15–17].

The social, family, and community contexts and beliefs do influence preparation for childbirth either positively or negatively [18]. The attitude of expecting couples, their understanding of the social pressure to prepare for childbirth, and whether they feel able to prepare for childbirth all contribute to their intention to prepare for childbirth. Increasing core knowledge about the components of birth preparedness is key strategy to ensure that birth preparedness intention translates into the actual practice of preparing for birth. As such, the aim of this study was to use the *Theory of Planned Behavior* to explain birth preparedness intention among expecting couples in the rural setting of Rukwa Region Tanzania.

2. Methods

2.1. Study Design and Setting. A community based cross-sectional study was conducted in Rukwa Region from June 1st to October 30th, 2017, among expecting couples from forty-five villages in Rukwa Region in the Southern Highlands of Tanzania. The region had a population of 1,004,539 people: 487,311 males and 517,228 females. The forecast for 2014 was 1,076,087 persons with a growth rate of 3.5%. The region has the lowest mean age at marriage where males marry at the age of 23.3 years and 19.9 years for females and fertility rate of 7.3 [19].

2.2. Sampling Method and Sample Size

2.2.1. Sampling Technique. Two districts (Sumbawanga Rural District and Kalambo District) were conveniently selected from the four districts of Rukwa Region. Three-staged multistage cluster sampling technique was used to obtain study participants. During first-stage random samplings, all wards (12 wards of Sumbawanga Rural District and 17 wards of Kalambo District) in each district were listed and by the use of the lottery method of random sampling, five wards from Sumbawanga District and ten from Kalambo District were picked. During second-stage random samplings, all villages in the selected wards were listed and another simple random sampling was conducted to select fifteen villages from Sumbawanga rural district and thirty villages from Kalambo District. The third-stage sampling was a systematic sampling used to obtain households with pregnant women of 24 weeks of gestation or less and living with a male partner. At each visited household, a female partner was interviewed for the signs and symptoms of pregnancy. A female partner who had missed her period for two months was requested to complete a pregnancy test. Those with positive tests who gave consent to participate were enrolled in the study. If a selected household had no eligible participants, the household was skipped and researchers entered into the next household.

2.2.2. Sample Size Calculation. The sample size for couples who were involved in the study was calculated using the following formula [20]:

$$n = \frac{\left\{ Z\alpha \sqrt{[\pi o (1 - \pi o)]} + 2\beta \sqrt{[\pi 1 (1 - \pi 1)]} \right\}^2}{(\pi 1 - \pi o)^2} \quad (1)$$

where

n is the maximum sample size,

$Z\alpha$ is the standard normal deviation (1.96) at 95% confidence level for this study,

2β is the standard normal deviate (0.84) with a power of demonstrating a statistically significant difference before and after the intervention between the two groups at 90%,

πo is the proportion at preintervention (use of skilled delivery in Rukwa Region 30.1%) [3],

$\pi 1$ is the proportion after intervention (proportion of families which would access skilled birth attendant 51%) [3],

$$n = \frac{\left\{ 1.96 \sqrt{[0.301 (1-0.301)]} + 0.84 \sqrt{[0.51 (1-0.51)]} \right\}^2}{(0.6-0.51)^2} \quad (2)$$

n = 162 couples + 10% = 180

Therefore, the required sample size in the intervention group is 180 couples.

Intervention: control ratio is 1:2. Therefore sample size in the control group is 360 couples.

2.3. Data Collection Procedure. Data was collected using self-administered questionnaires. Four trained research assistants (two from each district) were recruited, trained, and participated in data collection. Questionnaires on testing birth preparedness intention were developed using a Theory of Planned Behavior. The questionnaire had two parts: (i) the social demographic characteristics and (ii) a Likert scale where respondents were supposed to strongly agree, agree, neutral, strongly disagree, and disagree. There were three subparts of the statements in the Likert scale which were (i) attitudes towards birth preparedness, (ii) perceived subjective norms towards birth preparedness, and (iii) perceived behavior control towards birth preparedness.

2.4. Data Processing and Analysis. The data was checked for completeness and consistencies, then it was coded and entered into computer using statistical package IBM SPSS version 23. Descriptive statistics were used to generate frequency distribution and cross tabulation was used to describe the characteristic of the study participants. Logistic regression was done to determine the predictors of intention to prepare for childbirth.

2.5. Ethical Consideration. The proposal was approved by Ethical Review Committee of the University of Dodoma. A letter of permission was obtained from the Rukwa Regional

TABLE 1: Sociodemographic characteristics of respondents.

Character	Male (n_1, %) (n_1=546	Female (n_2, %) (n_2=546)	Total (n_1+n_2) 1092	p-value
Age (years)				
Less than 20	27 (4.9)	167 (30.6)	194 (17.8)	
21 to 25	143 (26.2)	156 (28.6)	299 (27.4)	
26 to 30	146 (26.7)	105 (19.2)	251 (23.0)	* * *
31 to 35	87 (15.9)	55 (10.1)	142 (13.0)	
36 and above	143 (26.2)	63 (11.5)	206 (18.9)	
Age at Marriage (years)				
Less than 18	71 (13.0)	395 (72.3)	466 (42.7)	
19 to 24	353 (64.7)	147(26.9)	500 (45.8)	
25 and above	122 (22.3)	4 (0.7)	126(11.5)	* * *
Ethnic group				
Fipa	367 (67.2)	322 (59.0)	689(63.1)	* * *
Mambwe	118 (21.6)	120 (22.0)	238 (21.8)	
Others	61 (11.2)	104 (19.0)	165 (15.1)	
Marital status				
Cohabit	154 (28.2)	156 (28.6)	310 (28.4)	
Married	392 (71.8)	390 (71.4)	782 (71.6)	
Number of wives				
Monogamous	467 (85.5)	469 (85.9)	936 (85.7)	
Polygamous	79 (14.5)	77 (14.1)	156 (14.3)	
Education level				
Non-formal	155 (28.4)	230 (42.1)	385 (35.3)	
Primary School	353 (64.7)	299 (54.8)	652 (59.7)	* * *
Secondary school or Higher	38 (7.0)	17 (3.1)	55 (5.0)	
Income per day				
Less than 1 dollar	382 (70.0)	399 (73.1)	781 (71.5)	
More than 1 dollar	164 (30.0)	147 (26.9)	311 (28.5)	
Own radio				* * *
Yes	308 (56.4)	253 (46.3)	561 (51.4)	
No	238 (43.6)	293 (53.7)	531 (48.6)	
Own mobile phone				
Yes	234 (42.9)	69 (12.6)	303 (27.7)	* * *
No	312 (57.1)	477 (87.4)	789 (72.3)	
Family members				
2	76 (13.9)	76 (13.9)	152 (13.9)	
3 to 5	250 (45.8)	249 (45.6)	499 (45.7)	
6 or more	220 (40.3)	221 (40.5)	441 (40.4)	
Adult female in the family				
None	315 (57.7)	318 (58.2)	633 (58.0)	
1 or more	231 (42.3)	228 (41.8)	459 (42.0)	
Covered by Health Insurance				
Yes	170 (31.1)	177 (32.4)	347 (31.8)	
No	376 (68.9)	369 (67.6)	745 (68.2)	
Health facility				
Dispensary	452 (82.8)	452 (82.8)	904 (82.8)	
Health centre	94 (17.2)	94 (17.2)	188 (17.2)	
Approximately distance to reach to the health facility (Km)				
Less than 1	259 (47.4)	258 (47.3)	517 (47.3)	
1 to 5	232 (42.5)	233 (42.7)	465 (42.6)	
More than 5	55 (10.1)	55 (10.1)	110 (10.1)	

Here, * * * indicates p<0.001.

TABLE 2: Frequency distribution table on attitudes, perceived subjective norms, perceived behavior control towards birth preparedness, and birth preparedness intention among expecting couples.

Variables	Pregnant women		Their partners	
	n	%	n	%
Attitude				
Positive attitude	537	98.4	528	96.7
Negative attitude	9	1.6	18	3.3
Subjective norms				
Positive subjective norms	495	90.7	526	96.3
Negative subjective norms	51	9.3	20	3.7
Perceived behavior control				
Positive behavior control	532	97.4	521	95.4
Negative behavior control	14	2.6	25	4.6
Intention to prepare for childbirth				
No	25	4.6	3	0.5
Yes	521	95.4	543	99.5

Administration. Both written and verbal consent were sought from study participants after explaining the study objectives and procedures. Their right to refuse to participate in the study at any time was assured.

3. Results

3.1. Sociodemographic Characteristics. A total of 546 couples were included in the study, with a response rate of 100%. The sample included 546 pregnant women (with gestational age of 24 weeks and below) and their partners. The mean age among the pregnant women was 25.57 years (sd=6.810) and the mean age of their partners was 30.65 years (sd=7.726). The majority of the couples were married (390, 71.4%), were monogamous (469, 85.9%), live on less than 1 dollar per day (382, 70.0%), and receive their basic obstetric care services from dispensaries (452, 82.8). Ninety-five percent of the cohort had completed primary school or less (Table 1).

Overall, the majority of study participants had the intention to prepare for childbirth. This included 521 (95.4%) pregnant women and their partners 543 (99.5%). Similarly, 537 (98.4%) pregnant women and 528 (96.7%) of their partners had positive attitudes towards birth preparedness. On perceived subjective norms, 495 (90.7%) pregnant women and 526 (96.3%) of their partners had positive perceived subjective norms about birth preparedness. Positive perceived behavior control was also present among 532 (97.4%) of pregnant women and 521 (95.4%) of their partners (see Table 2).

Among pregnant women, attitude (p<0.001), perceived subjective norms (p<0.01), perceived behavior control (p<0.001), ethnic group (p<0.05), ever heard about birth preparedness (p<0.001), economic status (p<0.05), and owning a mobile phone (p<0.05) had statistically significant relationship to birth preparedness intention. Among male partners only attitude (p<0.01), perceived subjective norms (p<0.01), and owning a mobile phone (p<0.05) had statistically significant relationship with birth preparedness intention (see Table 3).

After adjusting for the confounders (other variables which showed significant relationship with intention to prepare) among pregnant women, the model contained three components of Theory of Planned Behavior (attitude, subjective norms, and perceived behavior control). The full model containing all predictors was statistically significant (X^2 (3, N=546)=41.481 p<0.001) (see Table 4). The mode as a whole explained between 7.3% (Cox and Snell R square) and 23.6% (Nagelkerke R squared) of the variable birth preparedness intentions. The strongest predictor of birth preparedness intention was attitude towards birth preparedness. Respondents who had positive attitudes were 70.134 times more likely to have birth preparedness intention than those with negative attitudes towards birth preparedness. Another component of Theory of Planned Behavior which showed statistical significance was a perceived behavior control. Pregnant women who felt they have ability to prepare for childbirth were 7 times more likely to have birth preparedness intention than those who felt they were not capable.

Among male partners, the full model containing all predictors was statistically significant (X^2 (3, N=546)=8.548 p<0.05). The mode as a whole explained between 1.6% (Cox and Snell R square) and 23.6% (Nagelkerke R squared) of the variable birth preparedness intention. As shown in Table 5, attitudes towards birth preparedness intention made a significant contribution to the model. Male partners who had positive attitudes are 31.315 more likely to have birth preparedness intention than male partners with negative attitudes. Both subjective norms and perceived behavior control did not show statistical significant impact to birth preparedness intention.

4. Discussion

According to the *Theory of Planned Behavior*, birth preparedness intention is influenced by the attitude the individual has about birth preparedness, the perceived subjective norms this particular individual has, and the perceived control on performing the behavior [13]. In this study, the behavior of

TABLE 3: Distribution of participants by birth preparedness intention and the potential factors affecting birth preparedness intention (Chi-Square).

Variable	Intention to prepare Pregnant women (N=546)			Intention to prepare Their partners (N=546)		
	Yes n(%)	No n(%)	p-value	Yes n(%)	No n(%)	p-value
Attitude						
Positive attitude	519(96.65)	18(3.35)	0	526(99.62)	2(0.38)	0.003
Negative attitude	2(22.22)	7(77.78)		17(94.44)	1(5.56)	
Subjective norms						
Positive subjective norms	476 (96.16)	19(3.84)	0.01	524(99.62)	2(0.38)	0.006
Negative subjective norms	45(88.24)	6(11.76)		19(95.00)	1(5.00)	
Perceived behavior control						
Positive behavior control	512(96.24)	20(3.76)	0	518(99.42)	3(0.58)	0.704
Negative behavior control	9(64.29)	5(35.71)		25(100)	0(0.0)	
Age groups						
Less than 20	159(95.21)	8(4.79)		26(96.30)	1(3.70)	
21 to 25	150(96.15)	6(3.85)	0.799	141(98.60)	2(1.40)	0.064
26 to 30	98(93.33)	7(6.67)		146(100)	0(0.0)	
31 to 35	53(96.36)	2(3.64)		87(100)	0(0.0)	
36+	61(96.83)	2(3.17)		143(100)	0(0.0)	
Ethnic group						
Fipa	302(93.79)	20(6.21)	0.051	364(99.18)	3(0.82)	0.479
Mambwe	119(99.17)	1(0.83)		118(100)	0(0.0)	
Others	100(96.15)	4(3.85)		61(100)	0(0.0)	
Education Level						
No Formal	216(93.91)	14(6.09)	0.277	154(99.35)	1(0.65)	
Primary School	288(96.32)	11(3.68)		352(99.72)	1(0.28)	0.174
Secondary School or Higher	17(100)	0(0.0)		37(97.37)	1(2.63)	
Ever heard about birth preparedness						
Yes	441(97.57)	11(2.43)		442(99.55)	2(0.45)	
No	80(85.11)	14(14.89)	0	101(99.02)	1(0.98)	0.514
Economic status						
Less than one dollar/dollar	376(94.24)	23(5.76)		381(99.74)	1(0.26)	0.165
At least one dollar/day	145(98.64)	2(1.36)	0.029	162(98.78)	2(1.22)	
Own a mobile phone						
Yes	69(100)	0(0.0)		231(98.72)	3(1.28)	
No	452(94.76)	25(5.24)	0.052	312(100)	0(0.0)	0.045
Knowledge of birth preparedness components						
Not knowledgeable	482(95.26)	24(4.74)	0.514	511(99.42)	3(0.58)	0.665
Knowledgeable	39(97.5)	1(2.5)		32(100)	0(0.0)	
Parity						
Para 0	112(93.33)	8(6.67)				
Para 1-4	306(95.62)	14(4.38)	0.374			

TABLE 3: Continued.

Variable	Intention to prepare Pregnant women (N=546)			Intention to prepare Their partners (N=546)		
	Yes n(%)	No n(%)	p-value	Yes n(%)	No n(%)	p-value
Para 5+	103(97.17)	3(2.83)				
Have a prior pre-term delivery			0.765			
Yes	28(96.55)	1(3.45)				
No	493(95.36)	24(4.64)				
Prior C Session			0.424			
Yes	13(100)	0(0.0)				
No	508(95.31)	25(4.69)				

TABLE 4: The logistic regression predicting the likelihood of components of Theory of Planned Behavior to influence birth preparedness intention among pregnant women.

Variables	B	S.E	Wald	df	p	Odds Ratio	Lower	Upper
Attitude	4.250	.878	23.410	1	.000	70.134	12.536	392.360
Subjective norms	.291	.699	.174	1	.677	1.338	.340	5.269
Perceived behavior control	1.992	.794	6.286	1	.012	7.327	1.545	34.761

TABLE 5: The logistic regression predicting the likelihood of components of Theory of Planned Behavior to influence birth preparedness intention among male partners.

Variables	B	S.E	Wald	df	p	Odds Ratio	Lower	Upper
Attitude	3.444	1.551	4.928	1	.026	31.315	1.497	655.149
Subjective norms	2.842	1.538	3.416	1	.065	17.153	.842	349.308
Perceived behavior control	-20.437	6815.8	.000	1	.998	.000	.000	.

interest was birth preparedness. We found that the majority of study participants had birth preparedness intention (99.5% among male partner and 95.4% among pregnant women). The birth preparedness among male partners was found to be higher than their female partners. The reason for the difference could be due to the concern the two groups put on the issue of birth preparedness. Pregnant women being the one going through pregnancy and childbirth may put big weight on the issue of birth preparedness to an extent of feeling unable to prepare for childbirth.

Using the Theory of Planned Behavior framework, this study identified that attitude influenced birth preparedness intention among both pregnant women and their partners. This finding is in line with findings from previous study which reported attitude predicting intention to the choice of method of delivery [21].

The study also found that perceived behavior control significantly influenced birth preparedness intention among pregnant women. Pregnant women who felt they had ability to prepare for childbirth are more likely to had birth preparedness intention compared to those who felt they do not have ability to prepare for childbirth. Similar findings was reported in a previous study by Bahareh et al. [21]. Perceived behavior control was not a significant factor among male respondents.

Subjective norms were not a significant predictor of birth preparedness intention among both pregnant women and their partners. The finding is in line with a previous study by Kalolo and Kibusi [22] and contrary to a study done by Bahreh et al. [21]. The possible reason for the difference could be the study respondents in this study who were from similar environment sharing similar norms.

Maternal and neonatal mortality rates in Rukwa Region remain high, reinforcing the tremendous vulnerability of both women and babies at the time of birth [19]. Using the three-delay model as a framework, it is clear that health system strengthening is needed to reduce delays at each juncture. A key strategy for improving health outcomes includes strengthening community demand and mobilization. One wonders about the potential positive impact that deeper preparation of both men and women might have on both intention and action in this setting. The findings from this study recommend innovative interventions which will boost attitudes towards birth preparedness and perceived behavior control.

This study is not without limitations. The key information gathered from the study participants was self-reported which is subject to under- or overreporting. Attitudes can be difficult to ascertain. Despite the systematic data collection approach, there may have been some intrinsic bias in the questionnaire or manner in which questions were asked that affected the responses.

5. Conclusion

Birth preparedness intention among male partners was higher compared to their female partners. The reason for the difference could be the concern each group puts on the issue of birth preparedness. Among the three domains of intention, attitude and perceived behavior control were statistically significant predictors of birth preparedness intention among pregnant women. Attitude was the only domain which influenced birth preparedness intention among male partners. Therefore, interventional studies are recommended targeting attitudes and perceived behavior control in order to boost birth preparedness intention.

Additional Points

Limitation. This study may have its limitation that the study population is much older than the stated regional age of pregnancy which could have affected the reported findings.

Authors' Contributions

Fabiola Moshi led the conception, design, acquisition of data, analysis, interpretation of data, and drafting of the manuscript. Stephen Kibusi and Flora Phabian guided the conception, design, acquisition of data, analysis, interpretation, and critical revising of the manuscript for intellectual content and have given final approval for the version to be published. All authors read and approved the final manuscript.

Acknowledgments

The authors thank the University of Dodoma for providing ethical clearance for this study. We also gratefully acknowledge the University of Dodoma's financial support. We are grateful to the administration of Rukwa Region for allowing us to conduct the study and to each of the study participants for their participation in this study. We also thank Elisa Vandervort and Saada Ally for their kind review and language editing before submission.

References

[1] WHO., "WHO, UNICEF, UNFPA, World Bank Group, and United Nations Population Division Trends in Maternal Mortality: 1990 to 2015 Geneva: World Health Organization, 2015," 2014, http://apps.who.int/iris/bitstream/10665/112682/2/9789241507226_eng.pdf?ua=1.

[2] Ministry of Health and Social Welfare, "Health Sector Strategic Plan IV, Vol. 2020. 2015".

[3] National Bureau of Statistics., "Tanzania Demographic and Health Survey, Dar es Salaam, Tanzania; 2010," http://www.measuredhs.com.

[4] "Ministry of Health, Community Development, Gender, Elderly and Children (MoHCDGEC) [Tanzania Mainland], Ministry of Health (MoH) [Zanzibar], National Bureau of Statistics (NBS), Office of the Chief Government Statistician (OCGS) and I. Tanzania Demographic and Health Survey and Malaria Indicator Survey 2015-2016, Tanzania Demographic and Health Survey and Malaria Indicator Survey (TDHS-MIS) 2015-16. Dar es Salaam, Tanzania, and Rockville, Maryland, USA," 2016, https://www.dhsprogram.com/pubs/pdf/FR321/FR321.pdf.

[5] United. nation, *The Millenium Development Goals Report*, United Nations, 2014, http://www.un.org/millenniumgoals/reports.shtml.

[6] J. K. Kabakyenga, P-O. Östergren, E. Turyakira, and K. O. Pettersson, "Knowledge of obstetric danger signs and birth preparedness practices among women in rural Uganda," *Reprod Health*, vol. 8, no. 1, p. 33, 1972, http://www.pubmedcentral.nih.gov/articlerender.fcgi.

[7] K. C. Teela, L. C. Mullany, C. I. Lee et al., "Community-based delivery of maternal care in conflict-affected areas of eastern Burma: Perspectives from lay maternal health workers," *Social Science & Medicine*, vol. 68, no. 7, pp. 1332–1340, 2009.

[8] F. August, A. B. Pembe, R. Mpembeni, P. Axemo, and E. Darj, "Effectiveness of the Home Based Life Saving Skills training by community health workers on knowledge of danger signs, birth preparedness, complication readiness and facility delivery, among women in Rural Tanzania," *BMC Pregnancy and Childbirth*, vol. 16, no. 1, article no. 129, 2016.

[9] D. N. Bhatta, "Involvement of males in antenatal care, Birth preparedness, Exclusive breast feeding and immunizations for children in Kathmandu, Nepal," *BMC Pregnancy and Childbirth*, vol. 13, 2013.

[10] Z. Iliyasu, I. S. Abubakar, H. S. Galadanci, and M. H. Aliyu, "Birth preparedness, complications readiness and fathers' participation in maternity care in northern Nigerian community," *African Journal of Reproductive Health*, vol. 14, no. 1, pp. 21–32, 2010.

[11] O. Kakaire, D. K. Kaye, and M. O. Osinde, "Male involvement in birth preparedness and complication readiness for emergency obstetric referrals in rural Uganda," *Reprod Health*, vol. 8, no. 1, 2011, http://www.pubmedcentral.nih.gov/articlerender.fcgi?artid=3118172&tool=pmcentrez&rendertype=abstract.

[12] F. August, A. B. Pembe, R. Mpembeni, P. Axemo, and E. Darj, "Men's knowledge of obstetric danger signs, birth preparedness and complication readiness in Rural Tanzania," *PLoS ONE*, vol. 10, no. 5, 2015.

[13] R. Netemeyer, M. Ryn Van, and I. Ajzen, "The theory of planned behavior," *Organizational Behavior and Human Decision Processes*, vol. 50, pp. 179–211, 1991, http://linkinghub.elsevier.com/retrieve/pii/TAvailable from.

[14] M. Hailu, A. Gebremariam, F. Alemseged, and K. Deribe, "Birth preparedness and complication readiness among pregnant

women in Southern Ethiopia," *PLoS ONE*, vol. 6, no. 6, Article ID e21432, 2011.

[15] D. Bintabara, MA. Mohamed, J. Mghamba, P. Wasswa, and R. N. M. Mpembeni, "Birth preparedness and complication readiness among recently delivered women in chamwino district, central Tanzania: a cross sectional study," *Reprod Health*, vol. 12, no. 1, 2015, http://www.scopus.com/inward/record.url?eid=2-s2.0-84930206913&partnerID=tZOtx3y1.

[16] M. Kaso and M. Addisse, "Birth preparedness and complication readiness in Robe Woreda, Arsi Zone, Oromia Region, Central Ethiopia: a cross-sectional study," *Reprod Health*, vol. 11, no. 1, 2014, http://www.pubmedcentral.nih.gov/articlerender.fcgi?artid=4118259&tool=pmcentrez& rendertype=abstract.

[17] L. T. Martin, M. J. McNamara, A. S. Milot, T. Halle, and E. C. Hair, "The effects of father involvement during pregnancy on receipt of prenatal care and maternal smoking," *Maternal and Child Health Journal*, vol. 11, no. 6, pp. 595–602, 2007.

[18] D. Markos and D. Bogale, "Birth preparedness and complication readiness among women of child bearing age group in Goba woreda, Oromia region, Ethiopia," *BMC Pregnancy and Childbirth*, vol. 14, no. 1, 2014.

[19] National Bureau of Statistics, "Fertility and Nuptiality report 2015, Vol. IV," 2015, http://www.nbs.go.tz/nbs/takwimu/census2012/FertilityandNuptialityMonograph.pdf.

[20] C. I. Tobin-West and N. C. T. Briggs, "Effectiveness of trained community volunteers in improving knowledge and management of childhood malaria in a rural area of Rivers State, Nigeria," *Nigerian Journal of Clinical Practice*, vol. 18, no. 5, pp. 651–658, 2015.

[21] B. Soheili, A. Mirzaei, K. Sayemiri, and Z. Ghazanfari, "Predicting the behavioral intention of pregnant women's choice of delivery method based on the theory of planned behavior: A cross-sectional study," *Journal of Basic Research in Medical Sciences*, vol. 4, no. 1, pp. 37–44, 2017.

[22] A. Kalolo and S. M. Kibusi, "The influence of perceived behaviour control, attitude and empowerment on reported condom use and intention to use condoms among adolescents in rural Tanzania," *Reprod Health*, vol. 12, no. 1, p. 105, 2015, http://www.pubmedcentral.nih.gov/articlerender.fcgi?artid=4643513&tool=pmcentrez&rendertype=abstract.

Dietary Diversity and Associated Factors among HIV Positive Adult Patients Attending Public Health Facilities in Motta Town, East Gojjam Zone, Northwest Ethiopia, 2017

Addisu Tesfaw,[1] Dube Jara,[2] and Habtamu Temesgen ⓘ[3]

[1]Gendewoyin Health center, Gonchasiso Enese Woreda, North West Ethiopia, Ethiopia
[2]Department of Public Health, College of Health Sciences, Debre Markos University, Debre Markos, Ethiopia
[3]Department of Human Nutrition and Food Science, College of Health Sciences, Debre Markos University, Debre Markos, Ethiopia

Correspondence should be addressed to Habtamu Temesgen; habtamutem@gmail.com

Academic Editor: Giuseppe La Torre

Introduction. Dietary diversity is defined as the amount of different food groups or foods that are consumed over a specific reference time. The human immune deficiency virus problem remains one of the main public health challenges, especially in low and middle income countries. Nutrition has been linked to both the transmission of human immune deficiency virus and poor outcomes related to human immune deficiency virus. *Objective.* To assess dietary diversity and associated factors among human immune deficiency virus positive adult patients in Motta administrative town, Northwest Ethiopia, 2017. *Methods.* A facility based cross-sectional study design was conducted on 410 study participants selected using a stratified sampling technique with proportional allocation. The data were collected using semi-structured and pretested questionnaire. Data were entered into Epi-Data version 3.1 and analysis was performed using SPSS version 20. Descriptive statistics were used to describe the number and percentage of the study variables. The bivariate and multivariable logistic regression analyses were done to identify the independent factors associated with dietary diversity among adult human immune virus (HIV) positive patients. *Result.* A total of 410 study participants were included in the analysis. Of the total, 121 (29.5%) of adult HIV positive respondents consumed diversified diet with the mean dietary diversity score of 3.2 (SD±1.88). The predominant food item consumed during the study periods was starchy staples (96.1%) and legumes (81.7%). Having means of communication cell phone (mobile phone) [(AOR= 2.13 (1.16, 3.60)], media exposure status in the household [(AOR =1.95 (1.22, 3.11)] and nutrition counselling [(AOR =2.17 (1.09, 4.67)] were significant factors associated with dietary diversified feeding at 95% CI. *Conclusion.* The study revealed that low dietary diversity score was significant nutritional problem among HIV positive adults in Motta town health facilities. Having mobile cell phone, media exposure status and nutritional counseling were significantly associated with dietary diversity score. Therefore efforts should be strengthened to improve the counseling service at each health institution and encourage the patients to use media for the source of information.

1. Background

Dietary diversity is a quantitative number of food groups which is used extensively as a method of ascertaining variety and nutrient adequacy of diets. It is the number of different food groups consumed over a given reference period. Diversified diets that include a variety of foods from different food groups (vegetables, fruits, grains, and animal source foods) provide a balance of nutrients that promote healthy growth and development. It is indeed strongly associated with nutrient adequacy [1]. Increasing the variety of foods across and within food groups is recommended in most dietary guidelines. This explained that there is no any single food which contains all the required nutrients for optimal health [2].

Undiversified food and malnutrition are public health concerns worldwide, especially in developing countries [3]. In developing countries with high nutrient demands, chronic patients like HIV/AIDS are of high risk due to consumption of low-quality, monotonous food which leads to micronutrient and macronutrient deficiencies [4].

HIV/AIDS and malnutrition are both highly prevalent in many parts of the world, especially in Sub-Saharan Africa.

The effects are interrelated and exacerbate one another in a vicious cycle [5]. Both HIV and malnutrition can independently cause progressive damage to the immune system and increased susceptibility to infection, morbidity, and mortality through opportunistic infections, fever, diarrhea, loss of appetite, nutrient absorption, and weight loss. HIV speciïňĄcally affects nutritional status by increasing energy requirements, reducing food intake, and adversely affecting nutrient absorption and metabolism [6].

Nondiversified diet can have negative consequences on individuals' health, well-being, and development, mainly by reducing physical, social, cognitive, reproductive, and immunological capacities [2]. The level of dietary diversity and its determinant on HIV positive individuals will play a crucial role in improving quality of nutritional care and counseling provided by healthcare providers which in turn improves clients quality of life and physical and social capacity [7].

Dietary diversity problem in Ethiopia occurs at all times of the year. The number of relief dependent population has increased from time to time, which indicate that famine has become more prevalent than worse food diversity problems [8]. If adequate measures are not taken, the catastrophic nature of HIV will ground down the economic activities of countries because the global number of People Living with HIV (PLHIV) is seriously increasing [9]. Food diversity problem in Ethiopia derives directly from dependence on undiversified (monotonous) livelihoods style based on low-input, low-output rain fed agriculture and awareness problem [10, 11].

Inadequate dietary intake to meet the increased metabolic demands associated with HIV infection is likely to affect nutritional status in PLHIV, further lowering their immunity and hastening disease progression hence increased morbidity and mortality. The Ministry of Health has taken remarkable steps in addressing nutrition among PLHIV by developing the national nutrition in HIV/AIDS guidelines. Dietary diversity among HIV positive adults (18 years) is influenced by different factors. So, the current study assessed those factors which are significant for dietary diversity. There is also limited research document in Ethiopia and no published study conducted on this topic in the study area; therefore, it is essential to assess the current magnitude of dietary diversity and associated factors among People Living with HIV receiving care and support in the study area. Hence this study will be conducted to identify the level of dietary diversity and associated factors among PLHIV attending antiretroviral therapy (ART) clinics of Motta administrative town ART sites.

2. Methods

2.1. Study Design and Setting. Facility based cross-sectional study was conducted in Motta administrative town, East Gojjam zone, the Amhara Regional State from April 15 to 30, 2009 E.C. It is located 370 Km, Northwest of Addis Ababa, and the capital city of Ethiopia and 120 km Southwest of Bahir Dar city, the capital of the Amhara National Regional State,

respectively. The town had two ART sites. These were Motta Hospital and Motta Health Center. Motta Hospital started ART chronic care in 1998 E.C. and it served more than two thousands nearby woreda HIV patients. Motta Health Centre served about 355 HIV patients [12, 13].

2.2. Participants. The source population was all HIV positive adults aged 18 years and above registered for chronic medical care in Motta administrative town ART sites and those patients who were currently on ART attending Motta administrative town ART clinic during the data collection period were included in the study, while those respondents who were too sick and unable to communicate were excluded.

2.3. Sample Size Determination and Technique. The required sample size was calculated using a formula for the determination of sample size for a single population proportion, considering 58.8% [9] as the proportion of low dietary diversity (P) with 5% level of significance (α), at 95% level of confidence for two-tail test and a marginal error or level of precision (d)=5%. The sample size (n) then was calculated as follows:

$$n = \frac{(Z_{\alpha/2})^2 \, [P\,(P-1)]}{(d)^2} = \frac{(1.96)^2 \, [0.588\,(0.588-1)]}{(0.05)^2} \quad (1)$$
$$= 373$$

The final sample by adding 10% nonresponse rate becomes 410.

Stratified sampling was used to select the required samples. First classify the health institutions stratified into two strata. Those were Hospital and Health Centre. Sampling frame was constructed by using the list from daily patient flow from both health institutions and proportionally allocated sample for each health institution and then simple systematic random sampling technique was used to select study units (participants) at every K^{th} (4th) intervals (k was sampling fraction, which was calculated as N/n=1433/329≈4 for Motta Hospital and N/n=355/81≈4 for Motta Health Centre). The numerators 1433 and 355 were the number of HIV positive clients currently on chronic care at Motta Hospital and Motta Health Center, respectively. The starting sample was selected by lottery method among the first four clients. The procedure was continued until the required sample size was obtained.

2.4. Data Collection Tools and Procedures. Structured questionnaire and standardized individual dietary diversity score tool [14] were used to assess dietary diversity of adult PLHIV. The questionnaire was first prepared in English by reviewing literatures and translated into Amharic version, which later on translated to the English version to check its consistency and comparability of the finding. Four data collectors (diploma clinical nurses) and one supervisor (health officer) were recruited for data collection process in Motta town administrative ART sites. A one-day training was given for data collectors and supervisors on the objectives of the study, data collection methods, how to fill the information in the structured questionnaire, and the ethical aspect of how to approach the patient. Supervisors had checked completeness and consistency of the collected data by reviewing each completed questionnaire daily and onsite supervision was carried out during data collection periods.

2.5. Data Quality Control. The questionnaire was designed and modified into local context from previous related literatures. It was first prepared in English and then translated into the local language Amharic and then retranslated back to English by an expert who was fluent in both languages to maintain its consistency. Training was given for data collectors and supervisor. Pretesting of the questionnaire was made on 5% of sample size in the Gindewoyin Health Center prior to the actual data collection process. There after adjustments and corrections were effected to the tools after review following the pretest. The data collection process was strictly followed day to day by the supervisor and principal investigator.

2.6. Data Processing and Analysis. Data were coded and entered into Epi-data version 3.1 and were exported to SPSS version 20.0 for analysis. The data that needs coding were first recoded before analysis. Descriptive statistics like frequency and cross-tabulation was computed. The bivariate logistic regression analysis was used to assess the association between dependent and independent variables. Each independent variable was entered in the bivariate logistic regression. Finally, variables, which show associations in the bivariable logistic regression at P value of less than 0.2 with 95%CI, were entered into multivariable logistic regression and were declared statistically significant at P value of less than 0.05 with at 95% CI.

2.7. Ethical Consideration. Ethical clearance was obtained from Debre Markos University, College of Health Sciences, Ethical Review Committee, and letter of permission was obtained from Motta town administrative ART sites. The purpose of the study was explained to respondents and verbal informed consent will be obtained from participants. Confidentiality of information was maintained by omitting any personal identifier from the questionnaires. The collected data were kept in the form of file in secure place where no one can access it except the investigator.

3. Results

3.1. Sociodemographic and Economic Characteristics. 410 study participants were included in the analysis with overall response rate of 100%. The majority of the respondents, 150 (36.6%), belonged to age group of 35-44 years with the mean age of 37.0 (±9.63) years. Majority, 359 (87.6%), were Christian orthodox followers and 279 (68.0%) of the respondents were females. All of the respondents (100%) were Amhara and 192 (46.8%) were married. Majority, 214 (52.2%), of the respondents cannot read and write. Regarding to occupation, 125 (30.5%) of respondents were daily labourer and 315 (76.8%) of respondents' place of residence were urban (Table 1).

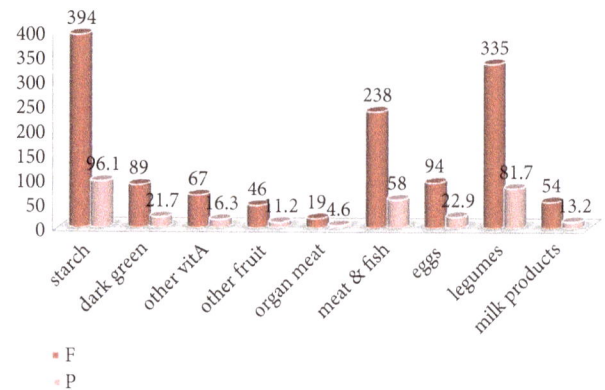

FIGURE 1: Twenty-four-hour food group consumption of adult HIV patients in Motta town public health facilities, April, 2017.

3.2. Behaviors Related Characteristics. Among the respondents, 140 (34.1%) were counseled about drugs, 23 (5.6%) about the illness, and 243 (59.3%) about feedings. Most patients 391 (95.4%) were counseled by healthcare providers whereas the others 17 (2.2%) were by case managers. One hundred twenty-three (30%) of the respondents were alcohol drunker and 11 (2.7%) were chat chewer.

3.3. Health Related Characteristics. Regarding working status, 405 (98.8%) of respondents could work their daily activities. One hundred seventy-three (33.4%) of respondents were taking Cotrimoxazole prophylaxis of which 116 (67.0 %%) of them took for less than six years. 5.4% of the patients developed side effect related to ARV drugs while 0.7% and 3.9% developed side effect related to INH and CPT, respectively. 192 (46.8%) of patients took AZT-3TC-NVP based regimens and 5 (1.2%) took second-line regimen. Among respondents 176 (42.9%) of them took ART for less than three and half years (42 months). 405 (98.8%) of respondents were currently under WHO clinical treatment stage one (T-1) and 230 (68.3%) had baseline CD4 count of less than 350 cells/mm3. Majority 376 (91.7%) of the respondents had monthly follow-up and 392 (95.6%) of the respondents had good adherence even if 2.9% of them lost due to their own reason (Table 2).

3.4. Level of Dietary Diversity. By considering the mean individual dietary diversity score, about 29.5% of HIV positive adults got diversified food. Starch staples (96.1%) and legumes were food groups predominantly consumed by the patients with 96.1% and 81.7%, respectively, whereas the least consumed food groups by the patients were organ meat (4.6%) and milk products (13.2%) (Figure 1).

3.5. Factors Associated with Level of Dietary Diversity. In multivariable logistic regression analysis, those patients who had cell phone means of communication were 2.13 times more likely to get diversified diet (AOR =2.13, 95% CI= 1.16, 3.60) compared to those who had not mobile cell phone. Those patients who had radio and television as means of source of information were 1.95 times more likely to get

TABLE 1: Sociodemographic characteristics of adult HIV positive patients in Motta administrative town ART sites, April, 2017.

Sociodemographic variables		Frequency (N=410)	Percent (%)
Sex	Male	131	32.0
	Female	279	68.0
Age of the respondent	<25 years	27	6.6
	25-34 years	139	33.9
	35-44 years	150	36.6
	≥ 45 years	94	22.9
Religion of the respondent	Orthodox	359	87.6
	Muslim	51	12.4
Educational status	Can't write and read	214	52.2
	Write and read	93	22.7
	Primary school	38	9.3
	Secondary school	54	13.2
	Certificate and above	11	2.7
Marital status	Single	34	8.3
	Married	192	46.8
	Divorced	152	37.0
	Widowed	32	7.8
Occupation	Farmer	109	26.6
	Government employed	54	13.2
	Merchant	90	22
	Daily laborer	125	30.5
	Student	9	2.2
	Others	23	5.6
Residence	Rural	95	23.2
	Urban	315	76.8
Family size	≤ 5 people	389	94.9
	> 5 people	21	5.1
Monthly income	<500 birr	105	25.6
	≥ 500 birr	305	74.4
Source of food	Farm/garden	118	28.8
	Purchase	279	68.0
	Relatives	13	3.2
Farmland ownership	Yes	122	29.8
	No	288	70.2
Livestock ownership	Yes	80	19.5
	No	330	80.5
Dummy cultivating land	Yes	65	15.9
	No	345	84.1
Milk in the house	Yes	28	6.8
	No	382	93.2
Chicken and eggs in the house	Yes	63	15.4
	No	347	84.6
Mobile phone	Yes	220	53.7
	No	190	46.3
Exposure to media sources	Yes	104	25.4
	No	306	74.6

TABLE 2: Health related information of adult HIV patients in Motta administrative town, April, 2017.

Health related variables		Frequency	Percent (%)
Working status of the respondent	Working	405	98.8
	Other	5	1.2
Taking Cotrimoxazole prophylaxis	Yes	137	33.4
	No	273	66.6
Duration of Cotrimoxazole	≤ 5 years	116	67.0
	>5years	21	33.0
Side effect of Cotrimoxazole	Yes	16	3.9
	No	121	29.5
INH preventive therapy	Yes	30	7.3
	No	380	92.7
INH side effect	Yes	3	0.7
	No	27	6.8
ART regimen	AZT-3TC-NVP	192	46.8
	AZT-3TC-EFV	30	7.3
	TDF-3TC-NVP	33	8.5
	TDF-3TC-EFV	148	36.1
	Other/second line	5	1.2
ART duration	6-18 months	50	12.2
	19-42 months	126	30.7
	≥43 months	234	57.1
Side effect of ART	Yes	22	5.4
	No	388	94.6
WHO stage	T-1	405	98.8
	T-2	4	1
	WHO-1	1	0.2
Opportunity infection	Yes	42	10.2
	No	368	89.8
Follow-up interval	Monthly	376	91.7
	Every 2 months	33	33.8
	Others	1	0.2
Supplementary feeding	Yes	57	13.9
	No	353	86.1
Baseline CD4	<200 cells/mm3	149	36.3
	200-349 cells/mm3	131	32.0
	350-499 cells/mm3	70	17.1
	≥500 cells/mm3	60	14.6
Current CD4	<200 cells/mm3	38	9.3
	200-349 cells/mm3	69	16.8
	350-499 cells/mm3	97	23.7
	≥500 cells/mm3	206	50.2
Adherence	Good	392	95.6
	Fair	10	2.4
	Poor	8	2.0

diversified diet (AOR =1.95, 95% CI= 1.22, 3.11) compared to those who had not media source and patients who got nutritional counseling were 2.17 times more likely to get diversified diet (AOR =2.17, 95% CI=1.09, 4.67) compared to counterparts (Table 3).

4. Discussion

This cross-sectional study was conducted to determine dietary diversity in adult HIV positive patients in Motta town public health institutions, North West Ethiopia. The

TABLE 3: Multivariate and bivariate logistic regression output showing factors associated with dietary diversity in adult HIV patients in Motta town public health facilities, April, 2017.

S. No.	Variables		Diversified diet		COR at 95% CI	AOR at CI 95%
			Yes	No		
1	Having media exposure	Yes	62	42	3.65(1.56,8.56)*	1.95(1.22,3.11)***
		No	227	79	1.00	1.00
2	INH preventive therapy	Yes	15	15	2.59(1.22,5.47)*	1.47(0.467,4.61)
		No	274	106	1.00	1.00
3	Cotrimoxazole	Yes	81	35	2.59(0.72,9.37)*	2.42(0.65,9.06)
		No	19	3	1.00	1.00
4	Availability of Mobile phone	Yes	138	8	2.30(1.47,3.59)*	2.13(1.16,3.60)***
		No	151	39	1.00	1.00
5	Food source	Farming	154	76	1.48(0.96,2.29)*	0.79(0.36,1.85)
		Other	135	45	1.00	1.00
6	Nutritional counseling	Yes	117	113	2.77(0.97,4.46)*	2.17(1.09,4.67)***
		No	172	8	1.00	1.00
7	Marital status	Married	127	65	1.48(0.967,2.27)*	1.20(0.53,2.72)
		Not ever married	162	56	1.00	1.00

*Significant at *p value<0.2 and ***p value < 0.05.*

finding of this study revealed that 29.5% of HIV positive adults have got diversified diet before 24 hours preceding the survey. This was in line with the study conducted in Hossana town, Ethiopia (32.1%) [15]. But it was lower than the study conducted in Metema Hospital (42.2%) [9], Jimma (44.2%) [16], Kenya (37.7%) [17], Eastern Uganda (41%) [18], and Butajira Hospital, Ethiopia (61.2%) [19]. This difference may be due to variations of study periods, geographical location, seasonal variability, and other sociodemographic factors.

Starch staples and legumes were food groups, predominantly consumed by the participants during the 24-hour recall, 96.1% and 81.7%, respectively, in Motta public health institutions. This finding is in line with the study conducted in Butajira, Metema Hospital, Nigeria [3, 19, 20]. On the other hand, organ meat, milk, and milk products were the least consumed food group during the study periods. This is in line with studies conducted at Butajira, Ethiopia, and Metema, Ethiopia. But in Metema in addition to milk, eggs were the least consumed food groups [3, 19]. The reasons might be due to the difference of socioeconomic status, study area, and periods and agrological differences.

This study finding revealed that adult HIV patients who had media exposure were two times more likely to get good diversified diet compared to counterparts. This finding is in line with studies done in central Uganda and South Gondar [15, 20]. The probable reason for this finding may be adult HIV patients who exposed to media sources might capture information about feeding from local media sources. Currently in Ethiopia there are local media that broadcast nutrition and health messages. On the other hand, this study also showed that those patients who had mobile cell phone were more than two times more likely to have got diversified diet as compared to those who had not mobile cell phone. This could be due to patients who had mobile access to close contact with the healthcare provider and could get counseling

and it is important for defaulter tracing mechanism to trace those defaulted individuals.

Those adult HIV patients who got nutritional counseling were more likely to have diversified diet as compared to those who did not get. The probable reason for this finding might be that those adult HIV patients who got nutritional counseling had higher chance to get advice about feeding pattern.

The study also showed that taking alcohol and smoking cigarettes had no association with dietary diversity which is in line with a study done in Uganda [21]. A finding in Botswana showed that age, marital status, and educational status affects the dietary diversity of the individual [22]. Other studies in Filipino [23] and Jimma [16] showed that household income had positive correlation with dietary diversity of the individual. Occupational status, sex, raring small animals, and cultivated dummy vegetables in the garden had significant association with an individual dietary diversity in Jimma [16] and South Gondar [24]. But the above listed variables did not show any association with dietary diversity in this study. A study finding in Metema Hospital also revealed that employment status, duration of anti-retro-viral treatment, and Cotrimoxazole prophylaxis had strong association with level of dietary diversity of an individual which is also in contrast with this study [3]. This may be attributed to many factors such as differences in the study area, study period, and study design.

This study may have certain limitations like recall bias and social desirability bias. And also since this is cross-sectional study design, it does not show real association.

5. Conclusion and Recommendations

The finding of this study revealed that diversified diet is a significant nutritional problem among HIV positive adults in public health facilities in Motta town. Nutritional counseling, having radio/television for source of information access, and having mobile were the factors contributing for dietary diversity. Therefore healthcare provider should focus on nutritional counseling and encourage the patients to use cell phone and increase awareness about the importance of media exposure.

Abbreviations

3TC: Lamivudine
AIDS: Acquired immune deficiency syndrome
AOR: Adjusted odds ratio
ART: Antiretroviral therapy
AZT: Zidovudine
CD4:   Cluster of differentiation 4
CI: Confidence interval
DDS: Dietary diversity score
EDHS: Ethiopian Demographic and Health Survey
PLWHIV: People Living with HIV AIDS
WHO: World Health Organization.

Authors' Contributions

Addisu Tesfaw was responsible for conceptualization. Addisu Tesfaw, Habtamu Temesgen, and Dube Jara were responsible for formal analysis; development or design of methodology; entering data into computer software; supervision; writing original draft; writing review and editing. Habtamu Temesgen and Dube Jara were responsible for validation. All authors read and approved the final manuscript.

Acknowledgments

We thank Debre Markos University, College of Health Science, for providing ethical clearance, data collectors, supervisors, Motta woreda administration, and study participants for their willingness to participate in the study.

References

[1] R. Jayawardena, N. M. Byrne, M. J. Soares, P. Katulanda, B. Yadav, and A. P. Hills, "High dietary diversity is associated with obesity in Sri Lankan adults: an evaluation of three dietary scores," *BMC Public Health*, vol. 13, no. 1, article 314, 2013.

[2] S. Drimie, M. Faber, J. Vearey, and L. Nunez, "Dietary diversity of formal and informal residents in Johannesburg, South Africa," *BMC Public Health*, vol. 13, no. 1, 2013.

[3] T. W. Amare, E. Y. Melkie, K. B. Teresa, and K. Y. Melaku, "Factors associated with dietary diversity among HIV positive adults (= 18 years) attending ART clinic at Mettema hospital, Northwest Ethiopia: cross-sectional study," *Journal of AIDS and Clinical Research*, vol. 6, no. 8, 2015.

[4] N. Nsele, "The effect of seasonal food variety and dietary diversity on the nutritional status of a rural community in KZN," 2014.

[5] A. C. Onyango, M. K. Walingo, G. Mbagaya, and R. Kakai, "Assessing nutrient intake and nutrient status of HIV seropositive patients attending clinic at Chulaimbo sub-district Hospital, Kenya," *Journal of Nutrition and Metabolism*, vol. 2012, Article ID 306530, 6 pages, 2012.

[6] R. K. Sachdeva, A. Sharma, A. Wanchu, V. Dogra, S. Singh, and S. Varma, "Dietary adequacy of HIV infected individuals in north India - A cross-sectional analysis," *Indian Journal of Medical Research*, vol. 134, no. 12, pp. 967–971, 2011.

[7] N. Mpontshane, J. Van Den Broeck, M. Chhagan, K. K. A. Luabeya, A. Johnson, and M. L. Bennish, "HIV infection is associated with decreased dietary diversity in South African children," *Journal of Nutrition*, vol. 138, no. 9, pp. 1705–1711, 2008.

[8] S. Drimie, G. Tafesse, and B. Frayne, *Renewal Ethiopia Background Paper: HIV/AIDS, Food and Nutrition Security*, International Food Policy Research Institute, Washington, DC, USA, 2006.

[9] P. K. Drain, R. Kupka, F. Mugusi, and W. W. Fawzi, "Micronutrients in HIV-positive persons receiving highly active antiretroviral therapy," *American Journal of Clinical Nutrition*, vol. 85, no. 2, pp. 333–345, 2007.

[10] T. D. B. Belachew and T. Temame, "Food insecurity and associated factors among people living with HIV attending ART clinic in Fitche zonal Hospital, Ethiopia," *Journal of Pharmacy and Alternative Medicine*, vol. 8, no. 3, pp. 408–411, 2015.

[11] T. Belachew, C. Hadley, D. Lindstrom, A. Gebremariam, C. Lachat, and P. Kolsteren, "Food insecurity, school absenteeism and educational attainment of adolescents in Jimma Zone Southwest Ethiopia: a longitudinal study," *Nutrition Journal*, vol. 10, no. 1, article 29, 2011.

[12] "Administrative Mt: Annual woreda base plan," Unpublished, 2016.

[13] "Hospital. M: Annual hospital based plan," Unpublished, 2016.

[14] G. Kennedy, T. Ballard, and M. C. Dop, *Guidelines for Measuring Household and Individual Dietary Diversity*, Food and Agriculture Organization of the United Nations, 2011.

[15] S. De Pee and R. D. Semba, "Role of nutrition in HIV infection: Review of evidence for more effective programming in resource-limited settings," *Food and Nutrition Bulletin*, vol. 31, no. 4, pp. S313–S344, 2010.

[16] B. T. Y. Tefera, "Dietary diversity among people 40 years and above in Jimma town, Southwest Ethiopia," *Ethiopian Journal of Health Sciences*, vol. 17, no. 3, pp. 115–119, 2014.

[17] M. L. Kemunto, "Dietary Diversity and Nutritional Status of Pregnant Women Aged 15-49 Years Attending Kapenguria District Hospital West Pokot County, Kenya," 2013.

[18] J. Bukusuba, J. K. Kikafunda, and R. G. Whitehead, "Food security status in households of people living with HIV/AIDS (PLWHA) in a Ugandan urban setting," *British Journal of Nutrition*, vol. 98, no. 1, pp. 211–217, 2007.

[19] D. Gedle, G. Mekuria, G. Kumera, T. Eshete, F. Feyera, and T. Ewunetu, "Food Insecurity and its associated factors among people living with HIV/AIDS receiving anti-retroviral therapy at butajira hospital, Southern Ethiopia," *Nutrition & Food Sciences*, 2015.

[20] S. R. Ajani, "An assessment of dietary diversity in six Nigerian states," *African Journal of Biomedical Research*, vol. 13, no. 3, pp. 161–167, 2010.

[21] D. Carol, "Factors associated with dietary intake among hiv positive adults (18-65 years) at the mildmay center, Kampala, Uganda," 2004.

[22] S. D. Weiser, K. Leiter, D. R. Bangsberg et al., "Food insufficiency is associated with high-risk sexual behavior among women in Botswana and Swaziland," *PLoS Medicine*, vol. 4, no. 10, Article ID e260, pp. 1589–1598, 2007.

[23] G. L. Kennedy, M. R. Pedro, C. Seghieri, G. Nantel, and I. Brouwer, "Dietary diversity score is a useful indicator of micronutrient intake in non-breast-feeding Filipino children," *Journal of Nutrition*, vol. 137, no. 2, pp. 472–477, 2007.

[24] N. M. E. Girma, T. Degnet et al., "Dietary diversity and associated factors among rural households in South Gondar Zone, Northwest Ethiopia," *Feed the Future*, vol. 5, no. 2, article 9, 2015.

3

Determinants of Focused Antenatal Care Uptake among Women in Tharaka Nithi County, Kenya

Eliphas Gitonga

School of Public Health, Kenyatta University, Nairobi, Kenya

Correspondence should be addressed to Eliphas Gitonga; eliphasg@gmail.com

Academic Editor: Ronald J. Prineas

Background. The health status of women is an important indicator of the overall economic health and well-being of a country. Maternal health is closely linked with the survival of newborns. For every woman who dies, about thirty others suffer lifelong injuries. Focused antenatal care is one of the interventions to reduce maternal morbidity and mortality. It recommends four targeted visits during pregnancy within which essential services are offered. The aim of the study was to assess the determinants of uptake of focused antenatal care among women in Tharaka Nithi County, Kenya. *Methods.* This was a descriptive cross-sectional survey. Stratified sampling was used to select the health facilities while systematic sampling was used to select the respondents. Chi square, Fisher's exact test, and logistic regression were used to analyse the data. *Results.* The level of uptake of focused antenatal care was slightly more than half (52%). The determinants of uptake of focused antenatal care are level of education, type of employment, household income, parity, and marital status of the pregnant women. *Conclusion.* Despite high attendance of at least one antenatal visit in Kenya, the uptake of focused antenatal care is proportionally low.

1. Introduction

The Sustainable Development Goals target a global maternal mortality ratio not greater than 70 maternal deaths per 100 000 live births by 2030. The maternal mortality is high in many countries to a point that in every minute a woman dies due to pregnancy related complications. Developing countries account for 99% of the global maternal deaths with sub-Saharan African region alone accounting for 62% [1]. Kenya's maternal mortality ratio is high at 362 maternal deaths per 100 000 live births. A ratio equal to or above 300 maternal deaths per 100 000 live births is considered high [1]. The Kenyan government at national and county level has put measures to improve maternal health. This includes setting up health facilities to offer perinatal care, training of staff, and provision of supplies. Policy guidelines have also been put in place for managerial and operational level.

Focused antenatal care (FANC) recommends that all health pregnant women should have a minimum of four scheduled comprehensive antenatal visits during pregnancy. It is guided by five principles which are quality of care rather than quantity of visits, individualized care, disease detection contrary to risk categorization, evidence based practices, and birth/complication readiness. During their visits, women are counselled on topics such as birth preparedness, complication readiness, danger signs, nutrition, exclusive breastfeeding, and family planning. Women are also immunised against tetanus. They are tested and treated for anaemia, malaria, human immunodeficiency virus/acquired immunedeficiency syndrome (HIV/AIDS), and sexually transmitted infections (STIs). The FANC model suggests that visits should take place before 16 weeks, between 16 and 28 weeks, at 28–32 weeks, and about 36 weeks [2]. Tharaka Nithi County is among the middle counties in uptake of focused antenatal care (FANC). Kenya is now governed through devolved units, counties. The uptake of FANC is the highest in Nairobi County at 73% while it is the lowest in west Pokot County at 18%. The uptake in the entire Tharaka Nithi County is 56%; it is lower in the subcounty of study (52%) [3].

2. Methods

2.1. Study Design and Target Population. A descriptive cross-sectional survey design was used. The target population was women who had delivered within one year prior to the study. This was estimated to be 4732 per year [4].

2.2. Setting. The study was conducted in Tharaka subcounty in eastern province, Kenya. It is in Tharaka Nithi County. Most of the subcounty is rural. The subcounty covers an area of $1569.5\,\mathrm{km}^2$. It has a total population of 130,098 people; among them 67,211 are women [4]. The subcounty has one subcounty hospital, one mission hospital, one sub-subcounty hospital, two health centres, and twenty dispensaries [5]. The number of women of reproductive age is estimated at 31,547. The estimated number of pregnant women is 4732 per year [4]. Only 39.2 percent of the women in the subcounty deliver under skilled attendance. The average distance to the nearest facility is 7 km. Most of the subcounty does not have good transport network [5].

2.3. Variables. The dependent variable was focused antenatal care uptake which was dichotomised as "uptake" for women who attended the four targeted antenatal care visits and "nonuptake" for the women who attended less than four antenatal care visits. The independent variables were age, level of education, marital status, type of employment, household income, gravida (number of pregnancies), and parity (number of births).

2.4. Sampling, Data Collection, and Data Analysis. Stratified sampling was used to select health facilities. Systematic sampling was used where every 14th client attending maternal/child health clinic in the sampled facilities was interviewed. The calculation is as follows $K\mathrm{th} = N/n$. N is the target population which is 4732, n is the sample size which is 345. $K\mathrm{th} = 4732/345 = 14$. The first respondent was picked by randomly picking the attendance number that the mothers were given when they arrived at the clinic. Sample size of 345 was calculated by Kothari method [6]. Semi-structured questionnaires were used to collect data.

Data was entered into STATA version 11. Descriptive statistics and chi square at 95% confidence interval were used to test the association of the independent and dependent variables. The variables that had statistically significant association using chi square and Fisher's exact test were subjected to logistic regression to generate the odds ratios. All results were interpreted as significant at a $P < 0.05$.

2.5. Ethical Considerations. Ethical approval was sought from Kenyatta University Ethics and Review Committee.

3. Results

Focused antenatal care encompasses at four targeted antenatal visits during the pregnancy period. The level of uptake of focused antenatal care is slightly higher than half (52%). Figure 1 shows the level of uptake of focused antenatal care.

3.1. Factors Associated with Antenatal Attendance. Women aged below 20 years were associated with least uptake (31%)

Focused ante natal care uptake

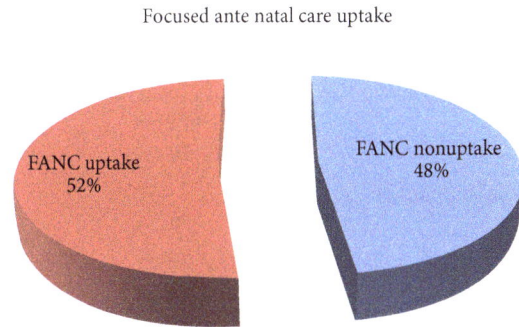

FIGURE 1: Uptake of focused antenatal care.

of FANC compared to women aged 30–34 years (63%). There was a significant association between FANC uptake and the level of education where women with secondary education had a higher uptake (78%) than those with a lower level of education. Having a partner during pregnancy was also associated with higher uptake of FANC (56%) compared with that of women without partners during the pregnancy period. Formal employment and more household income were associated with a higher uptake of FANC (90% and 77%, resp.). The number of pregnancies a woman has ever had and parity were associated with uptake of FANC where women with five or more pregnancies and births had the least uptake (33% and 31%, resp.). Table 1 shows the factors associated with antenatal attendance.

3.2. Determinants of Attendance of Focused Antenatal Care. A factor was deemed a determinant of focused antenatal care uptake if $P < 0.05$ on logistic regression. The likelihood of uptake of focused antenatal care is increased almost four times by attaining secondary education (odds ratio = 3.9). Being married increases the likelihood of FANC uptake by almost three time (odds ratio = 2.7). A formal employment increases by 8 times the likelihood of FANC uptake. An increase in household income increases the likelihood of FANC uptake by 2 times. An increase in parity reduces the likelihood of attending four or more antenatal visits by 0.7 times visits. The influence of age and number of pregnancies (gravida) was not statistically significant. Table 2 shows the determinants of attendance of focused antenatal care.

4. Discussion

Focused antenatal care provides a platform to offer a variety of services to pregnant women. It is one of the main indicators of safe motherhood. It was critical to determine the main factors that influence its uptake. This study found the level of education to be a determinant of uptake of focused antenatal care. An increase in the level of education was found to increase the likelihood of FANC uptake. Education is one of the factors that influence utilisation of health services. Women with higher level of education were more likely to attend more antenatal care visits and earlier in their pregnancy. Education is associated with more appreciation of the importance of antenatal care [7]. Concurring findings

TABLE 1

Variable	Group	Nonuptake of FANC	Uptake of FANC	Statistical values
Age in years grouped	Below 20	22 (68.75%)	10 (31.25%)	$\chi^2(5) = 12.104^*$ $P = 0.033$
	20–24	50 (48.1%)	54 (51.9%)	
	25–29	33 (40.7%)	48 (59.3%)	
	30–34	21 (36.8%)	36 (63.2%)	
	35–39	26 (55.3%)	21 (44.7%)	
	40–44	14 (58.3%)	10 (41.7%)	
Secondary school	No	155 (52.5%)	140 (47.5%)	$\chi^2(1) = 15.975^{**}$ $P < 0.0001$
	Yes	11 (22%)	39 (78%)	
Presence of a partner during pregnancy	No	43 (68.25%)	20 (31.75%)	$\chi^2(1) = 12.52^{**}$ $P < 0.0001$
	Yes	123 (43.6%)	159 (56.4%)	
Type of employment	Nonformal	164 (50.1%)	163 (49.9%)	Fishers exact = 0.001**
	Formal	2 (11.1%)	16 (88.9%)	
Income group in kshs.	Below 1000	84 (61.3%)	53 (38.7%)	$\chi^2(2) = 23.27^{**}$ $P < 0.0001$
	1000–5000	70 (44.9%)	86 (55.1%)	
	Above 5000	12 (23%)	40 (77%)	
Gravida	1-2	93 (48.7%)	98 (51.3%)	$\chi^2(2) = 18.609^{**}$ $P < 0.0001$
	3-4	28 (32.1%)	59 (67.9%)	
	5+	45 (67.2%)	22 (32.8%)	
Parity	1-2	92 (46.9%)	104 (53.1%)	$\chi^2(2) = 16.742^{**}$ $P < 0.0001$
	3-4	31 (35.6%)	56 (64.4%)	
	5+	43 (69.4%)	19 (30.6%)	

*Significant.
**Highly significant.

TABLE 2

Variable	Odds ratio	P value	Confidence interval
Secondary education	3.925**	<0.0001	1.936–7.961
Marital status during pregnancy	2.779**	0.001	1.556–4.966
Type of employment	8.049*	0.006	1.821–35.567
Household income	2.184**	<0.0001	1.575–3.028
Parity	0.738*	0.032	0.560–0.973
Gravida	0.802	0.111	0.613–1.051
Age	1.028	0.711	0.886–1.192

*Significant.
**Highly significant.

were found in study in Mwingi district (Kitui County), Kenya, where women with secondary level of education and above were more likely to attend ANC than those with lower levels of education [8]. In a study in the same area (Tharaka Nithi County), education was also found to influence the place of delivery where women with higher level of education were more likely to deliver in a health facility than those with lower level of education [9]. It was also noted among women in Tharaka subcounty (Tharaka Nithi County, Kenya), birth preparedness was more likely among the more educated than

the less educated [10]. This implies education has critical influence on many aspects of maternal health.

The marital status of women was found to determine uptake of FANC. Married women were more likely to attend the targeted visits as recommended compared to the unmarried. Married women have been found to attend the antenatal visits earlier than the unmarried. This concurs with other studies by Simkhada and colleagues that found that married women were more likely to attend antenatal clinics than the unmarried. This is partially secondary to support from partners and social acceptability of pregnancy. This is thought to encourage attendance of antenatal care [7]. Adolescents and unmarried younger women hid their pregnancy to avoid social embarrassment. This delayed their initiation of antenatal care visits [11]. In a study done in Ethiopia, however, single or divorced mothers more likely attended focused antenatal care than mothers who were married [12].

The type of employment strongly influenced the uptake of FANC. Women in formal employment were more likely to attend the stipulated antenatal visits compared to those in nonformal employment. FANC uptake was influenced by the level of household income. Women from households with higher income had a higher uptake than those from low income households. The economic status of households and individuals is a determinant of uptake of health services. High cost has been found to be a prohibiting factor to use of antenatal services. Women with high household economic status were noted to attend antenatal visits early and more frequently [8]. A lower wealth index was associated with underutilization of antenatal services in Indonesia [13]. This concurs with a Kenyan survey that found that women earning more than a dollar per day were more likely to attend at least four antenatal visits than those earning less than a dollar per day [8].

Parity is number of times a woman has given birth to a foetus above gestation of 24 weeks. The present study found that an increase in parity decreases the likelihood of uptake of FANC. This concurs with other studies that found that high parity has been found in many countries to be a barrier to utilisation of antenatal services [7].

5. Conclusion

Research has shown that the level of uptake of focused antenatal care is slightly above half of the respondents (52%). The main aim of the present study was to elucidate the determinants of focused antenatal care. This study concludes that it is critical to educate the girls in order to achieve the required uptake of focused antenatal care. In addition to education an increase in house hold income, securing more formal jobs, having support from partners during pregnancy, and reduction of the number of births (parity) lead to more likelihood of attending focused antenatal care.

Additional Points

Key Points. (i) Focused antenatal care reaches only about half of the women of reproductive age. (ii) Tharaka Nithi County ranks among the middle performers of uptake of focused antenatal care. (iii) The determinants of focused antenatal care uptake are increased level of education, type of employment, marital status, parity, and higher household income.

Recommendations. (1) This study found that about half of the samples have low uptake of focused antenatal care. In addition to the current strategies for improving maternal health, it is recommended that Kenyan Ministry of health and county governments increases the awareness of focused antenatal care among women of reproductive age. (2) This study found that an increase in the level of education increases the uptake of focused antenatal care. It is therefore recommended that the relevant government ministries and nongovernmental organisations should increase the education of girls (future mothers). (3) This study found that an increase in household income and securing formal employment improves the uptake of focused antenatal care. It is therefore recommended that the relevant government agencies should put in place strategies to increase the household incomes and stimulate formal employment. (4) This study found that an increase in parity lowers the uptake of focused antenatal care. This study therefore recommends to ministry of health targeting women with high parity during sensitization on focused antenatal care. (5) Marital status was found to influence the uptake of focused antenatal care. It is recommended that strategies to increase social support by the partners and relatives be put in place.

Competing Interests

There was no conflict of interests in the study.

References

[1] WHO, UNICEF, UNFPA, and World Bank and United Nations Population Division, *Trends in Maternal Mortality 1990–2013*, WHO, UNICEF, UNFPA, World Bank and United Nations Population Division, Geneva, Switzerland, 2014.

[2] Ministry of Health, *Focused Ante Natal Care*, Ministry of Health, Nairobi, Kenya, 2014.

[3] Kenya National Bureau of Statistics, *Kenya Demographic and Health Survey 20014-15*, KNBS, Nairobi, Kenya, 2015.

[4] Kenya National Bureau of Statistics, *The 2009 Kenya Population and Housing Census*, KNBS, Nairobi, Kenya, 2010.

[5] National Council for Population and Development, *Tharaka District Strategic Plan 2005–2010*, NCPD, Nairobi, Kenya, 2005.

[6] C. R. Kothari, *Research Methodology: Methods and Techniques*, New Age International, New Delhi, India, 2004.

[7] B. Simkhada, E. R. Van Teijlingen, M. Porter, and P. Simkhada, "Factors affecting the utilization of antenatal care in developing countries: systematic review of the literature," *Journal of Advanced Nursing*, vol. 61, no. 3, pp. 244–260, 2008.

[8] J. M. Nzioki, R. O. Onyango, and J. H. Ombaka, "Sociodemographic factors influencing maternal and child health service utilization in mwingi; A rural semi-arid district in Kenya," *American Journal of Public Health Research*, vol. 3, no. 1, pp. 21–30, 2015.

[9] E. Gitonga and M. Felarmine, "Determinants of health facility delivery among women in Tharaka Nithi County, Kenya," *The Pan African Medical Journal*, vol. 2, supplement 2, p. 9, 2016.

[10] E. Gitonga, M. Keraka, and P. Mwaniki, "Birth preparedness among women in Tharaka Nithi County, Kenya," *African Journal of Midwifery and Women's Health*, vol. 9, no. 4, pp. 153–157, 2015.

[11] C. Pell, A. A. Men, F. Were, N. A. Afrah, and S. Chatio, "Factors affecting antenatal care attendance: results from qualitative studies in Ghana, Kenya and Malawi," *PLoS ONE*, vol. 8, no. 1, Article ID e53747, 2013.

[12] T. G. Amanuel Alemu, "Focused antenatal care service utilization and associated factors in Dejen and Aneded Districts, Northwest Ethiopia," *Primary Health Care: Open Access*, vol. 4, no. 4, article no. 170, 2014.

[13] C. R. Titaley, M. J. Dibley, and C. L. Roberts, "Factors associated with underutilization of antenatal care services in Indonesia: results of Indonesia Demographic and Health Survey 2002/2003 and 2007," *BMC Public Health*, vol. 10, article 485, 2010.

4

Vaccination Coverage and Associated Factors among Children Aged 12–23 Months in Debre Markos Town, Amhara Regional State, Ethiopia

Tenaw Gualu and Abebe Dilie

Department of Nursing, College of Health Sciences, Debre Markos University, Debre Markos, Ethiopia

Correspondence should be addressed to Tenaw Gualu; tenawgualu@yahoo.com

Academic Editor: Ronald J. Prineas

Introduction. Vaccination is the administration of a vaccine or a biological substance intended to stimulate a recipient's immune system to produce antibodies or undergo other changes that provide future protection against specific infectious diseases. *Objective.* To determine vaccination coverage and associated factors among children aged 12–23 months in Debre Markos town 2016. *Methods.* Community-based cross-sectional study was employed among 288 mothers/caretakers to child (12–23 months) pair. Study populations were selected using systematic random sampling technique. Structured interviewer administered questionnaires were used to collect data. Variables with P value of less than 0.05 in multivariate analysis were considered as statistically significant at 95% CI. *Result.* About 264 (91.7%) of children were completely vaccinated. Male birth 3.24 (1.16–9.04), wanted pregnancy 2.89 (1.17–7.17), having at least two ANC follow-ups 4.04 (1.35–12.06), and short distance from vaccination site 3.38 (1.29–8.86) were found positively associated with complete immunization. *Conclusion and Recommendation.* There was relatively high immunization coverage in the study. Child's sex, ANC follow-up, type of pregnancy, and distance from health institution were factors associated with complete vaccination. Preventing unwanted pregnancy and promoting ANC and postnatal follow-up should be strengthened. Vaccination sites should also be further expanded.

1. Introduction

Vaccination is the administration of a vaccine, that is, a biological substance intended to stimulate a recipient's immune system to produce antibodies or undergo other changes that provide future protection against specific infectious diseases. Immunization is the stimulation of changes in the immune system through which that protection occurs [1].

The Expanded Program on Immunization (EPI) was established by the World Health Organization in 1974 to control vaccine preventable diseases. In Ethiopian, EPI program was launched in 1980 [2]. It was launched with the aim of reducing mortality and morbidity of children and mothers from vaccine preventable diseases. The target group when the program started were children under two years of age until it changed to under one year in 1986 to be in line with the global immunization target [3].

In a study conducted in Ethiopia, it was found that 73.2% of the children were fully immunized, 20.3% were partially immunized, and 6.5% received no vaccine [4]. In another study conducted, 76% of the children were fully immunized. Dropout rate was 6.5% for BCG to measles, 2.7% for Penta 1 to Penta 3, and 4.5% for Pneumonia 1 to Pneumonia 3 [5].

Vaccination is a highly effective method of preventing certain infectious diseases. Routine immunization programs protect most of the world's children from a number of infectious diseases that previously claimed millions of lives each year [6].

In Ethiopia, vaccine preventable diseases contribute substantially to under-five mortality as well as morbidity. Diarrhea (18%), pneumonia (18%), measles (1%), and meningitis are the leading causes of child mortality in the country [3].

Ten currently available EPI vaccines in Ethiopia include (BCG, measles, DPT-HepB-Hib or pentavalent, rotavirus, pneumococcus vaccine (PCV), and OPV. Moreover, it is directed in the implementation guideline to introduce Inactivated Polio Virus (IPV), measles-rubella, meningitis, and yellow fever vaccines for less than one-year-old children [2].

However, many factors are linked to un/undervaccinated children. In Ethiopia, living in rural area and distance to health clinic, mothers with limited education, and socioeconomic capital are linked to low vaccine uptake and placing children at risk for vaccine preventable diseases [7]. Mother education, mothers' perception to accessibility of vaccines, mothers' knowledge to vaccine schedule of their site, place of delivery, and living altitude were independent predictors of children immunization status [4].

As a result of the ten vaccines introduced, complementary with other interventions, many deaths due to vaccine preventable disease are being averted than ever before [3]. However, still related system-wide barriers are linked to incomplete vaccination or unvaccination of children.

As a result, childhood immunization and associated factors should be targeted through educational research. This study was conducted to identify the current gaps and supplement the past studies. Thus, this study can be used as a reference for health care providers, health care educators, policy makers, and future researchers in this and/or related fields.

2. Objectives

The main objective is to determine vaccination coverage and associated factors among children aged 12–23 months in Debre Markos town, Amhara Regional State, Ethiopia, 2016.

3. Methods

3.1. Study Area. The study was conducted in Debre Markos town. Debre Markos is found in East Gojjam Zone of Amhara Regional State of Ethiopia.

3.2. Study Period. The study was conducted from August to September, 2016.

3.3. Study Design. Community-based cross-sectional study design was used.

3.4. Source Population. The source population was all mothers/caretakers to children aged 12–23 months pair in Debre Markos town.

3.5. Study Population. The study population included all mothers/caretakers to children aged 12–23 months pair in Debre Markos town who fulfill the inclusion criteria.

3.6. Inclusion Criteria. The inclusion criteria were all mothers/caretakers to children aged 12–23 months pair who are permanent residents (for at least six months) in Debre Markos town.

3.7. Exclusion Criteria

(i) Mothers/caretakers with missed immunization card

(ii) Mentally/critically ill mothers/caretakers

(iii) Not volunteering to participate/being unable to give required information

3.8. Sample Size. The sample size was determined by using single proportion formula, by using prevalence of complete immunization coverage in children as 22.9% from previous study conducted in Ethiopia [8], 95% CI, and 10% nonresponse rate. Hence, the sample size calculated was 298.

3.9. Sampling Procedure. There were seven kebeles in the town. All the seven kebeles were included in the study. At each kebele, households are selected by using systematic random sampling. The sample in each kebele is allocated proportional to the number of households. When two or more eligible mothers/caretakers to child pair were found, only one was included by lottery method.

3.10. Instrument and Personnel. Structured interviewer administered questionnaire was used to collect the data. It was adapted from previous researches done on similar title [4, 7, 9]. The questionnaire was first prepared in English and translated to Amharic and back to English to maintain the consistency of the content of the instrument. Seven nursing students participated as data collectors.

3.11. Data Quality Control. Orientation and training were given to data collectors regarding purpose of study and ethical issues. Pretest was done on 5% of the actual study subjects out of the study area. After pretest, vague terms and questions were discarded. The result of pretest is not included in the study result.

3.12. Data Processing and Analysis. The data was cleaned, coded, and entered in EpiData version 3.1 and transferred to SPSS version 20.0 for analysis. Descriptive and inferential statistics were used to present the data. Descriptive statistics like frequency and percentage were used to summarize the sociodemographic characteristics of the study participants. Variables showed statistical significant in bivariate analysis, that is, P value < 0.05, and were entered in the final model of multivariate analysis. And P value of less than 0.05 in multivariate analysis was considered as statistically significant at 95% CI.

3.13. Operational Definitions

Complete Vaccination. A child who received ten basic vaccines (one dose of BCG, three doses each of the DPT-HepB-Hib (pentavalent), three doses of polio vaccines, three doses of PCV, two doses of Rota vaccine, and one dose of measles vaccine before first birth date) is considered to be completely vaccinated.

Incomplete Vaccination. A child who received some of the vaccines and/or not the full dose of the ten vaccines before

TABLE 1: Sociodemographic characteristics of parents in Debre Markos town, Amhara Regional State, North West Ethiopia, September 2016. ($N = 288$).

Variables	Frequency (N)	Percentage (%)
Relation of the respondent to the child		
Biological parent	269	93.4
Nonbiological parent	19	6.6
Age		
15–25	61	21.2
26–35	193	67
36–45	34	11.8
Religious affiliation		
Orthodox Christian	279	96.9
Muslim	5	1.7
Protestant	4	1.4
Marital status		
Not married	17	5.9
Married	254	88.2
Divorced	11	3.8
Widowed	6	2.1
Ethnicity		
Amhara	285	99
Oromo	1	0.3
Tigre	2	0.7
Educational status		
Not educated	25	8.7
Primary education	36	12.5
High school	164	56.9
College/university	63	21.9
Occupational status		
Employed	245	85.1
Non employed	43	14.9
Family size		
≤3	68	23.6
>3	220	76.4
Household monthly income in Ethiopian Birr		
<1000	18	6.3
1000–25000	42	14.6
>2500	228	79.1
Living condition		
Both parents are alive	257	89.2
Mother only	12	4.2
Both parents are not alive	19	6.6

first birth date is considered to have received incomplete vaccination.

3.14. *Ethical Considerations.* Ethical clearance was obtained from research and publication committee of Debre Markos University, College of Health Sciences. The purpose and importance of the study was explained to mothers and caregivers. And informed written consent was obtained from the mothers/caregivers of the children. Privacy and confidentiality was maintained throughout the study.

4. Result

4.1. Sociodemographic Characteristics of Parents. The study included a total of 298 eligible participants. Among this, 288 of participants voluntarily agreed to participate in this study. This made the response rate of the study to be 96.6%.

Majority of the participants, 193 (67%), were in age groups between 26 and 35. The mean age of the participants was 30.01. And about 279 (96.9%) of the participants were Orthodox Christian followers (Table 1).

TABLE 2: Characteristics of children aged 12–23 months in Debre Markos town, Amhara Regional State, North West Ethiopia, September 2016. (N = 288).

Variables	Frequency (N)	Percentage (%)
Sex of the child		
Male	130	45.1
Female	158	54.9
Average birth weight in grams		
<1500	22	7.6
1500–2500	36	12.5
≥2500–4000	230	79.9
Birth order		
First	131	45.5
Second	79	27.4
Third	64	22.2
Fourth	14	4.9

TABLE 3: Obstetrics history of the mothers in Debre Markos town, Amhara Regional State, North West Ethiopia, September 2016. (N = 288).

Variables	Frequency (N)	Percentage (%)
Gestational age in weeks		
<32	1	0.3
32–36	16	5.6
37–42	262	91
≥42	9	3.1
ANC follow-up (at least two)		
Yes	260	90.3
No	28	9.7
TT vaccination (at least two)		
Yes	250	86.8
No	38	13.2
Place of delivery		
Health institution	254	88.2
Home	34	11.8
Type of pregnancy		
Wanted	227	78.8
Unwanted	61	21.2

TABLE 4: Type of vaccines received by children aged 12–23 months in Debre Markos town, Amhara Regional State, North West Ethiopia, September 2016. (N = 288).

Variables	Frequency (N)	Percentage (%)
BCG		
Yes	278	96.5
No	10	3.5
Polio O		
Yes	273	94.8
No	15	5.2
Polio 1		
Yes	279	96.9
No	9	3.1
Polio 2		
Yes	269	93.4
No	19	6.6
Polio 3		
Yes	266	92.4
No	22	7.6
Penta 1		
Yes	279	96.9
No	9	3.1
Penta 2		
Yes	267	92.7
No	21	7.3
Penta 3		
Yes	265	92
No	23	8
PCV 1		
Yes	277	96.2
No	11	3.8
PCV 2		
Yes	267	92.7
No	21	7.3
PCV 3		
Yes	265	92
No	23	8
Rota 1		
Yes	278	96.5
No	10	3.5
Rota 2		
Yes	269	93.4
No	19	6.6
Measles		
Yes	264	91.7
No	24	8.3

4.2. Characteristics of the Child. About 158 (54.9%) of the children were females and majority were first in birth order (Table 2).

4.3. Obstetrics History. While about 260 (90.3%) of the mothers had ANC follow-up, 254 (88.2%) gave birth at health care institutions (Table 3).

4.4. Level of Vaccination. Among 288 children, 264 (91.7%) were completely vaccinated, 19 (6.6%) were partially vaccinated, and 5 (1.7%) were not vaccinated at all. The overall dropout rate was 5% (Table 4).

About 274 (95.1%) of the mothers/caretakers perceived vaccination as important. The main reasons that respondents vaccinated their children were protection, immunity, and good health, prevention of infections, advice from professionals, and being compulsory, 272 (96.1%), 247 (87.3%), 17 (6%), and 2 (0.7%), respectively.

4.5. Factors Associated with Complete Immunization. Relation to the child, occupational status, child's sex, type of

TABLE 5: Factors associated with complete immunization of children aged 12–23 months in Debre Markos town, Amhara Regional State, North West Ethiopia, September 2016. (N = 288).

Variables	Complete immunization				P value
	Yes	No	COR (95% CI)	AOR (95% CI)	
Relation to the child					
Biological parent	249	20	3.32 (1.00–1.95)		
Nonbiological parent	15	4	1		
Occupational status					
Employed	229	16	3.27 (1.30–8.21)		
Unemployed	35	8	1		
Child's sex					
Male	124	6	2.66 (1.02–6.91)	3.24 (1.16–9.04)*	0.025
Female	140	18	1	1	
Type of pregnancy					
Wanted	213	14	2.98 (1.25–7.10)	2.89 (1.17–7.17)*	0.022
Unwanted	51	10	1	1	
Place of delivery					
Health institution	236	18	2.81 (1.03–7.66)		
Home	28	6	1		
ANC (at least 2 follow-ups)					
Yes	242	18	3.67 (1.32–10.19)	4.04 (1.35–12.06)*	0.012
No	22	6	1	1	
Vaccination schedule					
I know	228	16	3.17 (1.26–7.94)		
I do not know	36	8	1		
Distance from vaccination site					
≤20 minutes	231	16	3.5 (1.39–8.82)	3.38 (1.29–8.86)*	0.013
>20 minutes	33	8	1	1	

1 = reference; *P value < 0.05 (significant).

pregnancy, place of delivery, ANC follow-up, knowledge of time of vaccination schedule, and distance from vaccination site were found to be significant on bivariate analysis. And child's sex, type of pregnancy, ANC follow-up and distance from vaccination site were found to be associated with complete vaccination on multivariate analysis (Table 5).

5. Discussion

In this study, it was found that 91.7% of children were completely vaccinated, 6.6% were partially vaccinated, and 1.7% were not vaccinated at all and there is 5% overall dropout rate. The result showed increased vaccination coverage when compared to previous studies done in different areas [4, 7]. This may be due to increasing access of vaccination and community awareness from time to time.

Adjusting for other factors, child's sex was significantly associated with complete immunization. Males were three times more likely to be completely vaccinated 3.24 (1.16–9.04) when compared to females. The result is in line with previous study done in northern Ethiopia [5]. But in a study done in Iran, no correlation was detected between gender and immunization status [10]. The difference might from cultural differences between study populations.

The type of pregnancy was another factor which predicts complete immunization. The odds of wanted pregnancy were two times more likely for complete immunization 2.89 (1.17–7.17) than unwanted pregnancy. The study is not congruent with previous study which showed no statistical association between immunization and wanted pregnancy [11].

Another factor that affects complete immunization was ANC follow-up during pregnancy. Mothers who had at least two ANC follow-ups during pregnancy were four times more likely to vaccinate 4.04 (1.35–12.06) their children when compared to mothers who did not have ANC follow-up during pregnancy. This is in line with a study done previously in which there was inverse correlation between delayed vaccination and the number of periodical visits of health centers [12]. This might be because mothers during ANC visit would receive counseling and education about the importance of postnatal visits and activities.

Distance of home from vaccination site was another predictive factor for children complete vaccination. Parents who are less than or equal to twenty minutes away from vaccination sites were three times more likely to vaccinate their children 3.38 (1.29–8.86) than parents who are more than twenty minutes away. But in a study done previously, no correlation was detected between vaccination delay time and distance from health centers [12].

6. Conclusion and Recommendation

There was relatively high immunization coverage in the study. About 91.7% were completely vaccinated, 6.6% were partially vaccinated, and 5 (1.7%) were not vaccinated at all and the overall dropout rate was 5%.

Child's sex, ANC follow-up during pregnancy, type of pregnancy. and distance from health institution were factors associated with complete vaccination of children.

Preventing unwanted pregnancy through family planning and promoting ANC and postnatal follow-up should be strengthened.

Vaccination sites should also be further expanded and accessible to the community. And health education should also be given largely to the community about the need to vaccinate all children.

Acknowledgments

The authors' gratitude is extended to Debre Markos University, Debre Markos town, administrators, data collectors, and study participants.

References

[1] P. Nieburg and M. Nancy, "Role(s) of vaccines and immunization programs in global disease control," Center for Strategic & International Studies, 2011.

[2] "Ethiopia National Expanded Programme on Immunization; Comprehensive Multi-Year Plan 2016–2020," Addis Ababa: Federal Ministry of Health, Ethiopia, 2015.

[3] "National Expanded Program on Immunization Implementation Guideline," 2015, Addis Abab: Federal Democratic Republic of Ethiopia Ministry of Health.

[4] W. Animaw, W. Taye, B. Merdekios, M. Tilahun, and G. Ayele, "Expanded program of immunization coverage and associated factors among children age 12–23 months in Arba Minch town and Zuria District, Southern Ethiopia, 2013," *BMC Public Health*, vol. 14, no. 1, article 464, 2014.

[5] M. B. Kassahun, G. A. Biks, and A. S. Teferra, "Level of immunization coverage and associated factors among children aged 12–23 months in Lay Armachiho District, North Gondar Zone, Northwest Ethiopia: a community based cross sectional study," *BMC Research Notes*, vol. 8, no. 1, article 239, 2015.

[6] "Vaccine-preventable diseases and vaccines," WHO, 2005.

[7] Control CfD Prevention, "Epidemiology of the unimmunized child: findings from the peer-reviewed published literature, 1999–2009," World Health Organisation, 2009.

[8] H. Mohammed and A. Atomsa, "Assessment of Child immunization coverage and associated factors in oromia regional state, Eastern Ethiopia," *Science, Technology and Arts Research Journal*, vol. 2, no. 1, p. 36, 2013.

[9] A. Negussie, W. Kassahun, S. Assegid, and A. K. Hagan, "Factors associated with incomplete childhood immunization in Arbegona district, southern Ethiopia: a case—control study," *BMC Public Health*, vol. 16, no. 1, article 27, 2016.

[10] N. Nisar, M. Mirza, and M. H. Qadri, "Knowledge, attitude and practices of mothers regarding immunization of one year old child at Mawatch Goth, Kemari town, Karachi," *Pakistan Journal of Medical Sciences*, vol. 26, no. 1, pp. 183–186, 2010.

[11] R. A. Brenner, B. G. Simons-Morton, B. Bhaskar, A. Das, and J. D. Clemens, "Prevalence and predictors of immunization among inner-city infants: a birth cohort study," *Pediatrics*, vol. 108, no. 3, pp. 661–670, 2001.

[12] J. Poorolajal, S. Khazaei, Z. Kousehlou, S. J. Bathaei, and A. Zahiri, "Delayed vaccination and related predictors among infants," *Iranian Journal of Public Health*, vol. 41, no. 10, pp. 65–71, 2012.

5

Parents' Experiences and Sexual Topics Discussed with Adolescents in the Accra Metropolis

Elizabeth AKu Baku (ID),[1] Isaac Agbemafle (ID),[2]
Agnes Millicent Kotoh (ID),[3] and Richard M. K. Adanu[4]

[1]School of Nursing and Midwifery, University of Health and Allied Sciences, Ho, Volta Region, Ghana
[2]Department of Family and Community Health, School of Public Health, University of Health and Allied Sciences, Ho, Volta Region, Ghana
[3]Department of Population, Family and Reproductive Health, School of Public Health, University of Ghana, Legon, Greater Accra Region, Accra, Ghana
[4]Office of the Dean, School of Public Health, University of Ghana, Legon, Greater Accra Region, Accra, Ghana

Correspondence should be addressed to Elizabeth AKu Baku; ebkpodotsi@uhas.edu.gh

Academic Editor: Carol J. Burns

Background. Traditionally, discussion about sexuality is subdued in proverbs and is earmarked for adults. However, adolescents also need information about their sexuality to make informed choices regarding sexual behaviours. This study, therefore, seeks to explore the experiences of parents discussing sexuality topics with adolescents in the Accra Metropolis, Ghana. *Methods.* This was a qualitative study that used focus group discussions (FGDs) and in-depth interviews (IDIs) to assess parents' experiences in discussing sexuality topics with adolescents. The FGDs, consisting of 8-12 parents each, were conducted for one "all fathers", then another "all mothers", and finally "fathers and mothers" groups. Parents who were not part of the FGDs were engaged in IDIs. The data was transcribed and analyzed manually. *Results.* Most of the parent-adolescent sexual discussions were based on physical changes, personal hygiene, abstinence, abortion, and saying "no" to forced sex. Parents discussed sexuality issues with adolescents to prevent them from premarital sex, pregnancy, and sexually transmitted infections. Parents sourced their knowledge about sexuality from books, television, radio, and personal experiences. Parents always seize opportunities such as television scenes to discuss sexual topics with their children. Although some parents expressed some level of comfort discussing sexual topics with adolescents, many still had difficulties explaining some terminologies related to sex. Preferentially, parents were protective of their girls than the boys when discussing issues on sexuality. Most parents received no sexuality education from their parents but a few reminisced precautionary advices on sex. Parents believed training on sexuality issues will help them to better discuss sexual topics with adolescents. *Conclusions.* Ghanaian parents preferentially discuss sex with their daughters as a protective tool against irresponsible sexual behaviours. Parents still have challenges discussing adolescent sexuality topics; hence equipping parents to effectively discuss such sensitive topics will improve adolescent reproductive health and sexual behaviour.

1. Introduction

Adolescence is a period of risk taking, particularly on sex, but many adolescents are not educated about their sexual and reproductive health issues by their parents (Arnett, 2003) [1]. Lack of education on sexual and reproductive health for adolescents may lead to increased risk of sexually transmitted infections (STIs), unintended pregnancy, and

other health problems [2]. Sedgh and Hussain noted that even though the importance of sexuality education is accepted, the intervention is opposed in many African countries, including Ghana, probably because of cultural beliefs and norms [3]. This stems from the fact that early introduction to information about sexuality and reproductive health could be seen as detrimental to adolescents than helping them to overcome sexual and reproductive health risks that they face in growing up. In Kenya, the main barrier to meaningful sex education between mothers and their daughters was taboos that prevent parents from discussing sex with their children [4]. In the Kenya study, most mothers had no sex education either from their parents or other family members and hence could not talk about sex to their own daughters. Similarly, parents in three cities in different regions of the United States complained that their parents never talked to them about sex; therefore it was difficult for them to know how to talk about sex to their own children [5]. Beyer reported that sex is still not discussed in certain localities in South Africa because adolescents in those localities were perceived as a high-risk group that could become curious about their sexual desires [6].

Although censored, the 2014 Demographic and Health Survey report indicated that about 42.7% of Ghanaian girls and 26.6% of boys become sexually active in their teens [7]. A 2004 national representative survey in Ghana indicated that nearly 75% of sexually active adolescent girls and 33% of sexually active boys reported receiving money or gifts in exchange for sex [8]. Indeed, this is a usual component of "boy-girl-friend" relationships in Ghana and other African countries. Irrespective of the risks associated with being an adolescent, talking about sex and sexual activities is not openly encouraged in Africa probably because sex is considered a sacred adult affair that is enshrined in secrecy. A negative effect arising out of secrecy could be incidence of teenage pregnancy that was recorded in many African countries including Ghana. For example in 2014 Ghana recorded teenage pregnancy rate of 11.8% [9] as compared to other African countries like Nigeria 23% [10], Kenya 18% [11], and South Africa 13.9% [12].

In Ghana, cultural taboos prevented education of adolescents on sexuality. Among the Akans, for instance it was a taboo to talk about sexual issues with a child because they believed that the child could be "spoilt". Even if the child wanted to find out certain things about sex, they would tell the child that he/she was not matured enough to know about such issues. Due to the taboos associated with sexuality education, some parts of the body could not be mentioned because it was considered a taboo to do so. For that matter, they expressed such things using euphemisms. For example, they prefer to call the penis "manhood". Some sexual discussions only took place with the girl after menarche. No education is given to boys on their sexuality [13].

Ghanaian culture considers sexuality as sacred; that is, it is something that should not be discussed with children and adolescents. In Ghana, teaching of sex education to children is generally seen as introducing them to early sexual intercourse and, subsequently, pregnancies. The understanding and tolerance for sex education among Ghanaian parents are nonexistent. Culture, thus, accounts for this intolerance for sex education[14].

However, there is some evidence of parent-adolescent sexuality discussion in some Ghanaian homes. A nationally representative data from Ghana showed adolescent communication with family and nonfamily members [15]. Traditionally, adolescents in Africa are rebuked for questioning their parents, particularly on issues concerning sex, and

they would be described as "spoilt children". Brocato and Dwamena-Aboagye documented that Ghanaian children, especially girls, are brought up with strict discipline and fear, making them timid to ask very sensitive questions on adolescent sexuality issues [16].

The Ghana Education Service has approved a cross-curricular method, in which some subjects related to sexual and reproductive health (SRH) have been included in specified school topics [17]. Basic SRH education topics are introduced in the fourth year of primary school, a level at which all subjects, including those that cover SRH topics, are required. However, in senior high school, the topics are included into two core, compulsory subjects (social studies and integrated science) and two elective subjects (biology and management in living). There are also two main cocurricular programs that offer additional activities outside of the regular curriculum, either during or after school: The School Health Education Programme (SHEP) and the HIV alert program. The goal of SHEP is to guide children in school to acquire the knowledge, skills and attitudes needed to achieve lifelong health [18]. The HIV alert programme, on the other hand, stresses the prevention of HIV infection and the significance of interrelated issues, such as chastity and abstinence. Both programs operate in all schools in Ghana and they target students in primary and junior high schools in particular. These are also offered in senior high schools with support from the Ministry of Health and the Ghana Health Service. The programme also exists in colleges of education as part of the preservice training for teachers who will teach this subject at the primary and junior high school levels [18].

In Ghana, religion and morality are considered as bed associates and study shows that religious teaching in Ghana from all the three major religious groups—Christianity, Islam, and traditional religions—forbids sex outside the background of marriage and, therefore, views it as a sin [19]. Religion has, therefore, been found to exercise the greatest effect on sexual socialization in Ghana than the state and society [19]. The moral structure religion produces seemed strong to the extent that parents saw it as substitute to the traditional system. When they could not exercise any meaningful influence on regulating their adolescents' sexual behaviours, they switch to religion for help [20]. The switch towards religion as a regulating moral mechanism over adolescents' sexual behaviour is validated on the perceived benefits from the moral system. Parents perceived religion as playing two major positive roles in regulating adolescent sexual behaviours. The first was the inhibition role. This is the view that religion values discourage children from certain immoral acts like sex. Secondly, religion was perceived to play a facilitative role. In this role, religious values, principles, ideals, and perhaps beliefs teach adolescents to make good choices. The role is best instigated by religious leaders in churches who basically become counsellors for adolescents. The talk therapy that is observed is reflective of religious directing the choice of adolescent behaviours [20].

In Africa, parent-adolescent communication on sexuality has turned sexuality discussion into forbidden subject for fear that adolescents may become curious about their sexual desires. On the contrary, there is considerable evidence that parent-adolescent sexuality communication is linked to reduction in risky adolescent sexual behaviours and delays in initiation of sexual intercourse [21, 22]. Success of parent-adolescent sexuality communication depends on parents as gatekeepers of sexuality information. At home, parents define content of adolescent sexuality discussion but there may be gaps between what they perceive that adolescents need and what adolescents themselves really need [23]. This creates conflict and leads to prevention of communication as many parents and adolescents do not have the ability to engage in active sexuality discussions. This present study, therefore, seeks to examine parents' opinions in relation to discussions with their adolescents about sexuality.

2. Materials and Methods

2.1. Study Design and Setting. A qualitative exploratory study design was used to explore the experiences of parents discussing topics on sex with their adolescent children in the Accra Metropolis, Ghana. The study has its research setting at the Osu Klottey and Ablekuma South submetropolises in the Accra Metropolis. The Accra Metropolis has 11 submetropolises, and the study was conducted in these two submetropolises because they are geographically far apart and very diverse. The Osu Klottey submetropolis is one of the oldest Ga communities along the coast in Accra and its inhabitants are mainly fishermen and fishmongers. Ablekuma South is a newly created submetropolis and it is cosmopolitan in nature.

2.2. Selection of Participants. Parent, defined as either the biological father or mother of the adolescent, was selected for the study if his/her adolescent child attends a public junior high school and has been living in one of the two areas for at least one year. The parents were recruited through their adolescent children in school using the simple balloting technique. A parent whose adolescent child picks "yes" from the ballot papers was given a letter inviting his/her parent to be part of the study. Parents who indicated their willingness to participate in the study signed informed consent forms and were recruited. The age range of the parents was between 25 and 55 years. Forty-four parents (6 teachers, 3 nurses, 2 mechanics, 1 pastor, 11 traders, 1 administrative officer, 2 record officers, 4 bankers, 12 artisans, and 2 hair dressers) were selected for the study. All the parents who were invited to take part in the study participated except one parent who travelled at the time of the study.

2.3. Data Collection. Focus group discussions (FGDs) and in-depth interviews (IDIs) were used to collect the data for the study. Four FGDs were held: 2 mothers' groups, 1 fathers' group, and 1 mixed group (both mothers and fathers). The IDIs were held with 6 mothers and 4 fathers (2 teachers, 1 nurse, 1 mechanic, 4 traders, 1 record officer, and 1 administrative officer). The FGDs were used because of the group dynamics that stimulate discussions, generate ideas, and provide the opportunity to explore sensitive issues or pursue a topic in greater depth. This produces results that are

peculiar to the mix of people and provides more insights into the subject of study. IDIs have the advantage of avoiding too much prejudgment, if the questions asked are not restrictive and can elicit information that reflects the interviewees' views and beliefs about an issue [24].

The in-depth interviews (IDIs) were conducted with parents in the comfort of their homes. The focus group discussions were held in a classroom at one of the study sites. A semistructured interview guide was used to conduct the interviews. Open ended questions were used to generate answers and these were probed until a full-understanding accomplished. The interviews were conducted in English and Twi and audiotaped with a digital voice recorder with the consent of participants. The interviews conducted in English were transcribed verbatim and those conducted in Twi were transcribed in English by the research assistants who understood the Twi language very well. The non-English transcripts were verified by the authors to further ensure the right content was reported. Each interview lasted between 30 and 60 minutes.

2.4. Data Quality Assurance. One facilitator and two observers who had worked with adolescents in health institutions were given a day's training. The training focused on the aim of the study, which is the process of conducting FGDs, the role of the facilitator and the observers in the FGD, and the topics to be discussed. Similarly, research assistants were taken through how to conduct IDIs. The interview guides for both the FGDs and the IDIs were pretested using three IDIs and one FGD in a different setting.

2.5. Data Analysis. The data were analyzed manually. The IDIs and FGDs were transcribed verbatim and processed using inductive thematic analysis [25]. Each of the tape recordings was separately transcribed by two independent research assistants and their scripts were compared. The transcriptions were compared and portions that differed significantly from each other were retranscribed by listening to those portions of the tape recording again. Thematic analysis was used to analyze the transcribed data and notes taken by the observer manually. First, the analysis of the data began with a search for similar ideas, thoughts, recurring words, and differences within the data. Second, codes were created manually based on the ideas, thoughts, and words. Similar and related codes were grouped to form themes and subthemes. The themes capture core issues discussed in relation to the overall research question. Third, as the analysis continued, related themes were clustered to form categories. The words representing the categories were written in the margin of the script where the theme or code was found and coloured. This was necessary to define and redefine logical connections between the themes for easy interpretation. Having developed the themes, the report was written verbatim, expressing the views and vivid thoughts of all the participants in the IDIs and FGDs.

2.6. Ethical Clearance. The study was approved by the Noguchi Memorial Institute for Medical Research Review

Board (IRB 097/11-12), University of Ghana, Legon. Permission was also obtained from the Accra Metropolitan Director of Education, and the head teachers of the selected junior high schools. Each parent selected for the study signed a consent form before taking part in the study. The parents were told that they could withdraw from the study at any point when they felt they were no more interested. Confidentiality and privacy were assured throughout the study. Anonymity was maintained by not linking responses to individual participants. All the parents who consented to the FGDs or IDIs participated in the discussions or in-depth interviews to completion. Thus, none of the parents withdrew from the study at any given time.

3. Results

3.1. Parents Discussing Sexuality Topics with Adolescents

3.1.1. Sexuality Topics Parents Ever Discussed with Adolescents. Many of the parents reported that they talked about menstruation, peer pressure to engage in sex, premarital sex, and HIV/AIDS. These responses were age-related as all the parents involved in this study had children between the ages of 12 and 17 years. Other parents talked about body changes, personal hygiene, abstinence, the consequences of getting pregnant, abortion, and how to say "no" if somebody wanted to force them to have sex.

> *"I always hammer on premarital sex because I have two girls. I tell them that premarital sex is not safe because they could get pregnant. And if they become pregnant, they would face the consequences alone while the boy would continue his education. She, the girl would be drawn back in the number of years she would spend in school because she must stop the school and have the baby before going back to continue or she might not continue the school at all. Secondly, she could get sexually transmitted diseases which could affect her reproductive life in future."* (a father who is an administrative officer, IDI)

> *"I talked to the children about the consequences of getting pregnant and abortion so that they will know exactly what to do and what not to do."* (a father who is a mechanic, IDI)

Even though many of the parents said they did not find it difficult talking about any sexual topics with their adolescents, a mother admitted having problem talking to her daughter about sexuality issues.

> *"I find it difficult talking with my daughter about sexual intercourse and kissing because she would not like me to talk about it. Sometimes you would be watching TV with her and you would see her covering her face during such scenes or she would walk out of the room. Sometimes I call her to come back and ask her to sit down and watch. Then I would tell her that it was just a film and they are*

> *just showing what people have been doing. It is when you practice what you see that you will have problems."* (a mother who is a data officer, IDI)

3.1.2. Gender and Age Disparities in Parent Discussion of Adolescent Sexuality. There were gender differences regarding communication among parents with their adolescents. The parents had diverse views about whether they should spend more time discussing sexual topics with boys or girls. Many of the parents would like to discuss more sexuality topics with their daughters because they perceived girls as more vulnerable than boys.

> *"...She is more gullible and easy to prey upon, so you have to give her the right information on sexual issues so that she can protect herself. Normally, it is the boys who are doing the chasing, so you must teach the girl to be assertive and how to say "no" to sex and she will be able to protect herself."* (a mother in Osu Klottey, FGD)

> *"...When girls start developing changes in their bodies, the girl will think she is matured and not listen to you. If you are not careful and monitor her, she may go out to bring problems to you. Let's say she got herself pregnant, at least people know that your daughter is pregnant but if the boy goes out and gets somebody pregnant, nobody will see that your boy is pregnant."* (a mother who is a teacher in Ablekuma South, IDI)

> *"...She is a girl and she is at the receiving end of any sexual action. She is the one who is going to suffer more be it her education, her life, or confidence level. It may affect her physically and psychologically. As for the boy, he can still go on with whatever he wants to do, even if he involves himself in sexual activity."* (a father who is an administrative officer in Osu Klottey, IDI)

On the contrary, few mothers prefer to talk to the boys rather than the girls while other parents would talk to both sexes because they are all vulnerable.

> *"I will talk to the boy because in recent times we are having problems with boys being abused by men and this is now a worrying issue."* (a mother in Ablekuma South, FGD)

> *"As a mother, I will start by talking with the two sexes together but as they grow, I will get the same gender that they can identify with to talk to them. This is because the boy has certain feelings that the mother doesn't know about but only hear of them. The boy and the father can talk as men and the mother can also talk with the girl."* (a mother in Osu Klottey, FGD)

There were disagreements with the age at which parents should start discussing sexual issues with their children in the

FGDs. Some of the parents believed that educating children about sexual issues should not be tied to age. Once the children understand what you are telling them, education can start.

> *"If a child asks a question, it is right for you to provide the right information to him/her and as he/she grows then you can be adding more information. We do not have to wait until a certain age before we start talking and if he/she comes with a question and you will say wait. No! We should provide the information as and when they need it."* (a mother in Osu Klottey, FGD)

Another mother in the FGD narrated her experience with her 6-year-old son about sexual issues and why it is important to start talking to them at a young age.

> *"My boy, before he turned 6 years of age, asked me why do boys urinate through the penis, but the girls do not? Does that mean that girls do not have penis? So, I must explain to him that the girls also urinate but through another place but not same as boys. You have to give an answer because they are inquisitive and observant."* (a mother, Osu Klottey, FGD)

Other parents were of the view that education on sexual topics should be age appropriate. Some of the parents would like to start talking to their children at the age of 10 years because there would be physical changes in their bodies at this time. Other parents would like to start talking to their children at 9 years because some of the girls may start having their period at this age.

> *"I would like to start talking to my children about sex when they are 10 years because at this time there are physical changes in their bodies which they will notice so whatever you tell them they will understand."* (a father who is a mechanic in Ablekuma South, FGD)

> *"I will like to start talking about sex with my child when my child is 9 years because these days some girls start having their period by this age. The hormones are working in them, so they are developing fast. When you see some of the adolescents you will think they are grownups and men usual approach them. So, when they are educated at this age they will know what to do in any situation."* (a mother who is a teacher at Osu Klottey, FGD)

> *"Parents should start talking to their children as early as 6 years because nowadays children are broad minded. Things that you think they do not know they have already heard or seen them somewhere and they will ask you questions. As soon as they start asking you those questions you must start talking to them about sex."* (a mother who is a trader in Osu Klottey, FGD)

3.1.3. Timing for Discussion of Adolescent Sexuality. Parents started talking to their adolescents about sexuality topics on different occasions. Some parents talked to their children when they watched an indecent television (TV) scene or indecent dressing on their way out with the children or used other peers' experiences as the basis to talk to their children.

> *"When I am going out with the children and we see dresses young girls wear, such as short skirts and dresses that expose their cleavage (space between her breasts), I use such things to start talking to them and tell them that wearing such dresses expose you to harm. Some men may take advantage of what you are wearing and lure you into sexual activity and that will result in all manner of consequences. Other times when we are watching films, for example African movies and a romantic scene appeared, I use that as an opportunity to start talking to them about sexual matters."* (a father who is a trader, IDI).

> *"Maybe something has happened to a family member and we are talking about it, I use such a channel to start talking with her. For example, I have a cousin who was about 16 years old and gave birth. Through that she could not continue with her schooling but the boy she had the baby with is still in school. That means that her future is curtailed but the boy will continue with school-ing."* (a mother who is a teacher, IDI).

3.1.4. Reasons for Parents' Discussion on Adolescent Sexuality. Parents from both the IDIs and FGDs confirmed discussing sexual topics with their adolescent children. However, there was no general agreement among the parents for the reasons of discussing sexual topics with their adolescents. The most important reason for discussing sexual topics with adolescents was to prevent them from engagement in early sexual activity.

> *"I talked about sexual issues with my daughter so that she would not be forced into sexual activity which would bring her problems. When girls associate with their friends, they try to learn bad things from their friends so you the parent must educate your child against such matters."* (a mother who is a teacher, IDI)

> *"I noticed that at the age of 10 years, my daughter was developing some reproductive features, so I told her when she sees them it means that she is growing up. I told her that those features are not there for nothing. They are there for a purpose; when the time comes she will use them for the purpose. I talked to her because I think she needs the information. Despite her age if she knows that there are some consequences in certain acts like sex, she will be careful."* (a father who is an administrative officer, IDI)

3.2. Parental Knowledge and Comfort Discussing Adolescent Sexuality

3.2.1. Sources of Parental Knowledge about Adolescent Sexuality. Parental knowledge about adolescent sexuality issues is important to ensure that adolescents get the facts right. Various strategies were used by parents to improve their knowledge on adolescent sexuality issues. Some parents in the FGD mentioned that they sourced knowledge on adolescent sexuality from reading books on such topics. Others reported using programmes they watched on television to educate their adolescents on sexuality issues. Others also used family members and friends as resource persons to educate their adolescent children.

> *"I read books on adolescents' sexuality. Sometimes, if I feel I cannot talk about a topic, I ask my friend to help me to educate my child on it."* (a mother who is a teacher, IDI)

> *"There is enough information on the television we watch, like HIV/AIDS so I call my daughter to come and watch and whatever advice I have I give her. Moreover, I work at the maternity department of a hospital and that has helped me to learn about what happens to young girls. Subsequently I advised her on situations I have seen at the hospital. Young girls come to the maternity department and I see them until they deliver. I see the problems they face, from start to the end."* (a mother who is a record officer, IDI)

3.2.2. Parents' Comfort Talking about Adolescent Sexuality Topics. During the IDIs, parents expressed diverse feelings about their comfort talking to their children about sexual topics. While many of the parents said they felt comfortable talking to their adolescents about sexual topics, some did not.

> *"I feel very comfortable when talking about sexual issues with my daughter and my friends' children because I have been trained on adolescent sexuality."* (a mother who is a nurse, IDI)

> *"I feel comfortable talking about any sexual topics with my children because I have four girls and I started with the most senior one and gradually the younger ones have also reached adolescence, so it made it very easy to talk to them about such issues as I have done so on several occasions."* (a father who is a mechanic, IDI)

> *"I don't feel comfortable because sometimes I think they may ask me questions that need to be answered and I may not have the answers to give them. I also think that if you give them too much information, adventurous as children are, they may want to try whatever you told them, for example, condom, when they see what it is they may like to try it."* (a father who is an administrative officer, IDI)

3.3. Challenges and Strategies to Improve Parent Communication on Adolescent Sexuality

3.3.1. Challenges to Parent Communication on Adolescent Sexuality. There was no agreement among the parents on challenges or difficulties they faced talking to their children about sexuality. Some parents opined that they have difficulties talking to their children about sexuality topics. Parents have problems with timing of the talk, terminologies they could not explain to the children, and health implications of certain issues like menstruation.

> *"The difficulties I faced talking about sexual topics with my children are: the appropriate time to provide the education. ii. There are also some terminologies that I am not able to provide an appropriate explanation for the children to understand me. iii. There are some health implications such as having menses which I could not explain e.g. why some girls have regular menses while others have irregular? I don't know whether that is normal or not. Why some girls have their menses early and others late. For instance, some girls start their menses at 10 years but others at 15 years of age."* (a father who is an administrator in Ablekuma South, FGD)

Other parents were worried because their children were not open to what they are telling them.

> *"Sometimes the children are not open to what you are saying to them. They will not like to listen to what you are saying. And if you force him/her, he/she will allow you to talk and after that he/she will ask you 'have you finished?' and he/she gets up and goes, that means he/she is not interested in what you told him/ her."* (a mother who is a teacher in Ablekuma South, FGD)

Some parents gave reasons why their parents did not educate them on sexuality topics.

> *"To be honest, I was not given any education on sex. You are even scared to go and ask questions on such things. My parents didn't educate me because it might be that they were themselves not educated by their parents and hardly had any exposure."* (a father in Osu Klottey, FGD)

> *"My parents never talked to me about sexual issues. I don't know whether or not they were feeling shy to talk to me about such issues."* (a father in Ablekuma South, FGD)

> *"My parents didn't talk to me may be because my father was a pastor and could not tell me anything on sexuality."* (a mother, Osu Klottey, FGD)

3.3.2. Strategies to Improve Parent Communication on Adolescent Sexuality. Many of the parents in the study believed that to improve communication between parents and adolescents, the former needs to start talking with their children at an early age because after a certain stage, it would be difficult to start talking to them. Other parents believed parents should have time with their children and talk with them regularly.

> *"We should start talking to our children early and make them our friends because if the children grow up to a certain stage it will be difficult to start talking to them about sexual issues. But if we are friends to them since childhood and they have confidence in us and confide in us, it will be easy for us to talk to them even when they are adolescents."* (a mother in Osu Klottey, FGD)

> *"Parents should have time to talk with their children, listen to them and answer their questions because if the children know that when they come to you, you will give them the right information even if they are not your friend they will come to you."* (a mother in Osu Klottey, FGD)

The parents also identified closeness to children, reading to acquire more knowledge on adolescent sexuality, and provision of educational programmes on adolescents' sexuality on television and radio to educate parents and help them discuss sexual topics with their children.

> *"I have to read more and have more knowledge about sexual issues to talk with my children. There should be an educational programme on adolescent sexuality on television and radio to educate parents. You must get closer to your child and find out what he/she is doing at a time, monitor him/her and where he/she goes, know his/her friends and take interest in him/her. Once he/she knows that you are interested in him/her, she can confine in you and tell you his/her problem then you can talk to him/her often about sexual issues."* (a mother who is a record officer, IDI)

3.3.3. Informal and Formal Sexuality Education. Parents expressed different opinions about the importance of informal and formal sex education as a strategy to improve parents ability to communicate effectively with adolescents on sexuality topics. Almost all the parents agreed that it would have been easier for them to communicate with their children on sexuality topics if they had received some form of education on these issues. Some parents mentioned that they received some talks on sexuality while they were adolescent, but it was only precautionary and to instil fear in you to avoid sex.

> *"I had some education, but it was precautionary. If you go and sleep with a girl she will get pregnant and they will come and arrest you. Such was the education."* (a father who is an administrator, IDI)

> *"My mother never educated me on sex. She will not tell you that if you have sex you will be get*

> *pregnant. She will tell you if a man touches you, you will be pregnant, so I had that in my mind so whenever a boy approaches me I will ask him not to touch me because I do not want to be pregnant. I do not want my mother to see that I am pregnant."* (a mother who is a record officer, IDI)

Parents believed that informal education from their parents will have enabled them to communicate with their adolescent children on sexuality topics better than what they are currently doing.

> *"If I had been educated when young I would have improved on what I am telling my children now because I would have gained more knowledge and experience than I have. Even the system we have now, you are bit restricted as what to educate our kids because you are not sure about what you are going to tell them. In effect you are reluctant when you want to give certain information to the children."* (a father, Ablekuma South, FGD)

> *"It would have been far easier because I have the knowledge but how to impact the knowledge to my children is the problem. Probably, if my parents had talked to me I could have used the experience I had from them to talk with my child."* (a mother, Ablekuma South, FGD)

> *"Yes, it would have contributed a lot. You know parents are the first teachers and before I grew up if I were to have some information on sexuality, wherever I go with a little top up will ameliorate what I have learnt. I would have had the understanding very well. So, when parents educate their children before they grow up it will help very much."* (a father and an administrative officer, IDI)

Parents were asked if they thought formal training of parents on adolescent sexuality would help them talk to their children about the subject. Many of them were of the view that if parents were trained on adolescents' sexual issues, it would help them to know the appropriate ways to talk to their children about their sexuality.

> *"Training of parents will help because you see, education on adolescent sexuality is a sensitive topic which requires some formal training. You must find the appropriate time, put the message into appropriate language and the children should be in a right mood to receive the message. For that matter, parents need to be taught how to give the education."* (a father who is an administrator, IDI)

> *"...Some parents have no knowledge about sexual issues or how to go about it. Therefore, if parents are trained, they will have the knowledge to educate their children and their children will, in*

turn educate their own children in future and they will be better than the present generation. I told my sister that "something" like blood is coming from my vagina when I had my first menses and she told my mother. When she told my mother about my experience, my mother said to me 'that is what we call 'period', don't you know, and I said I didn't. And she said that is what when a man calls you and you go you will become pregnant'. So, how will a man call me, and I will go'. You are afraid to go." (a mother, who is a record officer, IDI)

Parents expressed different opinions when they were asked about the impact of sex education on adolescent engagement in premarital sex. Most of the parents posited that adolescent sex education would not lead to premarital sex. However, other parents thought it could lead to premarital sex.

"Yes, because if you educate adolescents, out of curiosity, they would like to find out whether whatever you have told them is practicable or works depending upon the sort of groups they find themselves." (a mother, Ablekuma, FGD)

"No, educating them puts fear in them. Educating them will prevent them from indulging in early sexual activities, leading to a healthy sexual life now and in the future. But if we do not educate them now, when they grow up, they would become ignorant about a lot of things and they may find themselves wanting." (a father, Osu Klottey, FGD)

"I think it depends on how you go about the education. Because some of the adolescents are adventurous, and when you talk to them about sex, they will really want to find out what it is about. So, it is better we educate them, but we should let them know the dangers associated with indulging in sexual activity. Most of the adolescents indulge in sex because they may learn about it at school, but the teacher probably did not educate them about the dangers associated with indulging in sex. So, they want to experience it." (a mother, Osu Klottey, FGD)

4. Discussion

4.1. Parents Discussing Sexuality Topics with Adolescents. This study focused on parents' experiences discussing sexuality topics with their adolescent children. In agreement with previous studies in Ghana [15, 26] and in sub-Saharan Africa [22], parents reported talking to their adolescent children on various sexuality topics. Regarding sexual topics discussed with the adolescents, the parents reported that they discussed menstruation, peer pressure, premarital sex, HIV/AIDS, boy/girl relationships, personal hygiene, pregnancy, abstinence, sexually transmitted infections (STIs), abortion, and how to say "no" to forced sex. Previous studies have reported

similar range of sexual topics discussed by parents with their children, such as physical development, abstinence, unplanned pregnancy, HIV/AIDS, sex/intercourse, STIs, and safe sex [5, 22]. Among the topics discussed, abstinence was a major topic. Parents were particularly concerned with their female adolescents' indulgence in premarital sex since the outcomes of such actions are normally disastrous. It is important to note that these discussions tend to be precautionary as documented in previous studies from sub-Saharan Africa in which sexual discussions were authoritative and characterized by vague warning [22]. In this study, parents did not mention that they talked about contraceptive and condom use with their adolescents. This finding is consistent with previous studies in Tanzania and Nigeria that reported these topics as the least talked about by parents with their children during sexual discussions [27, 28]. On the contrary, a study in the United States indicated that parents often discuss issues such as condom use and protection with their adolescents [29]. Parents in Nigeria did not talk about contraceptives and condom use with their adolescents because they believed that such discussions would promote promiscuity [28]. Unacceptable opinions originating from cultural and religious beliefs may also underpin the low communication on contraceptive and condom use in the African setting compared to the United States and other developed countries.

The findings from this study also indicate that parents talk to their adolescents for various reasons; the most important is to prevent adolescent engagement in premarital sex. This supports earlier studies in the United States which observed that parent-adolescent communication about sex has been associated with delayed start of early sexual intercourse [21]. The benefits of sex education amassed by adolescents may be dependent on several factors, including timing of discussions as well as the nature of the discussion. While discussion of sexuality with adolescents has been a controversial issue, parents recounted that they started talking to their children on different occasions and on various topics. Many of them reported that they initiated discussions about sexuality topics with their adolescents while viewing television that showed romantic scenes. These views expressed by the Ghanaian parents is in consonance with previous studies of Caucasian, Latino-American, African-American, African, and Asian parents particularly mothers who take advantage of events like watching television to talk about sex-related topics with their children [5]. It is worthy of note that parents also took advantage of life situations as a case study for sex education, especially in instances when an adolescent's family member gets pregnant. They used such happenings as an opportunity to initiate discussion on safer and more protective sexual behaviours so that younger siblings/children can identify problems and solutions as they watch the consequences that befell victims of early sexual activities and do not repeat the same mistakes.

4.2. Gender and Age Disparities in Parent Discussion of Adolescent Sexuality. Although parents have the responsibility of discussing sexuality topics with both sexes, higher priority is given to educating their daughters. This finding agrees with prior studies that more mothers would like to talk with their daughters than with their sons about sex-related topics [4, 22]. Parents may be more concerned with the welfare of their daughters rather than sons as they would not like their daughters to indulge in early sex. This may be because parents are protective of their daughters as in any event, such as pregnancy, the daughter bears the greatest consequences. Regarding the suitable age at which parents could instigate conversation on sex-related discussions with their adolescents, parents wanted to start talking to their children about sexual topics as early as 10 years. This age estimate is identical to what parents in the United States and Greece opined; that is, their children should be educated about sexuality topics during the primary school years (between 10 and 12 years) [5, 30]. Among the parents who indicated a desire to educate children on sexuality topics at 10 years or younger (during the preadolescence stage), their reason was the desire to provide their children with the right information before they become sexually active. This is because it would be easier to start talking to children when they are preadolescent since they are more likely to listen and adopt it than when they grow older. If parents do not talk to their children about sex, it will mean that they will not have control over what their children learn about sex. Children are generally exposed to sexual issues from peers, sexual images, and sexual content in magazines, television, radio, and movies. Since parents cannot prevent adolescents from accessing sexual information, no matter how hard they try, they must provide them with education to make the right sexual decisions.

4.3. Parental Knowledge and Comfort Discussing Adolescent Sexuality Topics. Parents' knowledge about sexual topics motivates them to discuss sexuality topics with their adolescents. The more knowledgeable a parent is about sexuality topics, the more comfortable he or she feels about discussing such topics with his/her adolescent. A study in Bangladesh reported lack of knowledge among parents on basic understanding of adolescent reproductive and sexual health issues [31]. In the case of Ghana, parents showed varied levels of knowledge on adolescent sexual topics and this has been reported elsewhere [26]. A study among Australian parents also confirmed that parents felt generally knowledgeable about educating their children about sexuality [32]. In Ghana, mothers and aunties are mostly the main educators of children about sexuality issues. Evidence in an earlier study in Ghana indicated that the mother is the main resource person on sexual communication with adolescents [15]. Mothers may view the education of adolescents as their responsibility and, therefore, make more effort to acquire knowledge to enable them to discuss these issues with their adolescents. Fathers may not be so interested in adolescent sexuality topics because they may think that it is the mothers' duty. Some fathers may also genuinely not have the knowledge about sexual topics and need to be motivated to learn more about sexual topics in order to educate their children about such issues.

Although these parents generally reported feeling knowledgeable, they still resort to improve their knowledge by reading books on sexual topics. Other parents also reported buying books for their children to read themselves. Parents watching TV programmes and advice from friends were other sources of knowledge for parents about adolescent sexual and reproductive health issues. A similar finding was reported in a study in the United States in which parents used available resources such as books on sexuality topics (that is, for themselves and their children), TV programmes, and advice from parents and friends to improve their knowledge and ability to communicate with their children on adolescent sexuality issues [5]. Parents reading books on sexual topics and buying books for their children to read suggest that they have realized the need for them and their children to have more information on sexual and reproductive health issues. Unfortunately, the purchasing of these books for their children to read to acquire information on sexuality issues may not be sufficient for some children who might have difficulty in understanding what they read. Such children may therefore need parental support. Beyond what may be read in the books, parents may need to adapt and interpret knowledge in relation to the context that their adolescent lives in. However, parental use of other parents as resource persons in educating their adolescents about sexual topics is commendable.

Parental fear of being unable to answer sex-related questions posed by their adolescents emerged during the in-depth interviews as a reason for discomfort in discussing sexual topics with adolescents. In a study in Ethiopia, fathers did not discuss sex and menses issues with their children because it made them uncomfortable, as it was not traditionally accepted [33]. Again, in the United States, Wilson et al. [5] had earlier identified parental inability to handle questions posed by their children due to lack of technical knowledge on sexual topics. In Ethiopia, it was mentioned that even though parents valued their knowledge about the adolescent sexuality, this was not accepted by their children. In other words, they did not know what to do in those circumstances [33]. Therefore, having knowledge alone may not be enough and it must be coupled with communication and comfort enhancement strategies. Evidence-based programmes aimed at improving parental knowledge on adolescent sexuality must include modules to enhance parental comfort so as to improve frequency of such communications with adolescent children.

4.4. Challenges and Strategies to Improve Parent Communication on Adolescent Sexuality. Many parents face difficulties while discussing sexuality topics with their adolescents. This is because either the parents have problems when talking to their children or the children are not prepared to listen to the parents. Some parents in the in-depth interviews confirmed that they had difficulties when talking about sexuality issues with their adolescents. In the United States, parents reported that they experienced some types of difficulty such as unease about physical development and embarrassment when discussing sexual issues with their children [34]. Another parent had difficulty with technical aspects of sexuality such as the terminologies which he could not explain to his/her children to understand him. In the United States, Latino parents had difficulties when talking about technical aspects of sexuality, including contraceptives as they require specialized knowledge [35]. Sexuality is a specialized area which needs expert knowledge; thus some parents find it difficult to talk about sexuality issues. The need for expert knowledge, therefore, is paramount for parents to communicate better. Nonetheless, parents can explore sexuality topics with their children and learn together. Another possible reason why parents had difficulties talking to their children could be the late start of sex education. As the children grew up parents felt uncomfortable to discuss sexuality issues with their adolescents. For such discussions to take place, a good parent-child relationship needs to be built with the child at a younger age. This would encourage parent-adolescent communication when the children become adolescents.

4.5. Informal and Formal Sexuality Education. Many of the parents complained that they were not educated on sexuality when they were young, and this has made it difficult for them to educate their children now. This is in keeping with a 2010 study in the United States which reported that parents complained about their inability to talk to their own children about sex because they were not educated by their parents [5]. In Kenya, Mbugua also observed that among mothers who had no sex education from parents, providing sex education to their own daughters became difficult [4]. Parents believed that if they had been educated on sexual issues when they were young, it would have been easier for them to educate their own children.

Some parents also mentioned that they were educated on sexuality, but it was just precautionary. Other parents said that they never had any education on sex from their parents but received metaphoric caution against sex. In a study in Nigeria, parents deliberately misinformed their daughters about the realities of sex in order to discourage them from being interested in sexual matters and put fear into them against premarital sex [28]. This trend of authoritative, vague warning rather than direct open discussion is a common theme as documented in a review of studies of parent-adolescent communication about sexuality in sub-Saharan Africa [22]. There should be mutual consent between parents and adolescents concerning sexuality discussions such that a dialogue may ensue rather than it being a unidirectional communication. It is significant for parents to talk with their adolescent children to break the tradition of silence of talking about sexuality.

It was evident from this study that just parental knowledge on adolescent sexuality topics may not be enough. Some parents had the knowledge, but how to communicate the information to their adolescents was a challenge since this was considered as a sensitive issue; hence they would prefer not to talk about it. Many of the parents in both the FGDs and IDIs asserted that if parents receive structured training on communication about adolescent sexuality, it would enable them to talk with their adolescents about sexuality. Other researchers have also reported similar views by parents in different countries [4, 5, 34, 35]. Training parents to talk to their children about sexuality has other benefits like improving their knowledge of sexuality topics, confidence,

ability, and comfort to discuss such sensitive topics with their children [26].

4.6. Limitations of the Study. This study was conducted among parents in urban settings; hence the findings cannot be generalized to parents in rural setting. However, it is important to note that these parents were originally not from the city and may have migrated from rural settlements into their present urban locations. Hence, it is possible that parents in rural settings can identify with most of the views expressed by these parents in the urban setting. Another limitation to this study is the lack of information on the cultural and religious barriers to sex education in an urban context. This limitation is the focus of another manuscript under revision elsewhere. It is likely that the parents who were most likely to agree to take part in the study were parents who felt the most comfortable talking about sexuality, which may have affected the results. The diversity of ethnic groups represented by the parents is a strength to the current study which implored both FGDs and IDIs to express parents' experiences discussing adolescent sexuality topics in the Accra Metropolis.

5. Conclusion

It is important for parents to discuss sexual topics with adolescents to prevent exposure to early sex, pregnancy, and sexually transmitted diseases. Although girls are more vulnerable than boys, both sexes need education on sexuality, and it will be much easier for such an education to be effective if parents get closer to their children and start discussions about sexuality issues with them at a younger age. In a nut shell, parents may need some form of education to be able to handle challenges of sexuality discussions with adolescents.

Abbreviations

IDI: In-depth interview
FGD: Focus group discussion.

Disclosure

The funding agency was not involved in the design of the study and data collection, analysis, and interpretation of the results. The views reflected in this manuscript are those of the authors and do not in any way reflect the views of the funding agency.

Authors' Contributions

Elizabeth AKu Baku and Richard M. K. Adanu conceived the study. Elizabeth AKu Baku and Isaac Agbemafle performed the data analysis. Elizabeth AKu Baku, Isaac Agbemafle, and Agnes Millicent Kotoh drafted the script. Isaac Agbemafle reviewed the scripts and made the necessary corrections. All authors read and approved the final manuscript.

Acknowledgments

The research was financed by the Ghana Education Trust Fund (GETFUND). We are grateful to all the parents who dedicated their time and resources to the in-depth interviews and focus group discussions.

References

[1] J. J. Arnett, "Conceptions of the transition to adulthood among emerging adults in American ethnic groups," *New Directions for Child and Adolescent Development*, vol. 2003, no. 100, pp. 63–75, 2003.

[2] M. Kirkman, D. A. Rosenthal, and S. S. Feldman, "Talking to a tiger: fathers reveal their difficulties in communicating about sexuality with adolescents," *New Directions for Child and Adolescent Development*, no. 97, pp. 57–74, 2002.

[3] G. Sedgh and R. Hussain, "Reasons for contraceptive nonuse among women having unmet need for contraception in developing countries," *Studies in Family Planning*, vol. 45, no. 2, pp. 151–169, 2014.

[4] N. Mbugua, "Factors inhibiting educated mothers in Kenya from giving meaningful sex-education to their daughters," *Social Science & Medicine*, vol. 64, no. 5, pp. 1079–1089, 2007.

[5] E. K. Wilson, B. T. Dalberth, H. P. Koo, and J. C. Gard, "Parents' perspectives on talking to preteenage children about sex," *Perspectives on Sexual and Reproductive Health*, vol. 42, no. 1, pp. 56–63, 2010.

[6] C. Beyers, "Sexuality education in south africa: a sociocultural perspective," *Acta Academica*, vol. 43, no. 3, pp. 192–209, 2011.

[7] Ghana Statistical Service, *Ghana Demographic and Health Survey (GDHS)*, Ghana, 2008.

[8] A. M. Moore, A. E. Biddlecom, and E. M. Zulu, "Prevalence and meanings of exchange of money or gifts for sex in unmarried adolescent sexual relationships in sub-Saharan Africa," *African Journal of Reproductive Health*, vol. 11, no. 3, pp. 44–61, 2007.

[9] *Report FHDA: Adolescent Health*, Ghana Health Service, Accra, Ghana, 2016.

[10] *Demographic and Health Survey: Teenage pregnancy in Nigeria: Facts and Truth*, Ministry of Health, Nigeria, 2013.

[11] *Survey KDaH: 18% The rate of teenage pregnancy and motherhood in Kenya*, Ministry of Health, Kenya, 2014.

[12] B. Masilela, *Teen Mothers contribute 13% to child birth in SA/IOL News*, Africa News Agency, South Africa, 2017.

[13] E. Baku, R. Adanu, and P. Adatara, "Socio-cultural factors affecting parent-adolescent communication on sexuality in the Accra Metropolis, Ghana," *NUMID HORIZON, International Journal of Nursing and Midwifery*, vol. 1, no. 2, pp. 1–10, 2017.

[14] S. A. Owusu, "Cultural and religious impediments against sex education," Feature Article, Wednesday, 5th December 2012, https://www.ghanaweb.com/GhanaHomePage/NewsArchive/Cultural-and-Religious-Impediments-against-Sex-Education-258360.

[15] A. Kumi-Kyereme, K. Awusabo-Asare, A. Biddlecom, and A. Tanle, "Influence of social connectedness, communication and monitoring on adolescent sexual activity in Ghana," *African Journal of Reproductive Health*, vol. 11, no. 3, pp. 133–149, 2007.

[16] V. Brocato and A. Dwamena-Aboagye, *Violence against Women and HIV/AIDS*, Y. Amissah, Ed., The Ark Foundation, Achimota, Ghana, 2007.

[17] M. Beasley, A. Valerio, and D. Bundy, *A Sourcebook of HIV/AIDS Prevention Programs*, vol. 2, Education Sector-Wide Approaches, World Bank, Washington, DC, USA, 2008.

[18] K. Awusabo-Asare, M. Stillman, S. Koegh, D. T. Doku, A. Kumi-Kyereme, and K. Esia-Donkor, *From Paper to Practice: Sexuality Education Policies and their Implementation in Ghana*, Guttmacher Institute, New York, 2017, https://www.guttmacher.org/report/sexuality-education-ghana.

[19] J. Anarfi and A. Owusu, "The making of sexual being in ghana: the state, religion and influence of society as agents of sexual socialization," *Sexuality and Culture*, vol. 15, pp. 1–18, 2011.

[20] J. Osafo, E. Asampong, and C. Ahiedeke, "Perception of parents on how religion influences adolescent sexual behaviours in two communities: implications for hiv and aids," *Journal of Religion and Health*, vol. 53, no. 4, pp. 959–971, 2014.

[21] J. D. Hanson, T. R. McMahon, E. R. Griese, and D. B. Kenyon, "Understanding gender roles in teen pregnancy prevention among american indian youth," *American Journal of Health Behavior*, vol. 38, no. 6, pp. 807–815, 2014.

[22] S. Bastien, A. Biddlecom, and W. Muhwezi, "A review of studies of parent-child communication about sexuality and HIV/AIDS in sub-Suharan Africa," *Reproductive Health*, vol. 8, no. 25, pp. 1–17, 2011.

[23] S. K. Henshaw, I. Adewole, S. Singh, A. Bankole, B. Oye-Adeniran, and R. Hussain, "Views of adults on adolescent sexual and reproductive health: qualitative evidence from Ghana," *Occasional Report*, vol. 34, no. 1, pp. 40–50, 2008.

[24] M. Walsh and L. Wigens, *Introduction to Research: Foundation in Nursing and Health Care*, Nelson Thomas Ltd, Delta Place, UK, 2003.

[25] V. Braun and V. Clarke, "Using thematic analysis in psychology," *Qualitative Research in Psychology*, vol. 3, no. 2, pp. 77–101, 2006.

[26] E. A. Baku, I. Agbemafle, and R. M. K. Adanu, "Effects of parents training on parents' knowledge and attitudes about adolescent sexuality in Accra Metropolis, Ghana," *Reproductive Health*, vol. 14, no. 1, 2017.

[27] J. Wamoyi, A. Fenwick, M. Urassa, B. Zaba, and W. Stones, "Parent-child communication about sexual and reproductive health in rural Tanzania: implications for young people's sexual health interventions," *Reproductive Health*, vol. 7, pp. 6–23, 2010.

[28] C. O. Izugbara, "Home-based sexuality education: Nigerian parents discussing sex with their children," *Youth and Society*, vol. 39, no. 4, pp. 575–600, 2008.

[29] E. I. Pluhar and P. Kuriloff, "What really matters in family communication about sexuality? a qualitative analysis of the effect and style among African American mothers and adolescent daughters," *Sex Education*, vol. 4, no. 3, pp. 3003–3321, 2004.

[30] A. Kakavoulis, "Family and sex education: a survey of parental attitudes," *Sex Education*, vol. 1, no. 2, pp. 163–174, 2001.

[31] U. Rob, T. Ghafur, I. Bhuiya, and M. N. Talukder, "Reproductive and sexual health education for adolescents in Bangladesh: Parents' view and opinion," *International Quarterly of Community Health Education*, vol. 25, no. 4, pp. 351–365, 2006.

[32] A. Morawska, A. Walsh, M. Grabski, and R. Fletcher, "Parental confidence and preferences for communicating with their child about sexuality," *Sex Education: Sexuality, Society and Learning*, vol. 15, no. 3, pp. 235–248, 2015.

[33] D. G. Yesus and M. Fantahun, "Assessing communication on sexual and reproductive health issues among high school students with their parents, Bullen, Woreda, Benishangul Gumuz Region, North West Ethiopia," *Ethiopian Journal of Health Development*, vol. 24, no. 2, pp. 89–95, 2010.

[34] P. Jerman and N. A. Constantine, "Demographic and psychological predictors of parent-adolescent communication about sex: a representative statewide analysis," *Journal of Youth and Adolescence*, vol. 39, no. 10, pp. 1164–1174, 2010.

[35] M. Raffaelli and L. L. Ontai, "'She's 16 years old and there's boys calling over to the house': An exploratory study of sexual socialization in Latino families," *Culture, Health and Sexuality*, vol. 3, no. 3, pp. 295–310, 2001.

6

IPV Screening and Readiness to Respond to IPV in Ob-Gyn Settings: A Patient-Physician Study

Katherine M. Jones [1,2] Laura H. Taouk,[1,2] Neko M. Castleberry,[1]
Michele M. Carter,[2] and Jay Schulkin[3]

[1]Research Department, American College of Obstetricians and Gynecologists (ACOG), 409 12th Street SW, Washington, DC 20024, USA
[2]Department of Psychology, American University, 4400 Massachusetts Avenue NW, Washington, DC 20016, USA
[3]Department of Obstetrics and Gynecology, University of Washington School of Medicine, Box 356460, Seattle, WA 98195, USA

Correspondence should be addressed to Neko M. Castleberry; ncastleberry@acog.org

Academic Editor: Ronald J. Prineas

Purpose. Intimate partner violence (IPV) is a serious, preventable public health concern that largely affects women of reproductive age. Obstetrician-gynecologists (ob-gyns) have a unique opportunity to identify and support women experiencing IPV to improve women's health. Considering recent efforts to increase IPV awareness and intervention, the present study aimed to provide a current evaluation of nationally representative samples to assess ob-gyn readiness to respond to IPV as well as patient IPV-related experiences. *Methods*. 400 ob-gyns were randomly selected from American College of Obstetricians and Gynecologists' (ACOG) Collaborative Ambulatory Research Network. Each physician was mailed one physician survey and 25 patient surveys. *Results*. IPV training/education and IPV screening practices were associated with most measures of ob-gyn readiness to respond to IPV. Among respondents, 36.8% endorsed screening all patients at annual exams; however, 36.8% felt they did not have sufficient training to assist individuals in addressing IPV. Workplace encouragement of IPV response was associated with training, screening, detection, preparation/knowledge, response practices, and resources. Thirty-one percent of patients indicated their ob-gyn had asked about possible IPV experiences during their medical visit. *Conclusion*. Findings highlight specific gaps in ob-gyns' IPV knowledge and response practices to be further addressed by IPV training.

1. Introduction

Intimate partner violence (IPV) is a serious, preventable public health concern. The Centers for Disease Control and Prevention (CDC) defines IPV as physical violence, sexual violence, stalking, and/or psychological aggression by a current or former intimate partner [1]. In the United States, approximately 4.8 million women are physically assaulted each year by an intimate partner [2], and 42.4 million women (35.6%) are victims of rape, physical assault, and/or stalking by an intimate partner in their lifetime [3]. IPV has serious health consequences, including physical injury, psychological trauma, chronic health problems, and death [3–5]. For women, IPV is most prevalent among those of reproductive age and contributes to gynecological disorders, pregnancy complications, unintended pregnancy, and sexually transmitted infections [6].

Given these serious health consequences and the threat to women's safety, the Institute of Medicine recommends that all women be screened and counseled for IPV [7]. Obstetrician-gynecologists (ob-gyns), who serve a vital role in women's healthcare, have a unique opportunity to identify and support women experiencing IPV. Annual prevalence of IPV in ob-gyn settings has been estimated to be 12.7% [8]. The American College of Obstetricians and Gynecologists (ACOG) recommends that ob-gyns screen all patients for IPV periodically at routine, family planning, preconception, prenatal (at least once per trimester), and postpartum visits [9]. Guidelines for response to IPV disclosure emphasize the importance of assessing the patient's immediate safety, developing a safety plan with the patient and offering information about appropriate community resources and referrals [9]. Physician screening increases rates of IPV identification [10, 11], which enables physicians to offer patients counseling interventions as well as referral to community resources. Benefits of counseling interventions include improved quality of life, improved birth outcomes, reduced IPV for new mothers, decreased pregnancy coercion, and fewer violence-related injuries [11]. Improved health outcomes for women confer positive benefits for children, families, and communities.

In light of recent efforts to increase IPV awareness and intervention [12, 13], the present study aimed to provide a current evaluation of ob-gyn readiness (i.e., how prepared ob-gyns are) to recognize and respond to IPV (based on responses to a validated survey tool) as well as patient experiences in nationally representative samples. More specifically, ob-gyn training, preparation, knowledge, screening, response practices, opinions, and practice-related factors/resources were assessed. Patients also responded to questions regarding past and present IPV, their ob-gyn's assessment of possible IPV during their visit, and their satisfaction with their ob-gyn's assessment of possible IPV.

2. Methods

2.1. Materials. For the physician component of the study, the Physician Readiness to Manage Intimate Partner Violence Survey (PREMIS) [14] was minimally adapted for use with an ob-gyn specialist population, with minute changes made only to the demographics portion. The PREMIS is a validated 67-item self-assessment tool that assesses demographics as well as IPV training, perceived knowledge, perceived preparation, objective understanding, opinions, screening/response practices, and practice resources. The instrument has demonstrated the capacity to discriminate trained from nontrained physicians, and scales have been found to be closely correlated with theoretical constructs and predictive of self-reported practices [15].

For the patient component of the study, the Patient Safety and Satisfaction Survey (PSSS) [16] was modified to evaluate patient perceptions of ob-gyn IPV assessment. Questions on the altered PSSS regarded demographics, experiences of IPV, and experiences with their doctor (screening for IPV, satisfaction with screening, and presence of IPV materials). Like the PREMIS, minor changes were made to the language of the PSSS to best represent ob-gyn practices.

2.2. Procedures and Participants. Institutional Review Board approval was obtained from American University. In December 2014, 400 ob-gyns were each mailed one physician questionnaire and 25 patient questionnaires along with a cover letter, instructions for patient recruitment, and patient resource cards. Ob-gyns were randomly selected members of the Collaborative Ambulatory Research Network (CARN). CARN is a representative group of ACOG Fellows who volunteer to participate in questionnaire studies without compensation. More than 90% of US board-certified ob-gyns are members of ACOG. For patient recruitment,

ob-gyn office staff were instructed to offer patient surveys to all English-speaking women after their appointments until either all 25 surveys had been completed or the study deadline had passed. Written information for informed participation was provided; physician consent was implied by return of a survey, while patients checked a box to certify consent. Four additional mailings were sent to nonresponding ob-gyns between February and July 2015; only the first reminder mailing included patient materials. Data collection ended on July 29, 2015.

2.3. Data Analysis. From the physician data, several scale scores were calculated based on published scoring instructions for the PREMIS [14, 15]. Since objective knowledge questions were informed by the IPV literature, a total score of correct items was obtained. All other scales were calculated as mean scores, and internal consistency was excellent ($\alpha \geq 0.909$). Although opinion subscales and a composite practice issues score were calculated by Short and colleagues [14, 15], we found that grouped items demonstrated poor internal consistency and exploratory factor analyses failed to yield meaningful subscales. Consequently, key items from those sections will be discussed separately and not as scale scores.

Since physicians returned their surveys with their patient surveys, patient and physician data could be linked. Patient responses were compared with physician practice characteristics (e.g., type of practice). Other comparisons of patient-physician data, which used higher-order predictive models, are reported elsewhere [17].

Data analysis was conducted using a personal computer-based software package (IBM SPSS Statistics® 23.0, IBM Corp©, Armonk, NY, USA). Data were examined descriptively, and response categories endorsed by <10% of participants were collapsed. Unless otherwise noted, response frequencies were reported as percentages with total number of participants in the sample as the denominator. Pearson correlations were used to examine associations between continuous variables. Relationships between categorical variables were evaluated with chi-square tests; tests with ≥25% of cells with an expected count of less than 5 were considered invalid and discarded. Independent samples t-tests and ANOVAs were used to evaluate mean differences in continuous variables grouped by categorical variables. Tests were considered significant at $p < 0.05$.

3. Results

Of the 400 physicians invited to participate, 48.5% ($n = 194$) responded (48 opt-outs, 21 retired), and 125 eligible participants completed the survey for a viable response rate of 31.2%. Practices were well-distributed across 41 US states. Male participants ($m = 30.6$; SD = 10.4) had been in practice for significantly longer than female participants ($m = 21.7$, SD = 8.7, $t = 5.23$, and $p < 0.001$). The physician sample is described further in Table 1. Of the patients whose physician responded, 981 patient surveys were returned (31.4%) and the patient sample is described in Table 2.

TABLE 1: Physician sample demographics ($N = 125$).

Characteristics n (%)	
Gender ($n = 125$)	
Female	63 (50.4)
Male	62 (49.6)
Years in practice ($n = 125$) (including residency)	26.1 ± 10.5
Ethnicity/race ($n = 124$)	
White, non-Hispanic	107 (85.6)
Asian	5 (4.0)
Black/African American	4 (3.2)
White, Hispanic	3 (2.4)
Multiracial	3 (2.4)
Others	2 (1.6)
Primary medical specialty ($n = 125$)	
General ob-gyn	89 (71.2)
Gynecology only	20 (16.0)
Maternal/fetal medicine	6 (4.8)
Others	10 (8.0)
Type of practice ($n = 124$)	
Ob-gyn partnership/group	58 (46.4)
University faculty practice	25 (20.0)
Solo private practice	22 (17.6)
Multispecialty group	12 (9.6)
HMO/staff model	5 (4.0)
Military/government	2 (1.6)
Practice location ($n = 125$)	
Suburban	49 (39.2)
Urban non-inner-city	38 (30.4)
Urban inner-city	20 (16.0)
Rural	18 (14.4)
Professional self-identification ($n = 124$)	
Both primary care provider and specialist	74 (59.2)
Specialist	46 (36.8)
Primary care provider	4 (3.2)

TABLE 2: Patient sample demographics ($N = 981$).

Characteristics n (%)	
Year of birth ($n = 967$)	1977 ± 13.3
Ethnicity/race ($n = 977$)	
White, non-Hispanic	618 (63.0)
Black/African American	143 (14.6)
White, Hispanic	130 (13.3)
Multiracial	44 (4.5)
Asian	27 (2.8)
Others	15 (1.5)
Education ($n = 979$)	
Less than a high school degree	47 (4.8)
High school degree	155 (15.8)
Some college, no degree	269 (27.4)
College degree	286 (29.2)
Graduate/professional degree	222 (22.6)
Home location ($n = 963$)	
Suburban	362 (36.9)
Urban inner-city	224 (22.8)
Rural	192 (19.6)
Urban non-inner-city	171 (17.4)
Military	14 (1.4)
Insurance type ($n = 967$)	
Private	734 (74.8)
Medicaid/Medicare	204 (20.8)
Uninsured	29 (3.0)
Relationship status ($n = 980$)	
Married	546 (55.7)
In an intimate relationship	247 (25.2)
Single/separated/widowed	187 (19.1)
Pregnancy status ($n = 977$)	
Pregnant	280 (28.5)
Not pregnant	682 (69.5)
Unsure	15 (1.5)
Perceived role of ob-gyn ($n = 971$)	
Doctor in addition to PCP	649 (66.2)
Main doctor for healthcare needs	322 (32.8)
Number of previous doctor visits ($n = 963$)	
1st visit	338 (34.5)
Two to three visits	275 (28.0)
Three to five visits	119 (12.1)
More than five visits	231 (23.6)

3.1. Physician Data (from the Modified PREMIS)

3.1.1. Training, Preparation, and Knowledge. Amount of previous IPV training ranged from 0 to 40 hours ($m = 5.8$; SD = 0.7). Ob-gyns with no training (20.8%) had been in practice longer ($t = 2.23$; $p = 0.028$) and had lower scores on the perceived preparation ($t = -4.38$; $p < 0.001$), perceived knowledge ($t = -4.99$; $p < 0.001$), objective knowledge ($t = -2.58$; $p = 0.011$), and questioning in specific situations ($t = -2.74$; $p = 0.007$) scales. Training was not related to the response practices scale. Physicians who had received classroom training (34.4%; $t = 5.31$ and $p < 0.001$) and postgrad training (26.4%; $t = 3.98$ and $p < 0.001$) had been in practice for fewer years; other sources of IPV training (e.g., attending a lecture or talk—48.8%) were unrelated to years in practice. Of ob-gyns in the sample, 36.8% agreed that they did not have sufficient training to assist individuals in addressing IPV.

Perceived preparation and perceived knowledge scores (see Table 3) were normally distributed and strongly correlated ($r = 0.901$; $p < 0.001$). Notably, most ob-gyns indicated that they felt *fairly* to *quite well prepared* to appropriately respond to disclosures of abuse (63.2%) and make appropriate referrals for IPV (57.6%), while only 30.4% felt *fairly* to *quite well prepared* to help an IPV victim make a safety plan. Additionally, most physicians reported that they knew a *fair amount* to *very much* about signs and symptoms of IPV (55.2%) and how to document IPV in patient charts (54.4%),

TABLE 3: PREMIS scales used in analyses ($N = 125$).

Scale	Description	N	Items	Mean ± SD	Range	Alpha
Perceived preparation	Ob-gyns rated how prepared they felt to assess for/respond to IPV on a scale from *not prepared* (1) to *quite well prepared* (7).	124	12	4.10 ± 1.38	1.00 to 7.00	0.946
Perceived knowledge	Ob-gyns rated how much they felt they knew about IPV and IPV response on a scale from *nothing* (1) to *very much* (7).	123	16	4.14 ± 1.41	1.00 to 7.00	0.968
Objective knowledge	Ob-gyns answered multiple choice, select all that apply, matching, and true/false/DK IPV knowledge questions.	124	38	26.51 ± 5.24	10.00 to 34.00	—
Questioning in specific situations	Ob-gyns rated how often in the past 6 months they asked patients with associated symptoms about IPV from *never* (1) to *always* (5). N/A responses excluded.	115	7	2.90 ± 0.99	1.00 to 5.00	0.921
IPV response practices	Ob-gyns who had identified IPV in the past 6 months indicated how often they performed response practices from *never* (1) to *always* (5). N/A responses excluded.	79	11	3.51 ± 0.97	1.00 to 5.00	0.909

A total score of correct items was obtained to represent criterion-referenced, objective knowledge; accordingly, "measurement of internal consistency . . . was not appropriate" [14, 15]. For the remaining scales, mean scores were calculated to account for missing items.

TABLE 4: Correlation matrix of scale scores ($N = 125$).

	(1)	(2)	(3)	(4)	(5)
(1) Perceived preparation ($n = 124$)	1 124				
(2) Perceived knowledge ($n = 123$)	0.901** 123	1 123			
(3) Objective IPV knowledge ($n = 124$)	0.267* 123	0.294** 123	1 124		
(4) Questioning in specific situations ($n = 115$)	0.644** 114	0.616** 114	0.145 115	1 115	
(5) IPV responses practices ($n = 79$)	0.432** 79	0.454** 79	0.454** 79	0.441** 76	1 79

*Correlation is significant at the 0.01 level. **Correlation is significant at the 0.001 level.

while only 34.4% felt they knew a *fair amount* to *very much* about their legal reporting requirements for IPV. Perceived preparation and perceived knowledge were both positively correlated with objective IPV knowledge (see Table 4).

Overall objective knowledge was high, such that 27 items were answered correctly on average (SD = 5.24) out of 38 possible. Objective knowledge scores were negatively correlated with years in practice ($r = -0.315$; $p < 0.001$) and lower among ob-gyns in solo private practice ($F = 9.33$; $p < 0.001$). In response to independent items, 64.8% of ob-gyns were "unsure" as to whether they were practicing in a state where it is legally mandated to report IPV cases involving competent nonvulnerable adults, and only 35.2% endorsed awareness of state legal requirements for reporting suspected cases of IPV.

3.1.2. IPV Screening and Diagnosis.
Physician-reported IPV screening practices are described in Table 5. Ob-gyns who did not screen for IPV were more likely to have no previous IPV training ($\chi^2 = 6.68$; $p = 0.010$) and score lower on the perceived preparation ($t = 3.13$; $p = 0.002$), perceived

TABLE 5: Physician IPV screening practices ($N = 119$).

n (%)	Screening practice
16 (12.8)	I do not currently screen
47 (37.6)	I screen all new patients
46 (36.8)	I screen all patients with abuse indicators on history or exam
46 (36.8)	I screen all patients at the time of their annual exam
39 (31.2)	I screen all pregnant patients at specific times of their pregnancy
24 (19.2)	I screen all patients periodically
25 (20.0)	I screen certain patient categories only

Responses to "Check the situation listed below in which you currently screen for IPV" *(check all that apply)*. Missing = 6.

knowledge ($t = 3.69$; $p < 0.001$), objective knowledge ($t = 3.66$; $p < 0.001$), and questioning in specific situations ($t = 4.22$; $p < 0.001$) scales. Similarly, ob-gyns who did not screen all new patients (37.6%) scored lower on the aforementioned scales ($t = -3.08$ and $p = 0.003$; $t = -3.83$ and $p < 0.001$; $t = -2.29$ and $p = 0.024$; $t = -3.966$ and $p < 0.001$, resp.) than those who did. Only screening patients during pregnancy was associated with fewer years in practice ($t = 2.41$; $p = 0.018$). On the questioning in specific situations scale, most ob-gyns indicated that they "always" or "almost always" asked about IPV when seeing patients with injuries (57.6%), whereas a minority did so when seeing patients with other associated symptoms (e.g., chronic pelvic pain; depression/anxiety).

Regarding new diagnoses of IPV in the past 6 months, 29.6% of ob-gyns had made none, while 65.6% had made at least one. Physicians who had made no new diagnoses were more likely to indicate that they did not screen for IPV ($\chi^2 = 6.55$; $p = 0.010$). In contrast, physicians who had made at least one new diagnosis were more likely to indicate that they screened all new patients ($\chi^2 = 5.41$; $p = 0.020$), all patients at annual exams ($\chi^2 = 9.12$; $p = 0.003$), and all pregnant patients ($\chi^2 = 6.90$; $p = 0.009$). Ob-gyns who had made no new diagnosis had been in practice longer ($t = 2.78$; $p = 0.006$) and had fewer hours of previous IPV training ($t = -2.71$; $p = 0.008$). They also scored lower on the perceived preparation ($t = -4.37$; $p < 0.001$), perceived knowledge ($t = -4.11$; $p < 0.001$), objective knowledge ($t = -2.37$; $p = 0.019$), and questioning in specific situations ($t = -5.48$; $p < 0.001$) scales.

3.1.3. IPV Response and Practice-Related Factors.
On the response practices scale, most ob-gyns who had identified IPV in the past six months reported that they had "always" or "almost always" documented patient statements (85.7%), provided referral and/or resource information (82.2%), and offered validating or supportive statements (78.4%). Around half "always" or "almost always" conducted a safety assessment (54.7%) and helped the patient develop a safety plan (45.8%). The response practices scale positively correlated with perceived preparation ($p = 0.43$; $p < 0.001$), perceived knowledge ($p = 0.45$; $p < 0.001$), and objective knowledge ($p = 0.45$; $p < 0.001$) scores.

Of ob-gyns in the sample, 50.4% agreed with the statement "my workplace encourages me to respond to IPV." Those who agreed had more hours of IPV training ($F = 6.97$; $p = 0.001$) and higher scores on the perceived preparation ($F = 19.15$; $p < 0.001$), perceived knowledge ($F = 20.65$; $p < 0.001$), questioning in specific situations ($F = 8.13$; $p = 0.001$), and IPV response practices ($F = 7.05$; $p = 0.002$) scales. Objective IPV knowledge scores were not associated with workplace encouragement. Agreement was also associated with a greater likelihood of screening new patients ($\chi^2 = 9.43$; $p = 0.009$) and having made at least one new IPV diagnosis ($\chi^2 = 17.52$; $p < 0.001$) as well as knowledge of mandated reporting for IPV in their state (20.8%; $\chi^2 = 13.24$ and $p = 0.010$), awareness of an IPV response protocol at their clinic/practice (30.4%; $\chi^2 = 20.41$ and $p < 0.001$), familiarity with their institution's policies regarding IPV screening/response (33.6%; $\chi^2 = 26.83$ and $p < 0.001$), and feeling that their site had adequate referral resources (30.4%; $\chi^2 = 13.74$ and $p = 0.008$).

3.2. Patient Data (from the Modified PSSS)

3.2.1. IPV Experiences.
A small percentage (0.6%) of patients reported that they had visited their doctor that day because they were hurt by a current or former partner. When asked about IPV experiences within the past year, however, a greater number of patients indicated that they had been physically hurt (5.1%; e.g., pushed, shoved, hit, slapped, and kicked) and/or forced into sexual activities (1.9%) by a current or former partner. Responses to these questions revealed that 6.0% had experienced a form of IPV within the past year. Additionally, nearly one in five patients (18.8%) indicated having ever been emotionally or physically abused by a current or former partner.

Married women were less likely to have experienced IPV within the last year (2.4%; $\chi^2 = 30.40$ and $p < 0.001$) or at any point in time (12.2%; $\chi^2 = 47.81$ and $p < 0.001$), compared to those who were in an intimate relationship (9.9%; 22.7%) or not in an intimate relationship (12.0%; 35.0%). Additionally, non-Hispanic White patients were less likely to report that they had experienced IPV within the last year (4.1%) compared to Hispanic (10.2%), Black (9.2%), Asian (7.4%), and multiracial (11.4%) patients ($\chi^2 = 12.56$ and $p = 0.028$). Additionally, patients with less than a high school degree were the most likely to report that they had ever experienced IPV (34.8%), while those with college or graduate/professional degrees were the least likely (16.0-17.0%; $\chi^2 = 11.31$ and $p = 0.023$). Finally, participants with a more recent year of birth ($m = 1981$ versus 1977) were more likely to indicate that they had experienced IPV within the last year ($t = 2.45$; $p = 0.014$). Neither location nor insurance type was associated with IPV experiences.

3.2.2. IPV Screening during Medical Visit.
One-third of patients in the sample (31.4%) reported that their physician had asked about possible IPV experiences during their medical visit that day. Among those who had been asked ($N = 308$), the vast majority were satisfied with the way their doctor had asked about IPV (98.5%), the amount of time their doctor had taken to talk about IPV (98.9%), the private environment their doctor had provided (96.5%), and the resources their doctor had provided on IPV (98.8%). Married women were less likely to be asked about their possible experiences with IPV (28.6%) than those in an intimate relationship (39.1%) or not in an intimate relationship (39.7%; $\chi^2 = 11.88$ and $p = 0.003$). Women who visited a solo private practice were less likely to be asked (25.8%) than those who visited a university faculty practice (31.5%) or an ob-gyn partnership/group (37.9%; $\chi^2 = 10.60$ and $p = 0.014$). Additionally, higher education trended towards being associated with a decreasing likelihood of being asked about possible IPV ($p = 0.063$). Neither race/ethnicity, location, year of birth, nor insurance type was associated with being asked about IPV experiences.

Importantly, patients who indicated that they had experienced IPV within the past year ($\chi^2 = 12.39$; $p < 0.001$) or at any point in time ($\chi^2 = 5.87$; $p = 0.015$) were more likely to have been asked about possible IPV experiences during their visit. Including the visit prior to survey completion, patients who had visited their ob-gyn more frequently (3 or more times) within the past year were less likely to have been asked about possible IPV experiences that day (24.9–27.6%), compared to those who visited less frequently (36.5–39.4%; $\chi^2 = 15.10$ and $p = 0.002$). Similarly, pregnant patients reported more frequent ob-gyn visits within the past year ($\chi^2 = 324.68$; $p < 0.001$) and were less likely to have been asked about possible IPV experiences that day ($\chi^2 = 6.98$; $p = 0.031$).

4. Discussion

The present study evaluated ob-gyn readiness to detect and respond to IPV as well as patient IPV-related experiences. To begin, we found that classroom and postgrad IPV training has increased such that ob-gyns who have been in practice for fewer years are more likely to have received such training. Despite this increase in training, one third of ob-gyns in this sample felt they did not have sufficient training to assist individuals in addressing IPV. Lack of medical training on IPV identification and response is a common physician-reported barrier [18, 19]. One in five ob-gyns had received no previous IPV training. While unrelated to response practices following IPV identification, no training was associated with lower likelihood of screening for and detecting IPV as well as lower perceived preparation, perceived knowledge, objective knowledge, and questioning in specific situations. Scales were interrelated and associated with IPV screening practices and identification, both of which were closely linked.

Consistent with these results, IPV screening among general physicians has been associated with prior IPV training/education, perceived knowledge, and perceived preparation [19, 20]. We also found that the percentage of ob-gyns who endorsed screening all patients at annual exams was consistent with existing research [20]. However, both physician endorsement and patient-reported data suggest that ob-gyns are still more likely to screen for IPV during new patient visits than during subsequent visits. This is significant as repeated physician inquiry improves the likelihood of patient disclosure [21].

Overall, 31.4% of patients reported that their physician had asked about possible IPV experiences during their medical visit that day, which is higher than past patient-reported screening rates (e.g., 7%) [22]. In line with these previous studies [22], we found that women who were married and more highly educated were less likely to be asked about IPV during their visit. Whereas non-White race/ethnicity, younger age, living in a rural area, and greater health care utilization have also been found to predict higher rates of IPV screening [22, 23]; these associations were not found in the current study. Though we found that patients who were married, White, college-educated, and older in age were less likely to report IPV experiences, which is consistent with previous reports [3, 24], IPV affects women of all backgrounds and is not accurately predicted by demographic factors [25]. Universal IPV screening on the part of ob-gyns is therefore recommended.

Ob-gyns demonstrated good objective knowledge and endorsed use of appropriate response practices recommended by ACOG. After IPV identification, a majority of ob-gyns "always" or "almost always" documented patient statements, provided referrals and/or resources, and offered validation or support; however, safety assessment and safety planning occurred less frequently. This could indicate that time is a barrier to enacting ACOG-recommended response practices. Importantly, workplace encouragement of IPV response was associated with increased IPV training, screening, diagnosis, perceived preparation/knowledge, response practices, and resources to facilitate response (e.g., a response protocol), but not objective knowledge about IPV support. The majority of ob-gyns were unaware of an IPV response protocol at their site. While this is in line with existing research [19, 20], ob-gyn offices and practices should increase awareness of their protocols. Finally, in contrast to previous reports [22, 26], gender was not related to IPV screening nor readiness to respond to IPV.

The present study assessed current readiness to detect and respond to IPV in a nationally representative sample of ob-gyns as well as IPV-related experiences in a large, diverse sample of patients. However, several limitations are noted. Since ob-gyns were aware of the study aims, it is possible that they altered their screening practices during the data collection period, which consequently could have impacted patient-reported screening rates. Additionally, ob-gyn responses may have been influenced by social desirability bias, while patient responses may have been influenced by self-selection bias. Ob-gyns and office staff may have deviated from the data collection protocol (e.g., provided patients with the survey before their appointment instead of after). The patient survey was also only offered in English, preventing generalization to non-English-speaking patient populations. Finally, causal relationships cannot be drawn from questionnaire-based data. In the future, the impact of education and training programs on IPV screening and response should be evaluated using experimental designs, allowing for causal conclusions to be drawn.

5. Conclusion

In conclusion, our findings highlight the need to improve IPV training and workplace support to facilitate ob-gyn screening of and response to IPV. Addressing IPV in healthcare settings can improve the reproductive and overall health of women, confer positive outcomes for children/families, and reduce the wide-reaching societal and economic consequences of IPV [9]. However, physicians generally report dissatisfaction with their IPV education and training [18]. Specific areas of uncertainty (e.g., state legal requirements) and underutilized response practices (e.g., safety planning) need to be further addressed. Furthermore, IPV training programs may be more effective if they were to aid ob-gyns in recognizing the importance of universal and routine screening of all patients, not just those at increased risk of victimization, so as to reduce missed opportunities for identifying survivors. Additionally, it should be emphasized that screening for

IPV is itself an intervention, as detection and referral to appropriate community resources have significant impact. Recent research indicates computer screening may increase IPV disclosures as well as IPV discussions between physicians and patients and the amount of services provided [27]. Perceived workplace support for IPV response as well as practice-related resources (e.g., community referrals, an IPV response protocol) appear to facilitate ob-gyn preparedness to respond to IPV.

Disclosure

The present address for Katherine M. Jones is as follows: Counseling Center, Johns Hopkins University, 3003 N. Charles St., Baltimore, MD 21218, USA. The funding source had no role in the study design; the collection, analysis, and interpretation of the data; nor the preparation, writing, or submission of this manuscript.

Acknowledgments

This work was supported by the Maternal and Child Health Bureau (Title V, Social Security Act, Health Resources and Services Administration, Department of Health and Human Services) (Grant UA6MC19010).

References

[1] M. J. Breiding, K. C. Basile, S. G. Smith, M. C. Black, and R. Mahendra, *Intimate Partner Violence Surveillance: Uniform Definitions And Recommended Data Elements, Version 2.0*, vol. 2.0, National Center for Injury Prevention and Control, Centers for Disease Control and Prevention, Atlanta, Georgia, 2015.

[2] Centers for Disease Control and Prevention, *Costs of intimate partner violence against women in the United States 2011*, Centers for Disease Control and Prevention, National Center for Injury Prevention and Control, Atlanta, Georgia, 2011.

[3] M. C. Black, K. C. Basile, M. J. Breiding et al., *The national intimate partner and sexual violence survey (NISVS)*, National Center for Injury Prevention and Control, Centers for Disease Control and Prevention, Atlanta, Georgia, 2011.

[4] M. Ellsberg, H. A. Jansen, L. Heise, C. H. Watts, and C. Garcia-Moreno, "Intimate partner violence and women's physical and mental health in the WHO multi-country study on women's health and domestic violence: an observational study," *The Lancet*, vol. 371, no. 9619, pp. 1165–1172, 2008.

[5] World Health Organization, *Global and Regional Estimates of Violence against Women: Prevalence and Health Effects of Intimate Partner Violence and Non-Partner Sexual Violence*, WHO Press, Geneva, Switzerland, 2016.

[6] A. L. Coker, "Does physical intimate partner violence affect sexual health?: a systematic review," *Trauma, Violence, & Abuse*, vol. 8, no. 2, pp. 149–177, 2007.

[7] Institute of Medicine, *Clinical Preventive Services for Women: Closing the Gaps*, National Academics Press., Institute of Medicine, Washington, DC, USA, 2011.

[8] L. A. McCloskey, E. Lichter, M. L. Ganz et al., "Intimate partner violence and patient screening across medical specialties," *Academic Emergency Medicine*, vol. 12, no. 8, pp. 712–722, 2005.

[9] American College of Obstetricians and Gynecologists, "Intimate partner violence committee opinion," *Obstetrics & Gynecology*, vol. 119, pp. 412–417.

[10] R. O'Reilly, B. Beale, and D. Gillies, "Screening and intervention for domestic violence during pregnancy care: a systematic review," *Trauma, Violence & Abuse*, vol. 11, no. 4, pp. 190–201, 2010.

[11] H. D. Nelson, C. Bougatsos, and I. Blazina, "Screening women for intimate partner violence: a systematic review to update the U.S. Preventive Services Task Force recommendation," *Annals of Internal Medicine*, vol. 156, no. 11, pp. 796–808, 2012.

[12] N. Durborow, *How to Create a Healthcare-Based Domestic Violence/Sexual Assault Program*, National Health Resource Center on Domestic Violence, San Francisco, CA, USA, 2013.

[13] Futures Without Violence, *Addressing Intimate Partner Violence Reproductive And Sexual Coercion: A Guide for Obstetric, Gynecologic, Reproductive Health Care Settings*, Futures Without Violence, Washington, DC, USA, 2013.

[14] L. M. Short, E. Alpert, J. M. Harris Jr., and Z. J. Surprenant, "A tool for measuring physician readiness to manage intimate partner violence," *American Journal of Preventive Medicine*, vol. 30, no. 2, pp. 173–180, 2006.

[15] L. M. Short, Z. J. Surprenant, and J. M. Harris Jr., "A community-based trial of an online intimate partner violence CME program," *American Journal of Preventive Medicine*, vol. 30, no. 2, pp. 181–185, 2006.

[16] J. C. Campbell, J. H. Coben, E. McLoughlin et al., "An evaluation of a system-change training model to improve emergency department response to battered women," *Academic Emergency Medicine*, vol. 8, no. 2, pp. 131–138, 2001.

[17] K. Jones, M. Carter, A. Bianchi, and J. Schulkin, "Obstetrician/gynecologists' readiness to manage intimate partner violence".

[18] J. S. McCall-Hosenfeld, C. S. Weisman, A. N. Perry, M. M. Hillemeier, and C. H. Chuang, "I just keep my antennae out: how rural primary care physicians respond to intimate partner violence," *Journal of Interpersonal Violence*, vol. 29, no. 14, pp. 2670–2694, 2014.

[19] S. Sprague, K. Madden, N. Simunovic et al., "Barriers to Screening for Intimate Partner Violence," *Journal of Women and Health*, vol. 52, no. 6, pp. 587–605, 2012.

[20] C. Alvarez, G. Fedock, K. T. Grace, and J. Campbell, "Provider screening and counseling for intimate partner violence: a systematic review of practices and influencing factors," *Trauma, Violence Abuse*, vol. 18, no. 5, pp. 479–495, 2016.

[21] J. McFarlane, B. Parker, K. Soeken, and L. Bullock, "Assessing for abuse during pregnancy: severity and frequency of injuries and associated entry into prenatal care," *Journal of the American Medical Association*, vol. 267, no. 23, pp. 3176–3178, 1992.

[22] R. Klap, L. Tang, K. Wells, S. L. Starks, and M. Rodriguez, "Screening for domestic violence among adult women in the United States," *Journal of General Internal Medicine*, vol. 22, no. 5, pp. 579–584, 2007.

[23] A. Kramer, D. Lorenzon, and G. Mueller, "Prevalence of intimate partner violence and health implications for women using

emergency departments and primary care clinics," *Women's Health Issues*, vol. 14, no. 1, pp. 19–29, 2004.

[24] M. J. Breiding, S. G. Smith, K. C. Basile, M. L. Walters, J. Chen, and M. T. Merrick, "Prevalence and characteristics of sexual violence, stalking, and intimate partner violence victimization - national intimate partner and sexual violence survey, united states, 2011," *MMWR Surveillance Summaries*, vol. 63, no. 1, pp. 1–18, 2014.

[25] K. M. Devries, J. Y. Mak, and L. J. Bacchus, "Intimate partner violence and incident depressive symptoms and suicide attempts: a systematic review of longitudinal studies," *PLoS Medicine*, vol. 10, no. 5, Article ID e1001439, 2013.

[26] J. A. Jonassen and K. M. Mazor, "Identification of physician and patient attributes that influence the likelihood of screening for intimate partner violence," *Academic Medicine: Journal of the Association of American Medical Colleges*, vol. 78, no. 10, pp. S20–S23, 2003.

[27] N. Hussain, S. Sprague, K. Madden, F. N. Hussain, B. Pindiprolu, and M. Bhandari, "A Comparison of the Types of Screening Tool Administration Methods Used for the Detection of Intimate Partner Violence: A Systematic Review and Meta-Analysis," *Trauma, Violence, & Abuse*, vol. 16, no. 1, pp. 60–69, 2015.

7

Childhood Mortality: Trends and Determinants in Ethiopia from 1990 to 2015

Yohannes Mehretie Adinew,[1] **Senafikish Amsalu Feleke,**[2]
Zelalem Birhanu Mengesha,[2] **and Shimelash Bitew Workie**[1]

[1]*College of Health Sciences and Medicine, Wolaita Sodo University, Wolaita Sodo, Ethiopia*
[2]*Department of Reproductive Health, Institute of Public Health, University of Gondar, Gondar, Ethiopia*

Correspondence should be addressed to Yohannes Mehretie Adinew; yohannes1979@gmail.com

Academic Editor: Jennifer L. Freeman

Background. Millennium Development Goal 4 calls for reducing under-five mortality rate by two-thirds between 1990 and 2015. The aim of this review was to assess trend of childhood mortality and its determinants from 1990 to 2015 in Ethiopia. *Methods.* A systematic literature search was conducted in the databases of PubMed and Ovid Medline, Cochrane Library, national medical journals, government websites, and Google Scholar. Original observational study designs and reports conducted entirely or in part in Ethiopia that included a primary outcome variable of childhood mortality and published between 1990 and 2015 were included. Ascertained relevant articles were appraised and the findings were integrated into a systematic review. *Results.* Childhood mortality has declined in Ethiopia with more pronounced reduction over the last 10 years. Under-five mortality is 72% lower now than it was 25 years ago, with the pace of decline in infant mortality (83%) somewhat faster than child mortality (76%). The corresponding decline in neonatal and postneonatal mortality over the same period was 64% and 68%, respectively. Parental sociodemographic, socioeconomic, and behavioral variables and nutritional, environmental, and sanitary factors have been identified to affect child survival. *Conclusion.* Ethiopia has successfully achieved the Millennium Development Goal 4 to reduce under-five mortality.

1. Background

The Millennium Development Goals (MDGs) were demarcated to be measured over the period from 1990 to 2015 [1]. The objective of MDG 4 was to reduce mortality in children under-five years of age by two-thirds. Attaining the MDGs was expected to be tough for the developing nations [2]. As global drive for improving child survival rises, monitoring global and country level progress has become critical. The limited availability of data poses a significant challenge on generating accurate estimates of under-five mortality (U5M), probability of dying between birth and the fifth birthday, for many developing nations [3].

Large and increasing differences are observed in childhood mortality among world regions. The rate of decline in childhood mortality (CM), the probability of dying between exact ages of one and five, has accelerated over the past fifteen years [4], but high rates remain in sub-Saharan Africa where one child in every eight dies before age of five [5].

Ethiopia is one of the high burden child mortality (CM) countries in Sub-Saharan Africa [6]. Few records available on CM in Ethiopia appear with different rates, underpinning the high CM burden. At the beginning of the MDGs (1990) neonatal mortality (NM), probability of dying within the first month of life, and postneonatal mortality (PNM), probability of dying between the 5th and 52nd week of life, were 63 and 70 while infant mortality (IM), probability of dying between birth and the first birthday, and U5M were 133 and 216 per 1000 live births, respectively [7, 8].

In contrast to the then set MDG 4 target of 68 deaths per thousand live births [9], there have been appreciable reductions in CM fifteen years down the road. Ethiopia appreciably performed well to cut child deaths. Despite the significant progress in reducing child deaths, children from poorer or rural households remain disproportionately vulnerable [3, 9], as child survival interventions are not reaching the children who need them most. Childhood infections, breastfeeding, health service take-up, and maternal sociodemographic characteristics are known to have proximal effect on child survival while hygiene practices, standard of living index, and residence have distal effect [5, 10, 11]. The identification of country specific determinants of CM is a crucial step in planning and implementation of interventions [4]. So the aim of this review was to assess national progress in reducing childhood mortality and identify factors favoring and constraining the overall trend.

2. Methods and Materials

This systematic review was conducted and reported according to the PRISMA (Preferred Reporting Items for Systematic Reviews and Meta-Analysis) statement checklist [12].

2.1. Eligibility Criteria

2.1.1. Type of Records. This review considers all observational study designs (cross-sectional, cohort, and case control studies) and government reports that assessed neonatal, postneonatal, infant, child, and under-five mortality and determinants of childhood mortality in Ethiopia. The records published between 1990 and 2015 were included. Meeting abstracts and editorial letters were excluded.

2.1.2. Type of Outcomes. This review considers records reported on primary outcome variable of neonatal, postneonatal, infant, child, and under-five mortality and cause and determinants of childhood mortality in Ethiopia.

2.2. Search Strategy.
Computer based literature searches were done up to December 30, 2015, by (YM, SA) in the databases of PubMed and Ovid Medline, the Cochrane Library, national medical journals, Google Scholar, and government websites. The literature search was more enhanced by browsing the websites of major publishers (Oxford University Press, Wiley-Blackwell, Elsevier, and Nature Publishing Group) and by searching the references of the obtained records. The website of MEASURE DHS was also visited for the final reports of Demographic and Health Surveys (DHS) of Ethiopia. For local grey literatures that were unavailable electronically, manual search was conducted in university libraries and health bureau. The following search terms were used: "MDGs", "Ethiopia", "NM", "PNM", "IM", "CM", and "U5M" using the Boolean logic (AND, OR) by both authors. The search was peer-reviewed by ZB to increase its comprehensiveness.

2.3. Study Selection and Identification.
Retrieved records were categorized as "eligible for full document review" and "ineligible for full document review" based on title and abstract assessment. Records that were grouped as "eligible for full document review" were fully reviewed to decide whether to include them in the review or not. Selection of records was independently done by YM and SA. Differences

between records were settled through discussion (based on inclusion and exclusion criteria), reexamining the specific records jointly and consulting ZB for arbitration.

2.4. Data Extraction. YM and SA extracted the data independently by using same data extraction tool. ZB and SB verified the extracted data in order to reduce selection bias and minimize individual errors. Differences among researchers were settled by reevaluating the records until agreement was reached. Extracted information included (i) name of the first author, (ii) year of publication, (iii) objective, (iv) study area, (v) sample population, (vi) neonatal mortality, (vii) postneonatal mortality, (viii) infant mortality, (ix) child mortality, (x) under-five mortality, and (xi) causes and determinants of CM (Table 1). In case of any missing information or uncertainty during records review, efforts were made to contact the authors for clarification.

2.5. Synthesis of the Results. Synthesis was done by constructing a clear descriptive summary of the included records. This was done by tabulating details about name of author, year of study or year of publication, number of participants, and major findings. Results were appraised in a descriptive way according to the facts extracted from each of the comprised records.

3. Results

3.1. Description of Records. We aimed to describe Ethiopia's childhood mortality trends and determinants in 1990–2015. Selection of records for this study is depicted in the flow chart (Figure 1). Among 142 records identified by manual search and online browsing, 48 were duplicates and discarded. Out of the remaining 94 records, 78 were excluded based on title/abstract. Sixteen records were selected for a full-text analysis. Of these fully reviewed records, seven were later excluded as they did not fulfill the criteria.

3.2. Trend of Childhood Mortality. Achieving the MDG 4 was always likely to be very difficult for low-income countries [2]. In 1990 U5MR in Ethiopia was about 216 per 1000 live births, and child survival MDG for Ethiopia was 68 deaths per 1000 live births [1].

In 1990–1995, neonatal mortality and PNM were 63 and 70, while infant mortality and CM were 133 and 96 per 1000 live births, respectively. U5M during the same period was 216 per 1000 live births [1, 7, 13, 14]. For the period 1996–2000, the age distribution of U5M was 29% NM, 29% PNM, and 42% CM. Ethiopia was among the top five nations in NM. In Ethiopia, NM accounts for a smaller (29%) share of U5M than the average for the developing world (36%) [9, 10].

In 2000 Ethiopian Demographic and Health Survey (EDHS), the IMR and U5M in the five years preceding the survey were 95 and 165 deaths per 1,000 live births. This means that one in every ten Ethiopian children dies before reaching age one, while one in every six does not survive to their fifth birthday [10].

The 2005 EDHS reported that IM has declined by 19% over the five-year period preceding the survey from 97 to 77,

TABLE 1: Characteristics of studies that met the inclusion criteria and were included in the systematic review.

Author	Study area	Objective	Population sampling	Findings
You et al., 2015 [1]	Global, regional, and national	To assess levels and trends in under-5 mortality between 1990 and 2015		The U5MR in Ethiopia in 1990 was 205, in 2000 was 145, and in 2015 was 59, which is lower than the target 68. The annual rate of reduction was 5
EDHS, 2005 [5]	Country-wide	To assess the demographic and health condition in the country	14,500 HH	NMR (39), PNMR (38), IMR (77), CMR (50), and U5MR (123)
Wang et al., 2014 [7]	Global, regional, and national	To assess levels of neonatal, infant, and under-5 mortality during 1990–2013		NMR (22.9), PNMR (23.3), CMR (23.2), and U5MR (74)
Ministry of Health, Family Health Department, 2005 [9]	Country-wide	National Strategy for Child Survival in Ethiopia	Document	Children in Ethiopia suffer from poor health. The national U5MR is about 140/1000, with variations among the regions from 114 to 233/1000. The levels of mortality are worsened particularly by poverty, inadequate maternal education, lack of potable water and sanitation, high fertility, and inadequate birth spacing
National Planning Commission and the United Nations in Ethiopia, 2014 [11]	Country-wide	To assess Ethiopia's progress towards the MDGs	Report	U5M declined to 60 per 1,000 live births in 2015, which is below the MDG target of 63 indicating that Ethiopia has achieved its target of reducing child mortality by two-thirds ahead of time. Similarly, the infant mortality rate declined from 123 (per 1000 live births) in 1990 to 97 in 2000, 77 in 2005, and 59 in 2011, but it is unlikely that the MDG target of 31 per 1,000 live births in 2015 will be attained. Neonatal deaths (per 1,000 live births) showed a decline over time from 54 in 1990 and 49 in 2000, to 37 in 2011
Oestergaard et al., 2011 [14]	Global, regional, and national	To assess neonatal mortality levels for 193 countries in 2009 with trends since 1990	Compiled a database of NMR and U5MR	NMR in 2009 was between 30 and 45
EDHS, 2000 [13]	Country-wide	To assess the demographic and health condition in the country	1,355 couples HH	NMR (49), PNMR (48), IMR (97), CMR (77), and U5MR (165)
EDHS, 2011 [14]	Country-wide	To assess the demographic and health condition in the country	More than 17,000 households	NMR (37), PNMR (22), IMR (59), CMR (31), and U5MR (88)
World Bank, 2014 [15]	Global, regional, and national			U5MR was 64.40 in 2013

NMR: neonatal mortality rate; PNMR: postneonatal mortality rate; IMR: infant mortality rate; CMR: child mortality rate; U5MR: under-five mortality rate; HH: household.

while U5M has gone down by 25% from 165 to 123 deaths per 1,000 live births. The corresponding decreases in neonatal mortality and PNM over the same period were 15% and 22%, respectively [5]. Infant mortality and U5MR attained for the five years preceding the two surveys confirmed declining trend in mortality [5, 9, 10, 13].

In 2011 EDHS, the IM and CM were 59 and 31 deaths per 1,000 live births, while the overall U5MR for the same period was 88. Neonatal mortality and PNM were 37 and 22 deaths per 1,000 live births, respectively. The survey showed a rapid decrease in infant mortality and U5M during the 5 years prior to the survey compared to the 2005 EDHS. For example, IM has decreased by 23%, from 77 to 59, while U5M has decreased by 28%, from 123 to 88 deaths per 1,000 live births [11].

In 2015 NM and PNM are 23 and 22 per 1,000 live births, respectively. U5M was also 59 per 1,000 live births, with one in every sixteen children dying before their fifth birthday [5, 15]. Generally, the trend analysis showed that Ethiopia has achieved MDG 4; U5M fell by 72% compared with 1990 figures, which is 2.88% annual decrease. IM reduced from 133 to 23 accounting for 83% reduction. The annual decrement for IM was 3.32%. CM reduced from 96 to 23 deaths per 1000 live births which is 76% reduction; this means CM was dropping by nearly 3% annually. Neonatal mortality and PNM dropped from 63 to 23 and 70 to 22, respectively, with respective annual fall of 2.2 and 2.7% (Figures 2 and 3).

3.3. Determinants of Childhood Mortality. Parental sociode-mographic, socioeconomic, and behavioral variables and

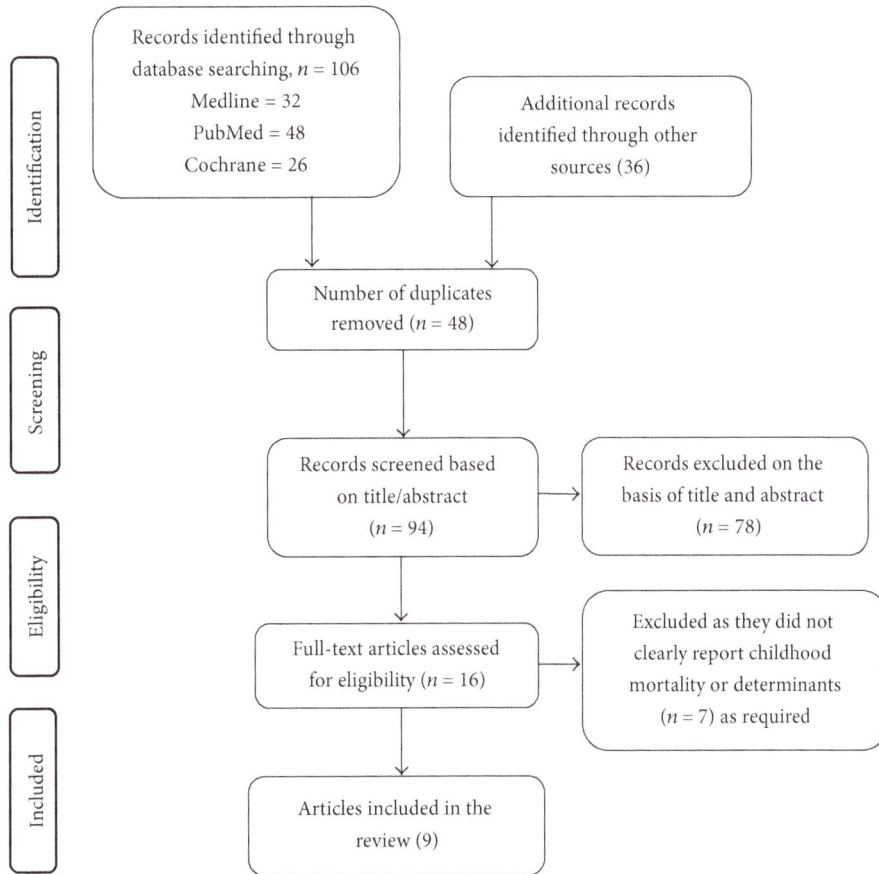

FIGURE 1: Flow diagram showing the procedure of selecting records for systematic review.

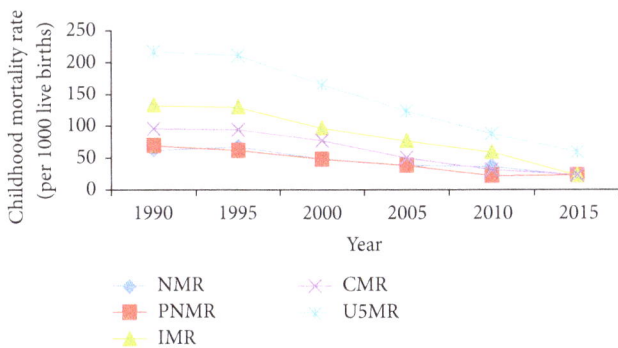

FIGURE 2: Overall trend on under-five mortality from 1990 to 2015 in Ethiopia [1, 5, 7, 9–13, 15].

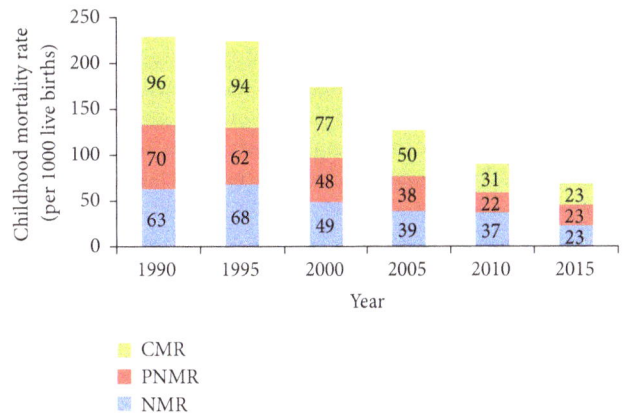

FIGURE 3: Progressive contribution of NM, PNM, and CM to U5MR from 1990 to 2015 in Ethiopia [1, 5, 7, 9–13, 15].

nutritional, environmental, and sanitary factors have been identified to affect child survival. Among identified determinants, maternal education, maternal age at first birth and mothers' marital status, preceding birth interval, birth order, breastfeeding, infections, healthcare, family income, and hygiene practice were found to be important determinants of childhood mortality.

3.4. Maternal Education. The review revealed important role maternal education played in the reduction of child mortality. One of the pathways by which mothers' education affects child survival is through improved child care [17]. Records revealed that neonatal mortality [18] and U5M [19] were associated with parental illiteracy; particularly maternal education has a strong relation with CM [20]. Children born to mothers with secondary education had a significantly reduced IM [16, 21]. Similarly in Jimma epidemiological assessment of determinants and causes of CM in 2004,

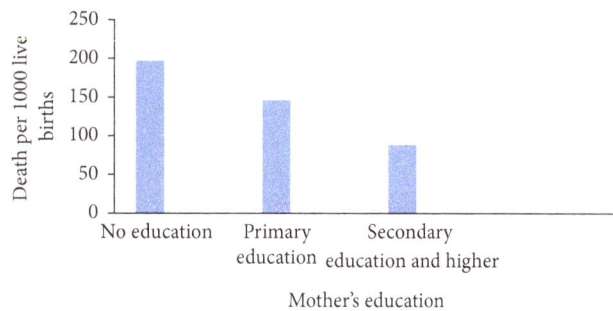

FIGURE 4: Under-five mortality by mothers' educational status in Ethiopia, 2011 [11].

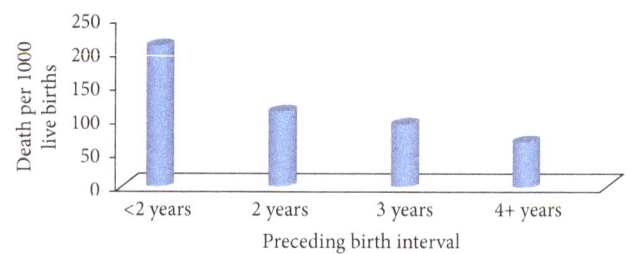

FIGURE 5: Under-five mortality by preceding birth interval in Ethiopia, 2000 [16].

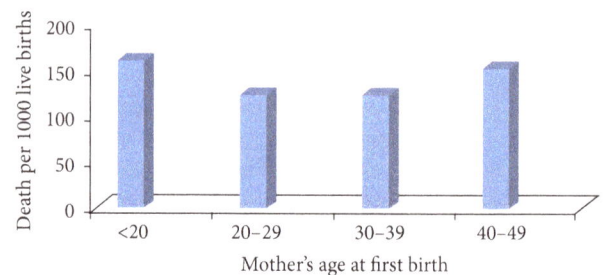

FIGURE 6: Under-five mortality by mother's age at first birth in Ethiopia, 2005 [5].

a reduction in death was observed in children of mothers with secondary or above level of education [22]. In Gilgel Gibe field research of determinants of U5M, children born to mothers whose educational level was below elementary were 14 times more likely to die compared to children whose mothers' education is above elementary [23].

Further analysis of the 2011 EDHS reveals that risk of dying for a child born to uneducated mother was 2.13 times higher compared to a child whose mother had primary and higher education [24]. In another study that analyzed birth history information of live births from the 2000, 2005, and 2011 EDHS to assess trends and determinants of NM in Ethiopia, neonates born to women with secondary or higher schooling had a lower risk of dying compared to neonates born to women with no education [25] (Figure 4).

3.5. Preceding Birth Interval.
Birth interval with previous child has a strong relationship with CM [20]. Analysis of the 1997 community and family survey data in Southern Ethiopia revealed that the risk of IM is significantly associated with short birth intervals of less than 18 months compared with an interval of 24–35 months [16]. In other records mortality among neonates [18, 25, 26] and infants [27] with a preceding birth interval of less than 24 months was found to be 2 times higher than those with a preceding birth interval of greater than 24 months. In epidemiological assessment of determinants of U5M in Jimma town, highest rate of death was observed in groups with short birth interval [22].

Data from EDHSs of 2000 and 2005 revealed higher IM among those with birth interval below two years [28]. In general, children born after long birth intervals (lasting three years or more) appear to have better survival chances in all these age periods [16]. This means that as the previous birth interval increased the risk of infant and child mortality decreased [29]. Age-specific mortality patterns indicate that the adverse effects of short interval are strongest in the infant period but appear to weaken in the 1–4 age categories [30]. Children from multiple births (twins, triplets, etc.) also experience much higher mortality than single births [28] (Figure 5).

3.6. Mother's Age at First Birth.
This review revealed that mother's age at first birth is negatively correlated with IM. Its effect (except children born to mothers older than 20

years of age at first births) has a significant impact on CM [29]. In particular, neonatal mortality and IM are very much influenced by the age of the mother [22]. Births to mothers in the age group of 15–19 face higher mortality risk than births to mothers in the age group of 25–29 or 30–34 [16]. The risk of IM has decreased as mother's age at first birth increased [29]; that is, the risk of IM has been high for mothers who had their first child at younger age [24, 26, 29]. Further analysis from the EDHS revealed that neonates born to mothers aged less than 18 years have higher mortality [25]. The risk of mortality is higher for children born from teenage mother and mothers aged 40–49 years (90 per 1000) [30] (Figure 6).

3.7. Marital Status of the Mother.
Single mothers had increased infant mortality compared to the married ones [22]. In both previous five-year periods of 2000 and 2005, children born to married women play a significant role in the reduction of IM in comparison to children born to other categories [29]. In study of determinants of mortality among one- to four-year-old children in Ethiopia, a child born to currently unmarried mothers had a 51.3% higher risk of dying than children born to currently married mothers [24].

3.8. Breastfeeding.
The role breastfeeding plays in prolonging birth intervals and reducing fertility which in turn reduces CM is critical [16]. Further analysis in both 2000 and 2005 EDHS confirmed that breastfeeding is the most important factor for reducing IM and death rate was lower for neonates who were put to breast immediately upon birth [29]. Children never breastfed had higher risk of dying than those who were breastfed [31]. The likelihood of death among children who were not breastfed was 6 times higher compared to their counterparts [23]. Infants not exclusively breastfed and given

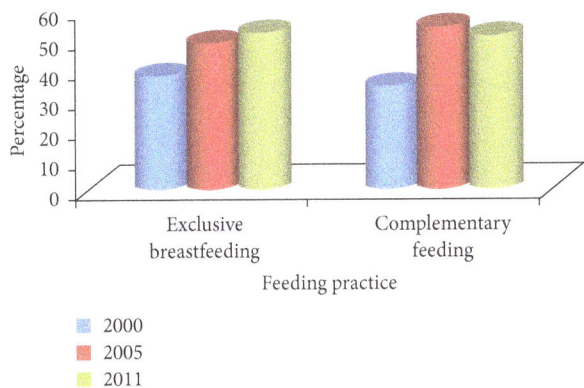

FIGURE 7: Trends in exclusive and complementary feeding in Ethiopia from 2000 to 2011 [5, 10, 11].

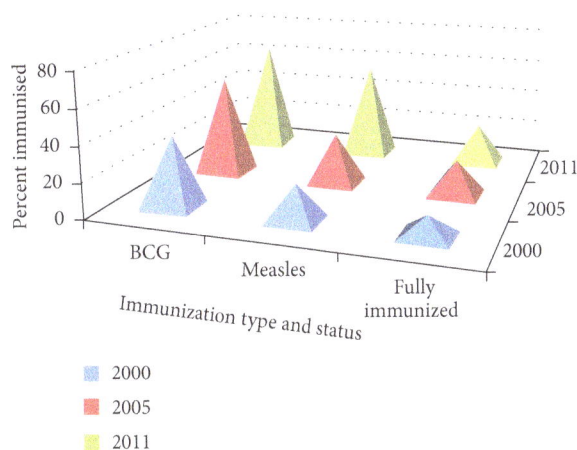

FIGURE 8: Trends of the common causes of under-five mortality in Ethiopia from 2000 to 2010 [5, 10, 11].

breast milk after 24 hours of birth had higher mortality than their counterparts with IRR = 7.86, 95% CI: (5.11, 12.10) and IRR = 4.84, 95% CI: (2.94, 7.99), respectively [32]. A community based study done using verbal autopsy method in Gondar revealed that malnutrition is one of the causes of childhood mortality [33]. Childhood wasting, underweight, and stunting were also the main risk factors for under-5 mortality, but all improved dramatically during the MDG era [34] (Figure 7).

3.9. Infections. Acute childhood diarrhea is the leading cause of death in children under five in Ethiopia, which is largely the result of lack of access to safe water, poor environmental condition, and crowded living conditions [35]. In Gilgel Gibe field research center 2005, the most common causes of neonatal deaths were prematurity (26.4%), pneumonia (22.6%), neonatal tetanus (9.4%), and sepsis (7.5%). The main reasons of postneonatal and child mortalities were malaria, diarrheal diseases, meningitis, and pneumonia. Diarrheal diseases were the primary cause of death for children above one year. Measles was an important contributing factor for 7% of PNM. Injury and HIV/AIDS were accountable for 5% of U5M [23]. Figures from the three EDHSs also confirm that malaria, diarrhea, and pneumonia are the common causes of under-five mortality [5, 10, 11] (Figure 8).

3.10. Health Service Utilization. One of the reasons behind the observed success in reducing under-five mortality has been the expansion of the coverage of health service. The health infrastructure and health extension programs have expanded significantly. As a result the ratio of health facilities to the population showed great improvements. For example, the ratio for health posts reached 1 : 5,352 while the ratio of health centers declined from 1 : 37,299 in 2009/10 to 1 : 27,706 in 2012/13. Primary health service coverage reached 93.4% of the population in 2012/13 and 94.0% in 2013/14 [13].

Another important element in the reduction of child mortality is immunization. Immunization for measles and DPT3 are important contributors to reducing child mortality. In 2013/14, pentavalent 3 immunization coverage was 91.1%, pneumococcal conjugate vaccine (PCV) immunization coverage was 85.7%, measles immunization coverage was 86.5%,

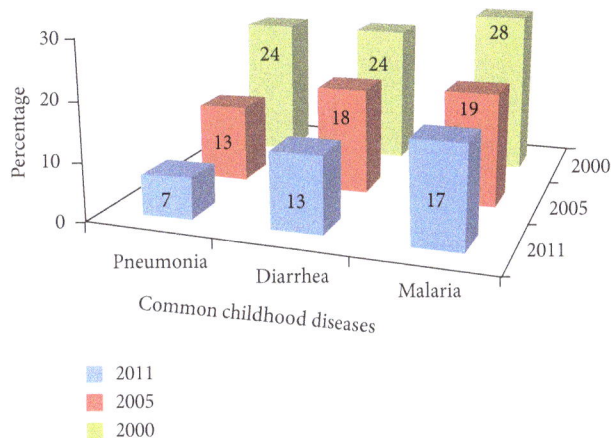

FIGURE 9: Trends of child immunization in Ethiopia from 2000 to 2011 [5, 10, 11].

and the percentage of fully immunized children was 82.9% [13].

A community based case control study conducted in Jimma revealed excess mortality among children who had never been immunized [31]. Unvaccinated children had highest U5M compared to those who were vaccinated at least once [36]. Neonates whose mothers attended antenatal visits exhibited lower risk of death than those whose mothers did not [26]. Mothers who did not attend antenatal care during their pregnancy had greater risk of experiencing infant death compared to those mothers who did at least once. In addition giving two tetanus toxoid injections to the mothers before childbirth decreased NM [25]. The EDHSs revealed improvement in utilization of child and maternal healthcare services [5, 10, 11] (Figures 9 and 10). High risk of U5M was observed when the mothers had no good practice of infection prevention and negative perception on severity of illnesses and modern treatment [23].

3.11. Birth Order. An increase in children birth orders showed a tremendous negative impact on IM in both 2000 and

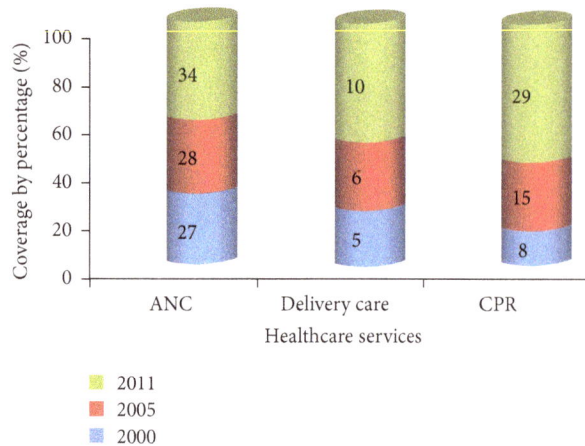

FIGURE 10: Trends in the use of healthcare facility services in Ethiopia from 2000 to 2011 [5, 10, 11].

2005 EDHSs; particularly the 2nd and 3rd birth order were dominant determinants [5, 7, 10]. The estimated hazard ratios of mortality were higher for first birth order compared to second and third ones [26]. In 2005 EDHS, IM among children born in 4th–7th birth order was low compared to those born in 2nd-3rd birth order. Therefore the U-shape relationship between birth order and IM confirmed that the risk of IM is higher for the first and for more than 7th birth order. A study based on the 2011 EDHS data reported that a first born child had a 2 times higher risk of dying than a child belonging to orders four and more [24]. As expected, multiple births were positively associated with CM in both 2000 and 2005 surveys [30].

3.12. Standard of Living Index. Standard of living index [SLI] is another important differential factor of CM [37]. Records showed that children in poor families have relatively higher risks of IM compared to those belonging to medium or rich families [16, 21], while higher level of wealth score has shown a significant reduction in CM [22, 36]. So, it is clear that the mother's SLI plays significant role in CM [37]. A prospective cohort study on trends and risk factors for NM in Butajira revealed that neonates born to poor mothers who had no oxen and lived in thatched houses conferred the highest risk of neonatal deaths [38]. In study done in Jimma from 2004 to 2005, higher level of wealth index was associated with a significant reduction in CM. Excess in mortality was observed in children who reside in household with a floor made of earth compared to that in a household with a floor made of cement [31].

Parental factors affected infants relatively more than the children, especially with regard to Acute Respiratory Infection (ARI) mortality. This was also noted with "absence of window," a proxy measure for evaluating the type of housing [29]. Birth cohort study in South West Ethiopia from 1992 to 1994 identified environmental factors like ventilation in the house and the type of roof and floor and sanitary factors like habit of soap use for hand washing and latrine facility to have association with IM [39].

3.13. Hygienic Practice. Maternal hygienic practice was found to have an association with child survival. Mothers who did not use soap for hand washing had higher infant death than those who used soap [39]. Infants whose mothers were not washing their hands with soap after visiting toilet and before feeding child had high mortality rate than their counterparts [IRR = 4.61, 95% CI: (2.24, 9.48)] [32]. In terms of etiological fractions, a greater number of U5M could be ascribed to parental compared to environmental conditions, with relatively more infants being affected than children [19].

3.14. Residence. According to EDHs childhood mortality in urban areas is consistently lower than in rural areas [5, 10, 11]. From EDHS 2011, infant mortality is 29 percent higher in rural areas (76 deaths per 1,000 live births) than in urban areas (59 deaths per 1,000 live births). Under-five mortality also had difference in urban and rural residence which was 83 deaths and 114 deaths per 1,000 live births [11]. Child mortality was also 34 percent lower in urban areas than in rural areas [10].

4. Discussion

The review showed a decreasing trend in childhood mortality. The identified determinants were parental sociodemographic, socioeconomic, and behavioral variables and nutritional, environmental, and sanitary factors.

Ethiopia, a low-income country in the sub-Saharan Africa, has achieved the MDG to reduce the mortality rate for children under the age of five. Sustained government drive brings down deaths among children by 72% compared with 1990 figures. U5M decreased appreciably well compared to NM. IM fell from 133 to 23 per 1000 live births, 83% reduction, and CM reduced from 96 to 23 deaths per 1000 live births which is 76% reduction. Neonatal mortality and PNM have dropped from 63 to 23 and 70 to 22 per 1000 live births, respectively. This means the risk of dying for any Ethiopian child is the same in the first month of life and in the remaining eleven months of the first year of life. Thus, 50% of infant deaths in Ethiopia occur during the first month of life; and almost one in every twenty babies born in Ethiopia (46.1 per 1,000) does not survive to celebrate their first birthday. Postneonatal and late neonatal deaths are amenable to public health interventions like immunization, breastfeeding, and improved hygiene. The achievement of major reductions in early neonatal deaths will depend on provision of individualized clinical care and quality of services which is much more challenging.

The 2013 progress report of the World Health Organization (WHO), World Bank Group, and UNICEF revealed Ethiopia's success of reducing under-five mortality by more than two-thirds over the past two decades. In 1990 Ethiopia had the seventh highest child death in the world, losing about 216 children in every 1,000 live births. By the year 2012 this rate had decreased to 68, an enormous 67% drop [6], which was further dropped to 64.4% in 2013 [15]. Under-five mortality was measured to be 59 deaths per 1000 live births at the end of the MDGs [1, 13]. This means preventable and treatable conditions are still killing more Ethiopian children in later childhood [9, 10].

Government commitment was central to the achievement. Implementation of the health extension program which deployed over 36,000 health workers to more than 15,000 health posts across the nation is believed to have a lion share in reduction of child deaths. The health extension workers, females who have completed tenth grade and trained in health extension program modules for one year, provide family planning and immunization services; they promote preparedness for birth and readiness for complications and active management of the third stage of labor among others [40]. To achieve these, they work on increasing knowledge and skills of communities and households and creating model families as role model. Since its establishment the HEP has created greater awareness of how to prevent communicable diseases. It also brought change in attitude and behavioral practices in preventive aspects of maternal and child health [41]. But further success in reducing under-five mortality will be very challenging to achieve.

Determinants during the late 20th century include sociodemographic, nutritional, healthcare, sanitary, and environmental factors. In addition within 21st century wealth index, utilization of family planning service, behavioral factors like child care practice, and negative perception on severity of illness were identified as determinants of U5M.

Education plays a great role in increasing awareness of healthcare. Mainly women's education results in more effective preventive and healthcare practices, which increases their productivity and affects infant mortality and CM [17].

Preceding birth interval was identified as a significant determinant of NM in both 2000 [10] and 2005 [5] EDHSs. The estimated result showed that the impact of preceding birth interval on CM is larger relative to the impact on IM. Short birth interval increases the risk of infant mortality and CM due to physiological and nutrition depletion of the mothers which relate to premature child birth and expose the mother to pregnancy complications [37]. As a result poor nutritional status is more common among children with short birth intervals. Thus the relative risk of being underweight is significantly higher for children of shorter birth intervals. The general trend also showed that children with long birth interval are less likely to face the problem of stunting and underweight [16, 28]. The proper spacing of births allows more time for childcare to make more maternal resources available for the care of the child and mother [28]. In addition households with maternal mortality had an increased risk of stillbirths and neonatal deaths [18].

Results by comparing 2005 [5] and 2000 [10] EDHS found that breastfeeding is the most important factor for reducing IM. Children breastfed for more than six months highly reduced the risk of IM. This is in line with the majority of Ethiopian mothers' economical statuses, being very poor and having no access to provide alternative nutrition choice for children, and therefore prolonged breastfeeding is common in Ethiopia.

In both periods of 2000 [10] and 2005 [5], children born to married women play a significant role in the reduction of IM in comparison to children born to other categories. This might be due to socioeconomic factors, traditions, and the lifestyle of the unmarried women.

As mother's age at first birth increased, the risk of IM was reduced and mothers who gave birth to their first child at younger age faced high IM risk due to social and reproduction immaturity. However, child gender and mother's age at first birth were significant only for the previous five-year period of 2005 [5] but not 2000 [10].

According to findings from the Global Burden of Disease Study in 2013, Child deaths due to diarrheal diseases that were attributable to unsafe water supply and sanitation declined by more than 60% between 1990 and 2013 [34]. The source of drinking water is another determinant that was consistently associated with child survival. The result revealed that children born in households with access to nonimproved source of drinking water (river or pond water) were (HR: 2.57, 2.01, and 2.14) more likely to experience the hazard of U5M compared with their counterpart [42].

5. Conclusion

Ethiopia has achieved the MDG goal set for child survival. U5M has dropped from 216 to 59, with 5% annual rate of reduction. The health extension program and the expansion of health facilities have played a significant part. Age, marital and educational status of mother, birth order, preceding birth interval, and family income were the dominant and the most significant determinants of childhood mortality. Other factors include nutritional factors like breastfeeding and healthcare factors like immunization, antenatal care, and delivery care. On the aspects of the environmental and sanitary factors, adequate ventilation, type of floor and roof of the house, availability of latrine facility, and habit of soap using for hand washing are associated with mortality. Regarding diseases, according to EDHS and WHO reports, the leading causes of this age group death are malaria, diarrhea, and pneumonia. Hence, it is worthwhile to address the appalling inequalities in the distribution and access to health services with a focus on service quality and improved sanitation to effectively mitigate childhood death and disease burden.

Abbreviations

ANC: Antenatal care
CM: Child mortality
CPR: Contraceptive prevalence rate
EDHS: Ethiopian Demographic and Health Survey
IM: Infant mortality
MDG: Millennium Development Goal
NM: Neonatal mortality
PNM: Postneonatal mortality
U5M: Under-five mortality
WHO: World Health Organization.

Disclosure

The current address of Zelalem Birhanu Mengesha is as follows: Translational Health Research Institute (THRI), School of Medicine, Western Sydney University, Penrith, NSW 2751, Australia.

Authors' Contributions

Yohannes Mehretie Adinew conceptualized the proposal, identified and reviewed all papers, and prepared the manuscript. Senafikish Amsalu Feleke participated in identification and review of the papers. Zelalem Birhanu Mengesha was reviewer and revised subsequent drafts of the paper. Shimelash Bitew Workie reviewed drafts of the paper and edited the manuscript. All authors reviewed the manuscript critically for content and approved the final version to be submitted.

References

[1] D. You, L. Hug, S. Ejdemyr et al., "Global, regional, and national levels and trends in under-5 mortality between 1990 and 2015, with scenario-based projections to 2030: a systematic analysis by the un Inter-agency group for child mortality estimation," *The Lancet*, vol. 386, pp. 2275–2286, 2015.

[2] UNICEF and WHO, "Fulfilling the Health Agenda for Women and Children: the 2014 Report," http://www.countdown2015mnch .org/documents/2014Report/The2014report/Countdown_The_ 2014_Report_final.pdf.

[3] Y. Danzhen, J. Gareth, and T. Wardlaw, "Levels & Trends in Child Mortality," *UN Inter-Agency Group for Child Mortality Estimation*, 2010.

[4] R. E. Black, S. S. Morris, and J. Bryce, "Where and why are 10 million children dying every year?" *The Lancet*, vol. 361, no. 9376, pp. 2226–2234, 2003.

[5] Central Statistical Authority [Ethiopia] and ORC Macro. Ethiopia Demographic and Health Survey,.

[6] World Data Bank, *World Development Indicators*, The World Bank Group, 2013, http://www.worldbank.org/en/country/ethiopia.

[7] Wang et al., "Global, regional, and national levels of neonatal, infant, and under-5 mortality during 1990–2013: a systematic analysis for the Global Burden of Disease Study 2013," *Lancet*, vol. 384, no. 9947, pp. 957–979, 2014.

[8] UNICEF, "Child mortality estimates," in *Estimates generated by the UN Inter-agency Group for Child Mortality Estimation (IGME)*, 2014, http://data.unicef.org.

[9] Ministry of Health: Family Health Department, "National Strategy for Child Survival in Ethiopia. Ministry of Health, Addis Ababa," https://extranet.who.int/nutrition/gina/sites/default/files/ETH% 202005%20National%20Strategy%20for%20Child%20Survival .pdf.

[10] Central Statistical Authority [Ethiopia] and ORC Macro, *Ethiopia Demographic and Health Survey*, 2000.

[11] Central Statistical Authority [Ethiopia] and ORC Macro, "Ethiopia Demographic and Health Survey," 2011.

[12] D. Moher, A. Liberati, J. Tetzlaff, and D. G. Altman, "Preferred reporting items for systematic reviews and meta-analyses: the PRISMA statement," *PLoS Medicine*, vol. 6, no. 7, Article ID e1000097, 2009.

[13] National Planning Commission and the United Nations in Ethiopia, "Millennium development goals report: Assessment of Ethiopia's progress towards the MDGs, Addis Ababa," 2014.

[14] M. Z. Oestergaard, M. Inoue, S. Yoshida et al., "Neonatal mortality levels for 193 countries in 2009 with trends since 1990: a systematic analysis of progress, projections, and priorities," *PLoS Medicine*, vol. 8, no. 8, Article ID e1001080, 2011.

[15] Trading economics, "Mortality rate - under-5 (per 1, 000) in Ethiopia," https://www.tradingeconomics.com/ethiopia/mortality-rate-under-5-per-1-000-wb-data.html, 2014.

[16] M. Ezra and E. Gurum, "Breastfeeding, birth intervals and child survival: Analysis of the 1997 community and family survey data in southern Ethiopia," *Ethiopian Journal of Health Development*, vol. 16, no. 1, pp. 41–51, 2002.

[17] D. Monica, "Death clustering, mothers' education and the determinants of child mortality in rural Punjab, India," *Population Studies*, vol. 44, no. 3, pp. 489–505, 1990.

[18] Y. Yaya, K. T. Eide, O. F. Norheim, and B. Lindtjørn, "Maternal and neonatal mortality in south-west ethiopia: estimates and socio-economic inequality," *PLoS ONE*, vol. 9, no. 4, Article ID e96294, 2014.

[19] D. Shamebo, A. Sandstrom, L. Muhe, L. Freij, I. Krantz, and S. Wall, *The Butajira Rural Health Project in Ethiopia: A Nested Case Referent (Control) Study of Under-5 Mortality And Its Public Health Determinants*, vol. 71, WHO, 1993.

[20] Dr. P. Prashanth Kumar and Gemechis, "Infant and child mortality in Ethiopia: a statistical analysis approach," *Ethiopian Journal of Education and Sciences*, vol. 5, no. 2, 2010.

[21] UNDP., "Sustainable development goals," http://www.et.undp .org/content/ethiopia/en/home/mdgoverview/overview/mdg4 .html, 2015.

[22] G. Belaineh, Epidemiological Assessment of Determinants and Causes of under-five Child Mortality in Jimma town: Is HIV/AIDS influencing the pattern of child mortality,.

[23] D. Amare, G. Belaineh, and T. Fasil, "Determinants of under-five mortality in Gilgel Gibe Field Research Center, Southwest Ethiopia," *Ethiopian Journal of Health Development*, vol. 21, no. 2, pp. 117–124, 2007.

[24] S. Seyoum and E. Wencheko, "Determinants of mortality among one to four years old children in Ethiopia: a study based on the 2011 EDHS data," *Ethiopian Journal of Health Development*, vol. 27, no. 1, pp. 8–15, 2013.

[25] Y. Mekonnen, B. Tensou, D. S. Telake, T. Degefie, and A. Bekele, "Neonatal mortality in Ethiopia: trends and determinants," *BMC Public Health*, vol. 13, no. 1, article 483, 2013.

[26] W. Negera, "Risk factors of neonatal mortality in Ethiopia," *Ethiopian Journal of Health Development*, vol. 27, no. 3, 2013.

[27] A. F. Dadi, "A systematic review and meta-analysis of the effect of short birth interval on infant mortality in Ethiopia," *PLoS ONE*, vol. 10, no. 5, Article ID e0126759, 2015.

[28] S. A. Sathiya, "Child mortality rate in Ethiopia," *Iranian Journal of Public Health*, vol. 41, no. 3, pp. 9–19, 2012.

[29] M. Desta, "Infant and Child Mortality in Ethiopia, The role of Socioeconomic, Demographic and Biological factors in the previous five years period of 2000 and 2005".

[30] J. E. Lawn, S. Cousens, and J. Zupan, "4 Million neonatal deaths: when? Where? Why?" *The Lancet*, vol. 365, no. 9462, pp. 891–900, 2005.

[31] B. Girma and Y. Berhane, "Children who were vaccinated, breast fed and from low parity mothers live longer: a community based case-control study in Jimma, Ethiopia," *BMC Public Health*, vol. 11, article 197, 2011.

[32] G. A. Biks, Y. Berhane, A. Worku, and Y. K. Gete, "Exclusive breast feeding is the strongest predictor of infant survival in Northwest Ethiopia: a longitudinal study," *Journal of Health, Population and Nutrition*, vol. 34, no. 1, 2015.

[33] M. Fantahun, "Patterns of childhood mortality in three districts of north gondar administrative zone. A community based study using the verbal autopsy method," *Ethiopian Medical Journal*, vol. 36, no. 2, pp. 71–81, 1998.

[34] A. Deribew, G. A. Tessema, K. Deribe et al., "Trends, causes, and risk factors of mortality among children under 5 in ethiopia, 1990-2013: findings from the global burden of disease study 2013," *Population Health Metrics*, vol. 14, no. 1, article no. 42, 2016.

[35] M. Asnake, C. Larson, and G. E. Teka, "Water handling practices and their association with childhood diarrhea," *Ethiopian Journal of Health Development*, vol. 6, pp. 9–16, 1992.

[36] M. Fantahun, Y. Berhane, S. Wall, P. Byass, and U. Högberg, "Women's involvement in household decision-making and strengthening social capital—crucial factors for child survival in Ethiopia," *Acta Paediatrica, International Journal of Paediatrics*, vol. 96, no. 4, pp. 582–589, 2007.

[37] G. T. Bicego and J. T. Boerma, "Maternal education and child survival: A comparative study of survey data from 17 countries," *Social Science and Medicine*, vol. 36, no. 9, pp. 1207–1227, 1993.

[38] M. Gizaw, M. Molla, and W. Mekonnen, "Trends and risk factors for neonatal mortality in Butajira District, South Central Ethiopia, (1987–2008): a prospective cohort study," *BMC Pregnancy and Childbirth*, vol. 14, article 64, 2014.

[39] M. Asefa, R. Drewett, and F. Tessema, "A birth cohort study in South-West Ethiopia to identify factors associated with infant mortality that are amenable for intervention," *Ethiopian Journal of Health Development*, vol. 14, no. 2, 2000.

[40] M. Koblinsky, F. Tain, A. Gaym, A. Karim, M. Carnell, and S. Tesfaye, "Responding to the maternal health care challenge: The Ethiopian Health Extension Program," *Ethiopian Journal of Health Development*, vol. 24, no. 1, pp. 105–109, 2010.

[41] H. Banteyerga, "Ethiopia's Health Extension Program: Improving health through community involvement," *MEDICC Review*, vol. 13, no. 3, pp. 46–49, 2011.

[42] B. Debebe and D. Tariku, "Trends and determinants of under-five mortality in amhara region, ethiopia using EDHS (2000 - 2011)," *Journal of Health, Medicine and Nursing*, vol. 28, 2016.

8

Perceptions, Practices, and Mother's Willingness to Provide Meconium for Use in the Assessment of Environmental Exposures among Children in Mukono and Pallisa Districts, Uganda

John C. Ssempebwa ⓘ,[1] Geofrey Musinguzi ⓘ,[1] and Simon Peter Sebina Kibira[2]

[1]*Department of Disease Control and Environmental Health, School of Public Health, College of Health Sciences,*
  Makerere University, Kampala, Uganda
[2]*Department of Community Health and Behavioural Sciences, School of Public Health, College of Health Sciences,*
  Makerere University, Kampala, Uganda

Correspondence should be addressed to John C. Ssempebwa; jssemps@musph.ac.ug

Academic Editor: Julio Diaz

Presence of biomarkers or metabolites is assessed in various human biospecimens including meconium in the investigation of exposures to environmental contaminants. This study gathered data on the perceptions and practices of mothers in two rural districts of Uganda concerning meconium and their willingness to provide meconium from their babies for research purposes. The study reveals a wide range of perceptions and beliefs around meconium as well as a number of associated taboos and practices. Many participants noted that meconium could be used to detect ailments among newborns based on its appearance. Practices and beliefs included using it to prevent stomach discomfort and other ailments of newborns, as a means to confirm paternity and initiate the child into the clan as well as facilitating father-child bonding that included ingestion of meconium by the fathers. Most mothers indicated scepticism in accepting to provide meconium for research purposes and had fears of unscrupulous people disguising as researchers and using meconium to harm their children. However, some were willing to provide meconium, if it helped to detect ailments among their children. These perceptions and practices may negatively influence mothers' willingness to participate in meconium study. However, through provision of educational and behaviour change interventions, mothers' willingness to participate in a meconium study can be improved.

1. Introduction

Presence of biomarkers and/or metabolites is assessed in various human tissues in the investigation of exposures to environmental contaminants. Among the human tissues are blood [1, 2], urine [3, 4], breast milk [5, 6], and meconium [7–9]. Meconium testing provides a more sensitive matrix to measure fetal exposure to toxicants, due to its ability to cover a longer period of exposure than other matrices such as infant hair and cord blood [10]. Meconium starts to accumulate in the 13-16th week of pregnancy and it is passed by a newborn within the first 24–48 hours soon after birth

[11, 12]. Meconium is composed of materials ingested during the time the infant spends in the uterus. It is a cumulative biological matrix of prenatal toxicant exposure, and its analysis has been documented as a sensitive, diagnostic tool to detect fetal exposure to heavy metals, pesticides, and other contaminants [10, 13, 14]. Meconium collection is easy and noninvasive; therefore it holds promise as a biological matrix for measuring the intensity and duration of environmental toxicant exposure.

Meconium provides key essential information about fetal exposure to toxic substances and may provide the groundwork for protecting the newborn from further damage [15, 16].

In many African countries, there are taboos associated with fecal matter and therefore the use of meconium as a biomarker would be faced with some cultural challenges. Communities, traditions, and cultures have different practices, values, and beliefs surrounding handling of meconium [17–19] and this might affect mothers' willingness to participate in meconium testing interventions or allow the use of meconium for research purposes. Culture plays a major role in the way a woman perceives and prepares for her birthing experience. Each culture has its own values, beliefs, and practices related to pregnancy and birth [20–22]. Meconium testing is feared to have social risks particularly for mothers, especially when it involves testing for alcohol and any other drug use [18, 23, 24]. Fear, embarrassment, and guilt have been reported to contribute to low consent rates of mothers to participate in meconium screening programs [8, 23].

Understanding whether mothers would be willing to allow the use of their newborn infant meconium for research purposes has the potential to inform future meconium studies especially in low income countries where there are many cultural beliefs and practices surrounding births [19, 25]. In this study, we explored mothers' perceptions, beliefs, practices, and willingness to participate in research where collection and use of meconium from newborns would be conducted in studying environmental exposures. The study was conducted in two districts of Uganda, Mukono in the central and Pallisa in the eastern part of the country.

The objectives of the study were to explore the sociocultural aspects including practices, perceptions, and beliefs surrounding meconium and to determine the willingness of mothers to participate in research where meconium would be used to assess exposure to environmental contaminants. The study findings may help identify reasons that could encourage or prevent mothers' participation in research where meconium is used to assess environmental exposures.

2. Methods

2.1. Study Design and Setting. This was an ethnographic study conducted in selected health centres (HC) and in the general community of Mukono and Pallisa districts among women of childbearing age. Mukono is located in central Uganda with 13 subcounties while Pallisa is located in eastern Uganda and has 14 subcounties (Figure 1). The study participants were recruited from four randomly selected subcounties in each of the two districts: Goma, Kyampisi, Mukono Town Council, and Nama in Mukono district and Butebo, Kibale, Pallisa Town Council, and Kakoro in Pallisa district.

The basic characteristics of the mothers who participated in the in-depth interviews are summarized in Table 1; majority of the mothers were aged 18-30 years, had no education or had only attained primary, were Catholics, and were married.

2.2. Data Collection, Management, and Analysis. Participants were purposely selected to provide details about their experiences. The team conducted 30 key informant (KI) interviews with health workers at selected health centres, Village Health Team (VHT) members, trained traditional birth attendants (TBAs), and community leaders. Forty-five (45) in-depth

TABLE 1: Sociodemographic characteristics of the mothers in the in-depth interviews.

Variables	Total Number (%)
Age Category	
18-24	14 (31.1)
25-30	14 (31.1)
31-35	13 (28.9)
36-40	4 (8.9)
Education level attained	
Primary/No education	33 (73.4)
Lower secondary (S.1-S.4)	7 (15.6)
Higher secondary (S.5-S.6)	2 (4.4)
Tertiary	3 (6.7)
Religion	
Catholic	14 (31.1)
Anglican	13 (28.9)
Moslem	12 (26.7)
Pentecostal/Born again	5 (11.1)
Others	1 (2.2)
Marital Status	
Married	43 (95.6)
Not married	2 (4.4)

interviews (IDIs) were also held with pregnant women and mothers who had birthing experience. The interviews lasted approximately 60 minutes. All the interviews were conducted in the local languages (Luganda in Mukono district and Lugwere in Pallisa district) and audio recorded. The KI and IDI guides were pretested in nonstudy villages in both Mukono and Pallisa to improve understanding and relevance and to elicit better responses. These were modified accordingly based on the feedback.

All audio files were transcribed verbatim and translated to English. The initial codes were derived from reading the transcripts and these were used to develop a codebook that was applied to all the transcripts. The new codes that emerged during the coding process were also added to the codebook. All codes were refined after consensus among the team. The codes were grouped into categories to give meaning to the data. These were then categorised under the relevant themes that reflected the objectives of the study.

2.3. Ethical Considerations. Approval to conduct the research was obtained from the Makerere University School of Public Health, Higher Degrees, Research and Ethics Committee and from the Uganda National Council for Science and Technology. Written informed consent was obtained from each participant, following a detailed explanation of the research purpose.

3. Results

3.1. Knowledge and Perceptions on Meconium. Mothers were asked to describe the baby's first stool (meconium) in terms of colour, smell, and texture. They described meconium as being blackish, charcoal black, greenish, or yellowish in

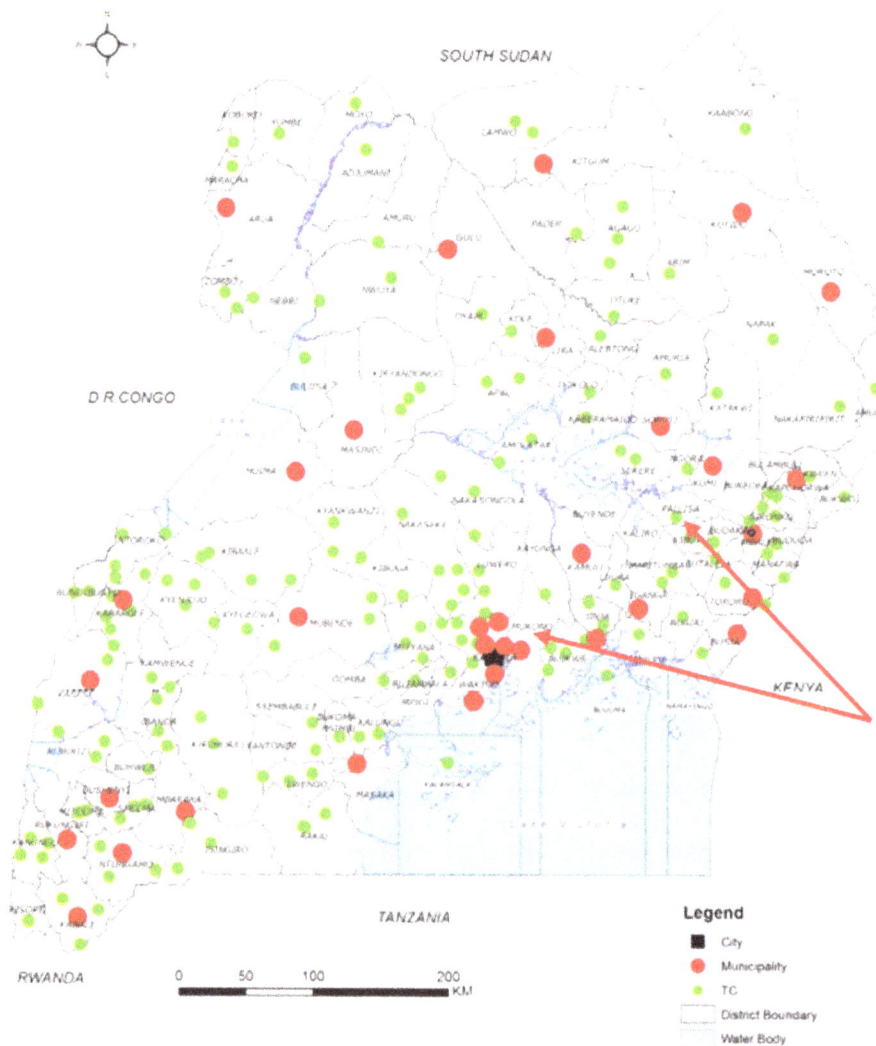

FIGURE 1: Map of Uganda showing Mukono and Pallisa districts.

colour. Some described it as a slippery and sticky substance with no smell. The textural descriptions were a sticky stool that appears like chicken dropping; a leafy like substance; a scrambled egg; or a tiny black mousse. Most mothers described meconium as waste that babies pass out at birth.

The majority felt that the colour and texture of meconium resulted from the food content the baby takes in during gestation or the substances the baby ingests at birth. However, the majority of those that thought meconium was ingested during delivery were not certain of how this occurs.

Some correctly reported that meconium was waste accumulated during gestation that passes out at birth. All key informants were of the view that meconium provides some clues about the health of the child at birth, and notably, meconium with high temperature was attributed to possibilities of a newborn having an infection. Similarly, TBAs mentioned that a strong meconium odour depicted that the newborn had fever associated illnesses.

3.2. Cultural Practices and Beliefs Associated with Meconium. Cultural practices that involve the use of meconium were investigated. Participants reported that meconium is used to prevent stomach discomfort and other ailments, as a means to confirm paternity, to initiate the child into the clan, and to facilitate father and child bonding. These categories are explained further below.

In both Mukono and Pallisa districts, meconium was widely used as a local remedy to alleviate abdominal discomfort that newborns experienced in the first three months of life. Mothers reported that a string made from a piece of cloth is smeared with meconium and then tied around the baby's waist. They believed that this relieves the baby's abdominal discomfort. Sources of such perception within the community were reported mainly by older mothers and TBAs. One TBA interviewed described how the procedure is performed: "All we do (among the Baganda ethnic group), we get a small piece of the baby stool and we wrap it in a small piece of paper making a ball shape, we again wrap it in a piece of cloth and then we tie it around the baby's waist so that the baby isn't disturbed by stomach discomfort (enjoka)" (KI_TBA_01).

It was also reported that as an alternative practice, meconium may be smeared on wall surfaces at a birth site. This was also believed to prevent baby abdominal discomfort and to enhance breast feeding.

Another TBA explained, "At the place where the mother has given birth from, I get a small portion of meconium and I smear it on the wall so that the baby does not fail to breast feed because of abdominal discomfort (obwoka)" (KI_TBA_02).

Mothers in Pallisa reported that meconium was a key item in rituals practiced in certain communities preceding the birth of a newborn. Specifically, they reported that meconium is very helpful in paternity verification and thus proof of the mother's fidelity to the husband. For example, they explained that, in some rituals, meconium is mixed in cooked millet and then served to both the baby's mother and the father. If the newborn is a biological child of the woman's partner as reported, it survives. If the mother lied about the paternity, it was believed that the newborn would die during the ritual. This was confirmed by some health workers in the area as well.

After fatherhood confirmation, they proceed with introductory practices that initiate the child into the father's clan. It was further reported that some mothers hide meconium, which they then take to their home villages for other cultural practices, which they did not substantiate.

It was also revealed that some mothers use meconium to facilitate bonding between children and their fathers. A participant noted that to achieve this, mothers get a piece of meconium, which they mix with a delicacy prepared for the child's father. When the father eats, it is believed that his love for the child increases and that such fathers tend to bond better with their children. A VHT member explained, "Women are the ones who use it (meconium) so much because they use it in food or tea and they serve it to their husbands. They say they want to create a close relationship between the father and the child" (KI_VHT- 10).

3.3. Meconium Disposal Practices. The mentioned common disposal sites included pit latrines, placenta pits that they use while the baby is still in hospital, the bushes, at open rubbish pits, dig-and-burry holes, and some at dedicated locations in banana plantations in their homes. Cultural beliefs were critical in determining where the disposal took place, with the disposal sites primarily being determined by mothers and their culturally grounded caretakers.

Those who disposed of meconium in pit latrines either were cautious of their household hygiene and sanitation status or had this as their only option. However, from KIs, it was also noted that fear of adversaries influenced choice of disposal into a pit latrine as explained in one of the meetings: "...another thing I know is that they do not want to pour meconium anywhere for reasons that someone may come and do something evil with it and the newborn gets problems. So, whenever they finish washing, they make sure that the water, which contains meconium, is poured into the pit latrine" (KII –Health Worker 8).

However, some participants indicated that it was a taboo in some communities to dispose of meconium into a pit latrine. They highlighted the existence of the following beliefs associated with disposal into a pit latrine: delayed growth of the baby's milk teeth or sometimes total inhibition of their growth; frequent childhood illness; and delayed commencement of breast feeding by the newborn. It was also reported that disposing meconium in pit latrines was equated to placing an omen on the newborn, and it should not be done so as to avoid the negative attributes. One KI explained, "Sometimes they (mothers) say that when a baby's stool mixes with adult faeces the child may develop illnesses. That's why they don't want to mix it with adult faeces to avoid frequent sickness of the newborn baby" (KI_VHT- 15).

When asked about the frequent childhood illness experienced, they pointed out abdominal discomfort, "mysterious traditional ailments", back pain, and fever. It was mentioned that it was better to dispose of stool into a pit latrine when the baby has started feeding on solid food.

Although it was recognized as taboo to dispose of meconium into pit latrines by some mothers, others perceived the practice as being protective of the baby especially from witchcraft. They reported that disposal into pit latrines denied access to those adversaries who would use the baby excreta to harm them. "My mother told me that I shouldn't dispose the baby's pooh anyhow; she told me to be throwing it in the pit latrine directly.... Asked why, she told me that it is not good because some people can do something bad with that pooh and your baby ends up falling sick" (IDI- 21).

Some mothers reported that they disposed of meconium at the base of a banana tree within their plantation and that the banana species chosen for this was dependent on the sex of the child.

This way of disposal was perceived to help the child grow with humility and to receive blessings. One KI narrated, "... Yes, they would dig a hole and place it there such that when the child grows up, she/he would be humble and blessed, and not wild" (KII- VHT10).

Mothers whose newborns passed out meconium while at the hospital disposed of the waste into the placenta pit. This was corroborated by KI health workers, who mentioned that they direct mothers to pour the waste in the placenta pit. However, it was stated that those mothers who were superstitious hid and took the meconium home for cultural use as already stated above.

The majority of the young mothers knew of the existence of the several cultural perceptions and practices associated with meconium, although they claimed they did not practice any themselves. Among these, it was reported that modernization and religion were the major reasons for not recognizing any cultural practices related to meconium. To affirm, a TBA reported that "...many mothers don't observe the cultural practices associated with meconium and many don't know the taboos associated with its use and disposal" (KI_TBA_01).

3.4. Influence on Willingness to Provide Meconium for Research Purposes. Mothers were asked about their willingness to provide meconium as a laboratory sample for research to inform future studies that could use meconium in investigating environmental exposures.

None of the mothers had ever participated in research that involved meconium collection and to most, the study would be very unusual. However, some indicated willingness to participate.

3.4.1. Perceived Benefits and Fears. The desire to detect possible ailments in their children would be a "pull factor" for mothers to participate and provide meconium for research. The mothers' love for their children's wellbeing was mainly expressed. The mothers indicated that if their newborns are diagnosed with potential for future ailments, healthcare providers would advise them accordingly. One mother reflected, "...maybe she could be having some ailment and they happen to advise me on how to treat the child and it saves me a lot in future" (IDI - 3).

Some mothers reported that they did not have any use for meconium and therefore, giving it away for research purposes would not be a problem. They noted that, instead of disposing of meconium, they would rather provide it for research as long as it would be useful in that perspective.

Although most participants indicated that they would be willing to participate and provide meconium for research purposes, some mothers expressed fears and uncertainties. The fears related to the credibility and intentions of researchers; use of meconium for witchcraft purposes; the feeling that meconium was disgusting to be given to researchers; uncertainties about why meconium was needed for research and what kind of research it would be; and the fears of spouses and/or elders not approving participation.

Some mothers were also afraid that unscrupulous people disguised as researchers could give meconium to sorcerers whose intentions might be to harm children. Mothers and KIs commonly reported fear of sorcery whose communities' sorcery practices were prevalent. A mother narrated, "Now the first challenge is that most mothers in this village believe so much in witchcraft that they would think that there is something wrong you are going to use that meconium for. It is because they hold the same perceptions that they fear you are probably going to do something evil with it. So, should her child fall sick, she will attribute that to the meconium that was collected simply because herself, practices witchcraft. So she may even fail to take the child to hospital for treatment thinking that; 'what I do is what these people also did'" (KI_VHT_10).

3.4.2. Uncertainty and Scepticism about Why Meconium Would Be Needed for Research. The participants noted that meconium was quite a rare specimen that was not requested in the past and therefore, they wondered why of all specimens a researcher would come requesting meconium. Most mothers noted that it was the first time to hear of a study that would request meconium and would therefore feel uncomfortable giving it away.

Some participants felt that meconium was filthy and that they would feel ashamed to participate in such research activities. One of the participants reflected, "The mother can feel ashamed to give someone such things (meconium) because they look bad." (IDI_03).

Mothers were sceptical that their spouses or family elders would not approve of their involvement in such a study. They indicated that they would have to seek authorization from their spouses or family elders, before providing meconium for research purposes.

Participants proposed recommendations to overcome the scepticism, where they indicated that like any other new health programme that faces similar challenges in communities, proper identification, sensitization, and liaison with local community leaders would be paramount in penetrating the community for such a study. It was also suggested that mothers should be informed of the purpose and procedure of the study well ahead of the newborn delivery. They further proposed that researchers would have to use midwives, VHT members, TBAs, and religious, cultural, and political leaders to raise awareness about the harmless nature and purpose of a meconium study. Additionally, they mentioned that researchers should make use of health programmes like antenatal care and immunization to raise awareness about the study. These programmes offer the opportunity to meet mothers in big numbers in a health setting. A participant in Mukono district advised that "You can use midwives to sensitize these people especially during antenatal visits- these can sensitize people about the research and ask the mothers to welcome the research." (IDI_03).

Another participant added, "They will accept if during antenatal the midwives inform them that when the baby passes out the first stool it will be required for investigation" (IDI_02). They argued that because mothers trust their health workers, it would be easier for samples to be collected by midwives or health workers at health facilities than from the communities. "It is because, they naturally have trust in these health workers even when they have not met them before but they have introduced themselves- like you have done - and you explained to them what they have come to do. Yeah somebody will be willing to give it to you" (KII –Health worker 9). Some mothers suggested that if meconium can be relied on to assess *in utero* exposures, then the Ministry of Health should make it a policy for mothers to provide meconium as the case is for antenatal care and immunization programmes attendance, so as to identify illnesses early in their babies. One participant views, "It should be a policy that when a baby passes out the first stool you have to give it to the health worker for assessment" (IDI_02).

4. Discussion

Our findings show that there exist a variety of perceptions, cultural practices, and beliefs around newborns that would greatly affect the acceptability of mothers to participate in studies assessing environmental exposures through examining meconium. The qualitative methods employed allowed gaining deeper insight into participants' practices, perceptions, and beliefs on meconium, as well as their willingness to participate in future research involving meconium to assess exposure to environmental contaminants. The idea of meconium as a medium that can be used to study *in utero* exposures to environmental contaminants was new among all the mothers interviewed in this study. This finding was consistent with those reported elsewhere [26].

A prevalent belief among mothers that meconium has a number of associated taboos was consistent with findings reported in another study in India [27]. In order to implement the use of meconium in research, there is need to assess knowledge and understanding of cultural perceptions and practices with regard to meconium. In any society, the birth experience is socially constructed, occurring within a cultural context and being shaped by the perceptions and practices of that culture [28]. Therefore, there are many beliefs and practices relating to the childbearing process that the woman and her family must observe to ensure the health and wellbeing of not only herself but also that of her newborn infant [28–30].

The practice of fathers unknowingly ingesting meconium via food or drink is a health hazard that mothers should be discouraged from practicing. Contaminants that are documented to be present in meconium include heavy metals [31–33], pesticides [31, 34], and phthalates [35, 36]. Therefore, fathers are potentially at risk of exposure to these contaminants. Mothers should be educated about the harmful effects of such a cultural practice that could potentially expose fathers to contaminants.

Addressing the perceptions and beliefs is important and can be tackled through the provision of education and behaviour change interventions. Majority of mothers (73.4%) had very low level of formal education or none at all, a situation that might present a challenge of how to explain the link between environmental exposures and meconium to such populations. However, education about beliefs may not be affected so much by the levels of education if it is done in the local languages with appropriate contextual factors in consideration. Future educational interventions prior to enrollment of mothers should understand and focus on dissuading misconceived beliefs and myths among the mothers. Although there was meconium related stigma that is multilayered, with cultural issues, fear, and ignorance, some mothers expressed willingness to participate in a study requiring meconium from their newborn infants.

Our findings suggest that involvement of health workers, particularly midwives in the collection of meconium while the newborn is still at the health facility would improve acceptability of mothers to the provision of meconium. Development of trust and confidence between the mothers, health workers, and the researcher would be key to the mothers' participation and consequently the success of a meconium study. Educating the health workers on environmental hazards and the benefit of collecting meconium would facilitate the recruitment process of mothers into studies where meconium is to be utilized [37].

An increasing number of studies have addressed the concern that environmental pollutants may contribute to the early origin of diseases [38–40]. Our findings show that mothers' knowledge that meconium could provide information about the potential of their child being at risk of developing adverse health outcomes would enhance their participation in a meconium study.

5. Conclusions

The study revealed that mothers in the two rural districts of Mukono and Pallisa in Uganda have cultural beliefs and practices, which might inhibit their willingness to participate in studies designed to assess environmental exposures using meconium from their babies. It was noted that the mothers' level of willingness to participate in a meconium study could be enhanced through educational and behaviour change interventions from their health workers during the entire pregnancy period. This study also brings forth a cultural practice that may expose the male spouses to environmental contaminants that could be contained in meconium and therefore must be abandoned. Since most mothers indicated willingness to participate in a meconium study if it could inform them of their newborns' health, research in low income countries ought to utilize this research opportunity among mothers.

Authors' Contributions

John C. Ssempebwa conceived the study and contributed to the design of the study. John C. Ssempebwa, Geofrey Musinguzi, and Simon Peter Sebina Kibira participated in writing and critical review of the manuscript. All authors read and approved the final manuscript.

Acknowledgments

This study was supported by the research grants from the U.S. National Institute of Health (Grant nos. [1R24TW009489] and [1R24TW009556]).

References

[1] R. B. Gunier, A. M. Mora, D. Smith et al., "Biomarkers of Manganese Exposure in Pregnant Women and Children Living in an Agricultural Community in California," *Environmental Science & Technology*, vol. 48, no. 24, pp. 14695–14702, 2014.

[2] M. Ratelle, J. Coté, and M. Bouchard, "Time profiles and toxicokinetic parameters of key biomarkers of exposure to cypermethrin in orally exposed volunteers compared with previously available kinetic data following permethrin exposure," *Journal of Applied Toxicology*, vol. 35, no. 12, pp. 1586–1593, 2015.

[3] S. T. Singleton, P. J. Lein, O. A. Dadson et al., "Longitudinal assessment of occupational exposures to the organophosphorous insecticides chlorpyrifos and profenofos in Egyptian cotton field workers," *International Journal of Hygiene and Environmental Health*, vol. 218, no. 2, pp. 203–211, 2015.

[4] G. Talaska, J. Thoroman, B. Schuman, and H. U. Käfferlein, "Biomarkers of polycyclic aromatic hydrocarbon exposure in

European coke oven workers," *Toxicology Letters*, vol. 231, no. 2, pp. 213–216, 2014.

[5] K. F. Arcaro and D. L. Anderton, "Potential of using breast milk as a tool to study breast cancer and breast cancer risk," *Future Oncology*, vol. 4, no. 5, pp. 595–597, 2008.

[6] A. J. Wheeler, N. A. Dobbin, M.-E. Héroux et al., "Urinary and breast milk biomarkers to assess exposure to naphthalene in pregnant women: An investigation of personal and indoor air sources," *Environmental Health: A Global Access Science Source*, vol. 13, no. 1, article no. 30, 2014.

[7] K. Delano and G. Koren, "Emerging Biomarkers of Intrauterine Neonatal and Pediatric Exposures to Xenobiotics," *Pediatric Clinics of North America*, vol. 59, no. 5, pp. 1059–1070, 2012.

[8] D. Chan, D. Caprara, P. Blanchette, J. Klein, and G. Koren, "Recent developments in meconium and hair testing methods for the confirmation of gestational exposures to alcohol and tobacco smoke," *Clinical Biochemistry*, vol. 37, no. 6, pp. 429–438, 2004.

[9] Z. Hong, M. Günter, and F. F. E. Randow, "Meconium: A matrix reflecting potential fetal exposure to organochlorine pesticides and its metabolites," *Ecotoxicology and Environmental Safety*, vol. 51, no. 1, pp. 60–64, 2002.

[10] E. M. Ostrea Jr., D. M. Bielawski, N. C. Posecion Jr. et al., "A comparison of infant hair, cord blood and meconium analysis to detect fetal exposure to environmental pesticides," *Environmental Research*, vol. 106, no. 2, pp. 277–283, 2008.

[11] R. M. Whyatt and D. B. Barr, "Measurement of organophosphate metabolites in postpartum meconium as a potential biomarker of prenatal exposure: A validation study," *Environmental Health Perspectives*, vol. 109, no. 4, pp. 417–420, 2001.

[12] C. F. Bearer, "Meconium as a biological marker of prenatal exposure," *Academic Pediatrics*, vol. 3, no. 1, pp. 40–43, 2003.

[13] E. M. Ostrea Jr., D. M. Bielawski, N. C. Posecion Jr. et al., "Combined analysis of prenatal (maternal hair and blood) and neonatal (infant hair, cord blood and meconium) matrices to detect fetal exposure to environmental pesticides," *Environmental Research*, vol. 109, no. 1, pp. 116–122, 2009.

[14] G. Turker, G. Özsoy, S. Özdemir, B. Barutçu, and A. S. Gökalp, "Effect of heavy metals in the meconium on preterm mortality: Preliminary study," *Pediatrics International*, vol. 55, no. 1, pp. 30–34, 2013.

[15] H.-C. Hsi, C.-B. Jiang, T.-H. Yang, and L.-C. Chien, "The neurological effects of prenatal and postnatal mercury/methylmercury exposure on three-year-old children in taiwan," *Chemosphere*, vol. 100, pp. 71–76, 2014.

[16] S. Narkowicz, Z. Polkowska, B. Kielbratowska, and J. Namiesnik, "Meconium Samples use to assess infant exposure to the components of ETS during pregnancy," *International Journal of Occupational Medicine and Environmental Health*, vol. 28, no. 6, pp. 955–970, 2015.

[17] M. McNeilly, M. Musick, and J. R. Efland, "Minority populations and psychophysiological research: challenges in trust building and recruitment," *Journal of Mental Health and Aging*, vol. 6, pp. 91–102, 2000.

[18] L. Marcellus, "Is meconium screening appropriate for universal use? Science and ethics say no," *Advances in Neonatal Care*, vol. 7, no. 4, pp. 207–214, 2007.

[19] S. Neelotpol, A. W. M. Hay, A. J. Jolly, and M. W. Woolridge, "Challenges in collecting clinical samples for research from pregnant women of South Asian origin: evidence from a UK study," *BMJ Open*, vol. 6, no. 8, p. e010554, 2016.

[20] L. C. Callister, M. N. Eads, and J. P. Yeung Diehl, "Perceptions of Giving Birth and Adherence to Cultural Practices in Chinese Women," *MCN, The American Journal of Maternal/Child Nursing*, vol. 36, no. 6, pp. 387–394, 2011.

[21] E. Naser, S. Mackey, D. Arthur, P. Klainin-Yobas, H. Chen, and D. K. Creedy, "An exploratory study of traditional birthing practices of Chinese, Malay and Indian women in Singapore," *Midwifery*, vol. 28, no. 6, pp. e865–e871, 2012.

[22] L. M. Vallely, P. Homiehombo, A. Kelly-Hanku, A. Vallely, C. S. E. Homer, and A. Whittaker, "Childbirth in a rural highlands community in Papua New Guinea: A descriptive study," *Midwifery*, vol. 31, no. 3, pp. 380–387, 2015.

[23] I. Zelner, S. Shor, H. Lynn et al., "Neonatal screening for prenatal alcohol exposure: Assessment of voluntary maternal participation in an open meconium screening program," *Alcohol*, vol. 46, no. 3, pp. 269–276, 2012.

[24] K. E. Wood, L. L. Sinclair, C. D. Rysgaard, F. G. Strathmann, G. A. McMillin, and M. D. Krasowski, "Retrospective analysis of the diagnostic yield of newborn drug testing," *BMC Pregnancy and Childbirth*, vol. 14, no. 1, article no. 250, 2014.

[25] N. Mohammadi, T. Jones, and D. Evans, "Participant recruitment from minority religious groups: The case of the Islamic population in South Australia," *International Nursing Review*, vol. 55, no. 4, pp. 393–398, 2008.

[26] G. Koren, J. Hutson, and J. Gareri, "Novel methods for the detection of drug and alcohol exposure during pregnancy: Implications for maternal and child health," *Clinical Pharmacology & Therapeutics*, vol. 83, no. 4, pp. 631–634, 2008.

[27] U. K. Choudhry, "Traditional practices of women from India: pregnancy, childbirth, and newborn care.," *Journal of Obstetric, Gynecologic, & Neonatal Nursing*, vol. 26, no. 5, pp. 533–539, 1997.

[28] S. Steinberg, "Childbearing research: A transcultural review," *Social Science & Medicine*, vol. 43, no. 12, pp. 1765–1784, 1996.

[29] B. Jordan, "Authoritative knowledge and its construction," in *Childbirth and Authoritative Knowledge: Cross-Cultural Perspectives*, R. E. Davis-Floyd and C. F. Sargent, Eds., University of California Press, Berkeley, California, CA, USA, 1997.

[30] P. Liamputtong, S. Yimyam, S. Parisunyakul, C. Baosoung, and N. Sansiriphun, "Traditional beliefs about pregnancy and child birth among women from Chiang Mai, Northern Thailand," *Midwifery*, vol. 21, no. 2, pp. 139–153, 2005.

[31] E. M. Ostrea, V. Morales, E. Ngoumgna et al., "Prevalence of fetal exposure to environmental toxins as determined by meconium analysis," *NeuroToxicology*, vol. 23, no. 3, pp. 329–339, 2002.

[32] C.-B. Jiang, H.-C. Hsi, C.-H. Fan, and L.-C. Chien, "Fetal exposure to environmental neurotoxins in Taiwan," *PLoS ONE*, vol. 9, no. 10, Article ID 0109984, 2014.

[33] S. Peng, L. Liu, X. Zhang et al., "A nested case-control study indicating heavy metal residues in meconium associate with maternal gestational diabetes mellitus risk," *Environmental Health: A Global Access Science Source*, vol. 14, no. 1, article no. 19, 2015.

[34] T. Berton, F. Mayhoub, K. Chardon et al., "Development of an analytical strategy based on LC-MS/MS for the measurement of different classes of pesticides and theirs metabolites in meconium: Application and characterisation of foetal exposure in France," *Environmental Research*, vol. 132, pp. 311–320, 2014.

[35] K. Kato, M. J. Silva, L. L. Needham, and A. M. Calafat, "Quantifying phthalate metabolites in human meconium and semen

using automated off-line solid-phase extraction coupled with on-line SPE and isotope-dilution high-performance liquid chromatography-tandem mass spectrometry," *Analytical Chemistry*, vol. 78, no. 18, pp. 6651–6655, 2006.

[36] C. Xie, R. Jin, Y. Zhao et al., "Paraoxonase 2 gene polymorphisms and prenatal phthalates' exposure in Chinese newborns," *Environmental Research*, vol. 140, pp. 354–359, 2015.

[37] M. Ondeck and J. Focareta, "Environmental Hazards Education for Childbirth Educators," *Journal of Perinatal Education*, vol. 18, no. 4, pp. 31–40, 2009.

[38] T. E. Arbuckle, "Maternal-infant biomonitoring of environmental chemicals: The epidemiologic challenges," *Birth Defects Research Part A: Clinical and Molecular Teratology*, vol. 88, no. 10, pp. 931–937, 2010.

[39] G. E. R. Schoeters, E. Den Hond, G. Koppen et al., "Biomonitoring and biomarkers to unravel the risks from prenatal environmental exposures for later health outcomes," *American Journal of Clinical Nutrition*, vol. 94, no. 6, 2011.

[40] T. Fernández-Cruz, E. Martínez-Carballo, and J. Simal-Gándara, "Perspective on pre- and post-natal agro-food exposure to persistent organic pollutants and their effects on quality of life," *Environment International*, vol. 100, pp. 79–101, 2017.

9

Loss to Follow-Up among HIV Positive Pregnant and Lactating Mothers on Lifelong Antiretroviral Therapy for PMTCT in Rural Uganda

Matilda Kweyamba [ID],[1,2] Esther Buregyeya,[2] Joy Kusiima,[3] Vianney Kweyamba [ID],[4] and Aggrey David Mukose[2]

[1]*Cornerstone Surgery, Kampala, Uganda*
[2]*School of Public Health, Makerere University College of Health Sciences, Kampala, Uganda*
[3]*FETP Fellowship Program, Uganda Cancer Institute, Kampala, Uganda*
[4]*Department of Surgery, Naguru Regional Referral Hospital, Kampala, Uganda*

Correspondence should be addressed to Matilda Kweyamba; mkweyamba@yahoo.com

Academic Editor: Julio Diaz

Background. Mother-to-Child Transmission of HIV accounts for more than 90% of all pediatric HIV infections. However, Prevention of Mother-to-Child Transmission (PMTCT) of HIV through provision of lifelong ART to HIV positive mothers faces various challenges which affect its success. One of such challenges is the loss to follow-up (LTFU) of mothers. *Methodology.* We conducted a cross-sectional study utilizing both quantitative and qualitative data collection methods. We were able to trace 279 HIV positive, pregnant, and lactating mothers among mothers who were initiated on lifelong ART for PMTCT in public health facilities in Ntungamo district, Western Uganda. The proportion of those who were lost to follow-up was determined, and Log binomial regression with stepwise backward elimination method was employed to identify factors associated with LTFU. Focus group discussions (FDGs) of women on lifelong ART and key informant interviews (KIIs) of peer educators were also performed. *Results.* Out of the 279 mothers that were successfully traced and interviewed, 103 (37%) were identified as lost to follow-up. The prevalence of LTFU was higher among those whose transport costs were above **$2.75, adj (adjusted) PR (Prevalence Ratio) 1.6 (95% CI; 1.02-2.55)**; those who waited beyond one hour before being attended to, **adj PR 1.74 (95% CI; 1.02-2.96)**; and those who assumed that their infant was already infected, **adj PR 1.76 (95% CI; 1.15-2.70)**. On interviews, LTFU in these mothers was attributed to fear of swallowing antiretroviral drugs, HIV related stigma and discrimination, inadequate facilitation of the peer educators, long patient waiting time, and transportation to the health facilities. *Conclusion.* More than one-third of mothers initiated on lifelong ART for PMTCT in Ntungamo district were lost to follow-up over a period of 25 months. *Recommendations.* Provision of regular and adequate pre-ART and ART adherence counseling and provision of routine health education would reduce LTFU.

1. Background

Mother-to-Child Transmission (MTCT) of HIV accounts for more than 90% of all new pediatric HIV infections [1]. It may occur in utero, during labor, during delivery, and/or during breastfeeding [1]. Without any intervention, the MTCT rate of HIV transmission would range from 25% to 45% [1]. The use of combined antiretroviral therapy (ART) and elective caesarean section has reduced MTCT rates to less than 2% in non-breastfeeding populations. Among breastfeeding populations, studies have demonstrated that timely antiretroviral therapy (ART) can reduce MTCT of HIV to 5% or less [2–4]. In view of these studies and more in 2010, UNAIDS set a target for member states to have virtual elimination of MTCT, defined as reducing MTCT to less than 5% and 90% reduction of new HIV infections among young children by 2015 [5]. However, poor uptake of Prevention of Mother-to-Child Transmission (PMTCT) of HIV services, Loss to Follow-Up (LTFU), and poor adherence to drugs are still a major challenge to achieving virtual elimination of

MTCT of HIV especially in Sub-Saharan Africa [6]. Reducing LTFU among mothers initiated on lifelong ART for PMTCT is therefore a crucial step towards elimination of MTCT of HIV.

In a 2014 Malawian study, 23.5% of the mothers who were initiated on lifelong ART at the antenatal clinic were lost to follow-up after one year [7]. Lifelong ART for PMTCT entails the use of HAART for all HIV positive pregnant and lactating mothers for life. The guidance on PMTCT is provided to countries by World Health Organization (WHO) and Ministry of Health of Uganda adapted these guidelines to eliminate MTCT of HIV in the country [8].

In 2002, Uganda adopted and began implementing the first National PMTCT guidelines. This came as recommendations from findings of the PMTCT pilot program of 2000 which had over time expanded to cover 56 districts by the end of 2003 [9]. The main drug that was being used for HIV positive mothers during labor was Nevirapine single dose tablet (SdNvp). In 2006, WHO recommended use of zidovudine (AZT) during pregnancy combined with SdNvp at delivery to the mother at onset of labor and to the newborn, then followed by two weeks of zidovudine and lamivudine (AZT/3TC) to the mother to reduce the risk of emergency resistant virus. Uganda as a country adopted these PMTCT guidelines and this treatment option was called Option A.

In 2010, Uganda adopted a third set of World Health Organization (WHO) guidelines. The recommendations were either use of Option A (maternal AZT during pregnancy plus SdNvp at delivery to the mother and the newborn and two weeks of AZT/3TC to the mother) or the use of highly active antiretroviral therapy (HAART) also known as Option B regimen [8]. In 2012, Uganda transitioned to the new (4th) set of WHO PMTCT guidelines with the implementation of Option B+ (lifelong ART). By 2013-2014, the rapid roll-out had covered all districts in the country.

According to the Ministry of Health of Uganda, these new policy guidelines focus not only on eliminating HIV transmission via mother to child, but also on reducing mortality and morbidity among HIV positive women and their HIV exposed or infected infants [8].

In Ntungamo district, the program was launched in March 2013 with the support of Elizabeth Glaser Pediatric AIDs foundation (EGPAF). EGPAF is a non-governmental organization (NGO) running HIV and TB services in the southwestern part of Uganda. Health facilities in Ntungamo district that were implementing the 2nd PMTCT guidelines (Option A) slowly transitioned to lifelong ART (the 4th PMTCT guidelines). EGPAF built capacity for health workers to provide lifelong ART services in high patient volume sites (health centre (HC) IVs and hospitals) and later scaled up to lower volume sites (HCIIIs). This was followed up with mentorships and provision of necessary logistics to enable a smooth transition.

However, several challenges have been noted in the implementation of the lifelong ART program and such challenges include mothers initiated on HAART either during pregnancy, delivery, or breastfeeding getting lost along the way and not returning to the clinic for monitoring [8]. Monitoring adherence and retention for mothers on Option B+ are still a big challenge and yet information has already shown that there is substantial LTFU [8].

We aimed at determining the proportion of those on lifelong ART for PMTCT in Ntungamo district who were lost to follow-up and associated factors.

2. Methods

2.1. Study Design. This was a cross-sectional study which employed both qualitative and quantitative methods of data collection.

2.2. Study Setting. The study was carried out in Ntungamo district, located in south western Uganda. The district has 42 health facilities of which one hospital and 16 health centres offer PMTCT. However, eight of these health facilities had adopted and were offering lifelong ART for PMTCT in the district, between September 1st, 2013, and September 30th, 2015. The study involved mothers who were attended to at these health facilities during this period. It also included peer mothers that were once enrolled on lifelong ART and were involved in the follow-up of mothers on PMTCT within the district.

2.3. Selection Criteria

Inclusion Criteria. All mothers who were identified as having been enrolled on lifelong ART for PMTCT from 1st September 2013 to 30th September 2015, as documented in the PMTCT and ART registers, were included.

Exclusion Criteria

(i) Mothers who had no telephone contact and/or no clear physical address.

(ii) Mothers who could not be traced to their physical address. That is, those who had either changed physical address or changed the telephone contact.

2.4. Sample Size Determination

Quantitative Component. All mothers that had a telephone contact or clear physical address were traced. Those successfully traced were included in the study.

Qualitative Study. Two focus group discussions (FGDs) with mothers initiated on lifelong ART and attending family support groups (FSGs) and fifteen key informant interviews (KIIs) with peer educators were conducted.

2.5. Sampling Procedure

Sampling for Quantitative Study. Names and contacts of mothers that were initiated on lifelong ART for PMTCT between 1st September 2013 and 30th September 2015 (period of study) were obtained from the ANC/PMTCT and ART clinic registers of the 8 health facilities that were offering lifelong ART for PMTCT at that time. These formed the sampling frame for the study. All mothers that had been enrolled on lifelong ART for PMTCT from 1st September 2013 to 30th September 2015 were considered. However, mothers that either did not have a clear contact address or had no telephone contact recorded in the individual ART card were disregarded. The selected respondents were physically identified using their telephone contacts and physical address as recorded in their individual ART cards and ANC/PMTCT/ART clinic registers, with the help of peer educators and or village health teams (VHTs), a method that has also been suggested by Gwadz [10].

Sample Selection for Qualitative Study. The respondents for qualitative data included peer educators and HIV positive pregnant and lactating mothers under care on lifelong ART. This was carried out in the five peer supported health facilities. These are facilities that have high volume with many HIV patients attending the HIV clinic. In each of the five facilities, 3 KIIs with peer educators were conducted.

Two focus group discussions were conducted at two facilities that had the highest patient volumes in the district. The FDGs were conducted among pregnant and lactating mothers on lifelong ART for PMTCT during clinic days.

2.6. Data Collection

Quantitative Data Collection. Records of mothers in the eight health facilities were extracted from the PMTCT and ART registers using abstraction forms that were developed to capture the names, telephone contacts, next of kin, and physical address. Information relating to the mothers' physical address and telephone contact was extracted from the ART card. Information on sociodemographic characteristics of the mothers was collected through a structured questionnaire that was administered to the mothers. Additional information collected through the structured questionnaire included information on individual and interpersonal factors, peer and family support, health provider attitudes, date of last clinic visit, transportation to health facility, stigma and discrimination, patient waiting time, and health beliefs.

Qualitative Data Collection. Qualitative data was collected through FGDs with mothers and KIIs with peer educators. These were conducted with the help of a focus group and key informant interview guides. The FGDs, consisting of 25–30 members each, explored perception towards PMTCT program, challenges in accessibility of PMTCT services, challenges faced because of being HIV positive, support of family members, reasons why mothers get LTFU, and proposed interventions to reduce LTFU of mothers.

Fifteen KIIs were held with peer educators who work with health workers and are assigned the duty of follow-up of mothers once enrolled into PMTCT care. During the FGDs, two research assistants were present: one is to facilitate the discussion while the other was taking notes. Audio recordings for both FGDs and KIIs were also taken by the PI during the interactions, with permission from the respondents.

2.7. Statistical Analysis. We analyzed data using STATA version 12. Percentages were used to determine the proportion

of HIV positive pregnant and lactating mothers enrolled on lifelong ART for PMTCT, who were lost to follow-up defined as HIV positive pregnant and lactating mothers initiated on lifelong antiretroviral therapy (ART) for PMTCT that had not returned to the clinic in > 90 days from their last scheduled appointment.

Log binomial regression was used to determine factors associated with LTFU among pregnant and lactating mothers initiated on lifelong ART. Prevalence ratios were used as the measure of association since the outcome (LTFU) was >10% (37%).

Following bivariable analysis, we selected variables with a significance level of 10% (P<0.1) for inclusion in the multivariable analysis. Multivariable analysis was done using the stepwise approach-backward elimination method. Statistical significance of variables for inclusion in the final model was set at a p value <0.05.

2.8. Ethics Considerations. This study was approved by Makerere University School of Public Health Higher Degrees Research and Ethics Committee and permission was obtained from the District Health Officer in Ntungamo. All respondents eligible for the study provided written consent. To ensure confidentiality, all interviews were conducted in privacy and respondent questionnaires were identified using unique identifiers.

3. Results

Overall 480 mothers were identified as having been initiated on lifelong ART for PMTCT between September 1st, 2013, and September 30th, 2015; of these 302 mothers met the inclusion criteria (had a clear physical address or a telephone contact). However, 279 mothers were successfully traced and these were included in the study. Out of these 279 mothers, 103 (37%) were identified as lost to follow-up.

3.1. Quantitative Findings

3.1.1. Demographics Characteristics of the Mothers and Their Individual Perceptions. The mean age (SD) was 28.2 (4.6) years and the median age (IQR) was 28 (25-30 years) and 106 (38%) of the mothers were in the age range of 24 to 28 years. 74% were married and 56% were subsistence farmers. Over 99% knew that the drug was safe for them and the baby and that the administered drug works. Majority of the mothers had positive perceptions towards the medication they were receiving; however, approximately one-third (29.3%) feared taking their medication, and a quarter reported having experienced side effects (25.9%) (Table 1).

3.1.2. Proportion of Mothers LTFU. We successfully traced and interviewed 279 HIV positive pregnant and lactating mothers. Of the 279 mothers interviewed, 103 (37%) were lost to follow-up (Figure 1)

3.1.3. Factors Associated with LTFU. From the bivariate analysis, variables that had a p value of < 0.1, such as fear of

TABLE 1: Social demographic characteristics of the mothers (N=279) and individual perceptions of HIV positive women towards highly active antiretroviral therapy (HAART).

Demographic characteristics	Frequency (n)	Percent (%)
Age		
Mean (sd)	28.2 (4.6)	
Median (IQR)	28 (25-30)	
Age_resp		
19-23	46	16.5
24-28 yrs	106	38
29-33 yrs	92	33
34-38 yrs	30	11
>38 yrs	5	1.8
Religion		
Catholic	79	27.9
Muslim	22	7.9
Evangelical	34	12.2
Anglican/Presbyterian	144	51.6
Tribe		
Acholi	3	1.1
Muganda	15	5.4
Mukiga	40	14.4
Munyankole	202	72.7
Munyarwanda	15	5.4
Other	4	1
Marital status		
Divorced	36	12.9
Married	207	74.2
single	18	6.5
Widowed	18	6.5
Occupation		
Subsistence farmer	156	56.5
House wife	43	15.6
Causal laborer	24	8.7
Professional	28	10.1
Business woman	25	9.1
Individual perceptions		
Perceive administered drug is safe for me and baby		
No	3	1.1
Yes	276	98.9
Perceive that administered drug works		
No	6	2.2
Yes	272	97.8
Fear swallowing ARVs		
No	198	71
Yes	81	29
Ever experienced side effects when swallowing ARVs		
No	206	74.1
Yes	72	25.9
Perceived ease of receiving ARVs		
No	5	1.8
Yes	274	98.2

Are ARVs offered free		
No	3	1.1
Yes	276	98.9
Do you think you can infect your child with HIV		
No	117	42.6
Yes	158	57.5
Do you think you need ARVS		
No	5	1.8
Yes	274	98.2

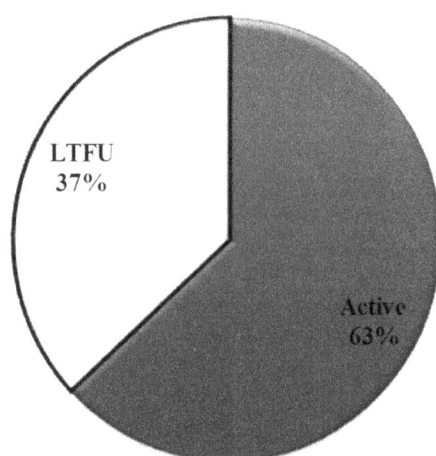

FIGURE 1: Proportion of mothers on lifelong ART for PMTCT who were lost to follow-up between Sept 2013 and Sept 2015, n= 279.

swallowing ARV drugs, perception that the mother can infect the child, disclosure to other relatives other than the spouse, and transport costs, were analyzed further in multivariable analysis.

At multivariable analysis, transport costs above $2.75 (**adj PR 1.6, CI: 1.02-2.55**), waiting time greater than 1 hour (**adj PR 1.74, CI: 1.02-2.96**), and perception that the child is already infected (**adj PR 1.76, CI: 1.15-2.70**) were the factors significantly associated with loss to follow-up, p value < 0.05. However, the mother knowing that ARV drugs work (**adj PR 0.35, CI: 0.23-0.56**) was protective (Table 2).

3.2. Qualitative Findings. Qualitative evaluation was done to explore further mothers views as to why women on lifelong ART get lost to follow-up. A total of two focus group discussions (FGDs) with mothers and 15 key informant interviews (KIIs) with peer mothers were conducted. The factors that were repeatedly common throughout these interviews were fear of swallowing ARV drugs, domestic violence following disclosure, HIV related stigma and discrimination, inadequate facilitation of peer educators and mothers, long patient waiting time, and cost of transportation to the health facilities.

4. Discussion

This study found that the proportion of mothers who get lost to follow-up from the PMTCT program was 37%. A study done in Malawi revealed the LTFU as 30% after 3 years of initiation on lifelong ART [11]. This is an indication that there is significant LTFU of mothers initiated on lifelong ART for PMTCT. Therefore, addressing the associated factors will go a long way to reduce this loss, hence leading to the sustainable achievement of elimination of MTCT.

Mothers who had to incur transport costs above $2.75 (adj PR 1.6, CI: 1.02-2.55) were more likely to be lost to follow-up. In a rural setting transport is costly because most mothers are subsistence farmers with a poor socioeconomic status. This forces mothers to resort to walking long distances. This finding is in agreement with other studies, where distance to the clinic and transport cost were found to be major barriers to retention in care in a wide variety of settings in Africa including Uganda [12].

Waiting at the health facility for more than an hour before being attended to by a health worker was a predictor of LTFU (adj PR 1.74, CI: 1.02-2.96). This may be a result of low staffing levels compared to the large volumes of patients, hence leading to the long waiting time. A study done in Northern Uganda also noted that high patient loads at the facilities caused long patient waiting times [13]. Preventing batching up, that is, having all patients flooding the clinic at the same time very early in the morning, synchronizing staff shifts so as to have more staff on duty during clinic days, triaging of the mothers in order to separate critically ill from those walking or for refill, and provision of health education may go far in reducing the waiting times or make them endurable [14].

Knowing that the mother could infect their baby was a predictor for LTFU (adj PR 1.76, CI: 1.15-2.70). This indicates that mothers are knowledgeable about the transmission of HIV to their babies. But, upon defaulting from the PMTCT, they perceive that their breastfed child is HIV positive and hence fear returning to the clinic to avoid being blamed by the health workers if the child turns out to be HIV positive on testing. Improving health provider attitudes and providing customer care training to health providers could help change the way patients perceive care and their choice on whether to continue receiving care or not.

Interviews from the qualitative evaluation also noted high transport costs and long patient waiting time as some of the predictors of loss to follow-up. Other factors that were

TABLE 2: Factors associated with LTFU among HIV positive pregnant and lactating mothers on lifelong ART for PMTCT.

	Proportion lost to follow-up	Crude PR (95% CI)	Adjusted PR (95% CI)	P value
Age (years)				
19-23	16/46	Ref		
24-28 yrs	39/106	1.05(0.66-1.7)		
29-33 yrs	31/92	0.96(0.59-1.58)		
34-38 yrs	16/30	1.53(0.91-2.57)		
>39 yrs	1/5	0.46(0.48-4.55)		
Religion				
Catholic	32/79	Ref		
Muslim	7/22	1.4(0.92-2.06)		
Evangelical	19/34	0.78(0.4-1.53)		
Anglican/Presbyterian	45/144	0.77(0.53-1.1)		
Marital status				
single	8/18	Ref		
Married	76/207	0.83(0.47-1.43)		
Divorced	15/36	0.94(0.49-1.79)		
Widowed	4/18	0.5(0.08-1.52)		
Occupation				
Subsistence farmer	62/156	Ref		
Home maker	17/43	0.99(0.65-1.5)		
Causal laborer	9/24	0.94(0.54-1.6)		
Professional	7/28	0.63(0.32-1.23)		
Self employed	6/25	0.6(0.29-1.24)		
Tribe				
Muganda	7/15	Ref		
Munyankole	75/202	0.79(0.45-1.41)		
Mukiga	16/40	0.86(0.44-1.66)		
Acholi	0/3	Omitted		
Munyarwanda	3/15	0.43(0.14-1.35)		
Other	1/3	0.7(0.31-3.8)		
Perceptions towards HAART				
Perceive admin drug is safe for me and baby				
No	1/3	Ref		
Yes	102/276	1.17(0.2-5.5)		
Perception that administered drug works				
No	**6/6**	**Ref**		
Yes	**97/272**	**0.35(0.30-0.42)**	**0.35(0.23-0.56)**	**0.00**
Fear to swallow ARVs				
No	62/198	Ref		
Yes	41/81	**1.62(1.19-2.18)**	**0.77(0.51-1.2)**	0.23
Ever experienced side effects after swallowing ARVs				
No	76/206	Ref		
Yes	27/72	1.02(0.72-1.44)	**0.84(0.45-1.57)**	0.59
Perceived ease of receiving ARVs				
No	3/5	Ref		
Yes	100/274	0.6(0.29-1.26)		

TABLE 2: Continued.

	Proportion lost to follow-up	Crude PR (95% CI)	Adjusted PR (95% CI)	P value
Is the drug easy to swallow				
No	7/18	Ref		
Yes	96/261	0.91(0.34-2.43)		
Are ARVs offered free				
No	1/3	Ref		
Yes	102/276	1.1(0.2-5.5)		
*Do you think you can infect your child with HIV****				
No	33/117	Ref		
Yes	66/158	**1.5(1.05-2.1)**	**1.72(1.13-0.62)**	**0.01**
Do you think you need ARVS				
No	2/5	Ref		
Yes	101/274	0.92(0.31-2.7)		
Mode of transport to facility				
Walking	29/71(40.8)	Ref		
Taxi	40/99(40.4)	0.98(0.68-1.43)		
Boda boda (motor cycle)	72/106(32.0)	0.78(0.53-1.16		
*Total Transport Cost****				
<5000 shs	30/99(30.3%)	Ref		
5001-10000 shs	25/73(34.2%)	1.13(0.7-1.74)	1.09(0.70-1.7)	0.7
>10001	18/34(52.1%)	**1.75(1.12-2.74)****	**1.57(1.002-2.4)**	**0.049**
Waiting time between arriving and receiving service				
<30 min	19/67(28.3%)	Ref		
30 min-1 hr	28/79(35.4%)	1.2(0.77-2.03)	1.5(0.83-2.7)	0.2
>1 hr	56/133(42.1%)	1.5(0.96-2.28)	**1.74(1.02-2.96)**	**0.04**
STIGMA				
Disclosed to spouse				
No	19/69	Ref		
Yes	81/199	1.48(0.97-2.28)		
*Does he support you?****				
No	32/68	Ref		
Yes	50/135	0.79(0.56-1.10)		
Disclosed to relatives other than spouse				
No	153	Ref		
Yes	126	**1.5(1.10-2.04)**	1.38(0.86-1.7)	0.4
Any one refused to offer any service to you because of your HIV status				
No	82/243	Ref		
Yes	20/35	**1.69(1.21-2.38)**	1.3(0.84-2.1)	0.2

PR: prevalence ratio.

mentioned as predictors of LTFU included fear of swallowing ARV drugs, domestic violence following disclosure of HIV status, stigma and discrimination, and inadequate facilitation of the peer educators.

Fear of swallowing ARVs as a reason for getting lost to follow-up needs to be recognized. The size and smell of the tablets, taking the medication without an assurance of a meal, and the anticipated side effects are some of the reasons mothers stopped taking the ARVs, hence self-censoring themselves from coming to the clinic. Studies have also shown that poor adherence to drugs is attributed to the feared side effects [15] and food insecurity [16, 17]. Health Education coupled with initial and ongoing HIV and adherence counseling especially with the help of peers will help dispel the myths that are associated with the taking of medication.

Mothers interviewed in this study expressed the fear of stigma and discrimination from the community and family members. This was attributed to the fear of domestic violence after disclosing their status to their spouses. Some quantitative studies have shown this to be true [18].

4.1. Limitation of the Study. The strength of this study is that women were traced to their physical addresses and therefore, we were able to know if a mother was lost to follow-up or active in care. However, this study had some important limitations that should be considered when interpreting the results. First the cross-sectional nature of the study design does not confirm definitive cause and effect relationship between dependent and independent variables. In addition, the study did not account for the mothers that could not be traced and hence could lead to underestimation of the LTFU. In order to get more insight of the study's third objective, we should have conducted in-depth interviews with mothers that we had found to be lost to follow-up as this would give a clear view of why mothers get lost to follow-up. The use of the definition of LTFU in this study as patients who were started on lifelong ART and not seen for more than 90 days after their scheduled appointment has a weakness as some mothers were found to have transferred to other facilities than the original facility where they were initiated on treatment. However, since mothers were being interviewed and had to recall some instances which were used to ascertain LTFU, this could have some recall bias.

4.2. Conclusions. There was substantial LTFU of mothers initiated on lifelong ART for PMTCT in Ntungamo district. Personal fears, wrong perceptions among patients, stigma, discrimination in the community, high transport costs, long patient waiting time, and inadequate facilitation of peer educators are some of the bottlenecks to achieving success desired from the provision of lifelong ART for PMTCT.

4.3. Recommendations. Focus should be directed to provision of regular quality pre-ART and ART adherence counseling, provision of routine health education, strengthening HIV awareness campaigns through local village authorities, increasing HIV outreach services, community engagement, and building community networks through peer support. Large scale research to look at the rates of LTFU at the different points of PMTCT cascade would inform targeted PMTCT interventions.

Abbreviations and Operation Definitions

Lifelong ART: This is an approach recommended by World Health Organization to prevent mother-to-child HIV transmission with which all HIV positive pregnant and lactating women are initiated on antiretroviral therapy (ART) for life regardless of CD4 count or WHO staging

Loss to follow-up: Patients who were started on lifelong ART and not seen within 90 days of their scheduled appointment

Peer educator: HIV positive patients who are trained to provide peer support and counseling to their fellow HIV positive patients and also follow up mothers by virtue of their good adherence and to some extent their level of education

ANC: Antenatal care

EGPAF: Elizabeth Glaser Pediatric AIDs Foundation

e-MTCT: Virtual Elimination of Mother-to-Child Transmission

HAART: Highly active antiretroviral therapy

HC: Health centre

HIV: Human immunodeficiency virus

LTFU: Loss to follow-up

MCH: Maternal and child health

MOH: Ministry of Health

PMTCT: Prevention of Mother-to-Child Transmission

UNAIDS: United Nations Joint Program on AIDS

VCT: Voluntary Counseling and Testing

WHO: World Health Organization.

Disclosure

The corresponding author had full access to all the data in the study and had final responsibility for the decision to prepare the manuscript and submit for publication.

Authors' Contributions

Matilda Kweyamba was responsible for the manuscript from its conception, analysis, and interpretation of data; she drafted the manuscript. **Joy Kusiima** participated in data analysis and review of the manuscript. **Esther Buregyeya** participated in the interpretation and review of the manuscript. **Aggrey Mukose** participated in the interpretation and review of the manuscript. **Vianney Kweyamba** participated in the drafting, interpretation, and review of the manuscript. All authors approved the final manuscript.

Acknowledgments

The authors would like to thank the study subjects for their willingness to participate in the study. They would also like to thank the district authorities and the various health workers working in the health facilities. Last but not least, heartfelt thanks are due to the research assistants.

References

[1] "M M. WHO updates HIV treatment guidance for pregnant women and preventing HIV infection in babies: Science Speaks: Global ID News," 2012, http://sciencespeaksblog.org/2012/04/09/who-updates-hiv-treatment-guidance-for-pregnant-women-and-preventing-hiv-infection-in-babies/.

[2] C. S. Chasela, M. G. Hudgens, D. J. Jamieson et al., "Maternal or infant antiretroviral drugs to reduce HIV-1 transmission," *The New England Journal of Medicine*, vol. 362, no. 24, pp. 2271–2281, 2010.

[3] Z. Namukwaya, P. Mudiope, A. Kekitiinwa et al., "The impact of maternal highly active antiretroviral therapy and short-course combination antiretrovirals for prevention of mother-to-child transmission on early infant infection rates at the mulago national referral hospital in Kampala, Uganda, january 2007 to may 2009," *Journal of Acquired Immune Deficiency Syndromes*, vol. 56, no. 1, pp. 69–75, 2011.

[4] R. L. Shapiro, M. D. Hughes, A. Ogwu et al., "Antiretroviral regimens in pregnancy and breast-feeding in Botswana," *The New England Journal of Medicine*, vol. 362, no. 24, pp. 2282–2294, 2010.

[5] Goals MD, Session UNGAS, and Organization WH, *PMTCT Strategic Vision 2010-2015: Preventing Mother-to-child Transmission of HIV to Reach the UNGASS and Millennium Development Goals: Moving Towards the Elimination of Paediatric HIV*, World health organization (WHO), 2010.

[6] M. Sidibé, Global Report: UNAIDS Report on the Global AIDS Epidemic: 2010, UN Joint Programme on HIV/AIDS (UNAIDS), 2010.

[7] H. Tweya, S. Gugsa, M. Hosseinipour et al., "Understanding factors, outcomes and reasons for loss to follow-up among women in Option B+ PMTCT programme in Lilongwe, Malawi," *Tropical Medicine & International Health*, vol. 19, no. 11, pp. 1360–1366, 2014.

[8] "G E. The New National Guidelines (2010) for PMTCT and Infant Feeding in the Context of HIV Kampala: MOH Uganda," 2010, http://library.health.go.ug/publications/service-delivery-diseases-control-prevention-communicable-diseases/hivaids/new-national.

[9] C. A. S. Karamagi, J. K. Tumwine, T. Tylleskar, and K. Heggenhougen, "Antenatal HIV testing in rural eastern Uganda in 2003: Incomplete rollout of the prevention of mother-to-child transmission of HIV programme?" *BMC International Health and Human Rights*, vol. 6, 2006.

[10] M. Gwadz, C. M. Cleland, H. Hagan et al., "Strategies to uncover undiagnosed HIV infection among heterosexuals at high risk and link them to HIV care with high retention: A "seek, test, treat, and retain" study," *BMC Public Health*, vol. 15, no. 1, article no. 481, 2015.

[11] A. D. Haas, L. Tenthani, M. T. Msukwa et al., "Retention in care during the first 3 years of antiretroviral therapy for women in Malawi's option B+ programme: an observational cohort study," *The Lancet HIV*, vol. 3, no. 4, pp. e175–e182, 2016.

[12] E. H. Geng, D. R. Bangsberg, N. Musinguzi et al., "Understanding reasons for and outcomes of patients lost to follow-up in antiretroviral therapy programs in Africa through a sampling-based approach," *Journal of Acquired Immune Deficiency Syndromes*, vol. 53, no. 3, pp. 405–411, 2010.

[13] Mugisha A. O. K., S. Edward, L. Ciccio, R. Muwanika, and O. James, "Retention of HIV Positive Persons in Antiretroviral Therapy Programs in Post-Conflict Northern Uganda-Baseline Survey of 17 Health Units," 2009.

[14] M. B. Mavuso, "Patient waiting time at a HIV Clinic in a Regional Hospital in Swaziland," 2008.

[15] M. Ngarina, R. Popenoe, C. Kilewo, G. Biberfeld, and A. M. Ekstrom, "Reasons for poor adherence to antiretroviral therapy postnatally in HIV-1 infected women treated for their own health: experiences from the Mitra Plus study in Tanzania," *BMC Public Health*, vol. 13, no. 1, article 450, 2013.

[16] W. M. Bezabhe, L. Chalmers, L. R. Bereznicki, and G. M. Peterson, "Adherence to antiretroviral therapy and virologic failure: a meta-analysis," *Medicine*, vol. 95, no. 15, 2016.

[17] S. D. Weiser, D. M. Tuller, E. A. Frongillo, J. Senkungu, N. Mukiibi, and D. R. Bangsberg, "Food insecurity as a barrier to sustained antiretroviral therapy adherence in Uganda," *PLoS ONE*, vol. 5, no. 4, Article ID e10340, 2010.

[18] F. W. Kalembo and M. Zgambo, "Loss to Followup: A Major Challenge to Successful Implementation of Prevention of Mother-to-Child Transmission of HIV-1 Programs in Sub-Saharan Africa," *ISRN AIDS*, vol. 2012, Article ID 589817, 10 pages, 2012.

10

Complementary Feeding Practice and Associated Factors among Mothers Having Children 6–23 Months of Age, Lasta District, Amhara Region, Northeast Ethiopia

Menberu Molla,[1] Tadese Ejigu,[2] and Girma Nega[3]

[1]Save the Children International, West Amhara, P.O. Box 993, Bahir Dar, Ethiopia
[2]School of Public Health (SPH), College of Medicine and Health Sciences, Bahir Dar University, P.O. Box 79, Bahir Dar, Ethiopia
[3]School of Food and Chemical Engineering, Department of Applied Nutrition, Bahir Dar University, P.O. Box 26, Bahir Dar, Ethiopia

Correspondence should be addressed to Tadese Ejigu; tade_et@yahoo.com

Academic Editor: Ronald J. Prineas

Introduction. The first two years of life are a critical window of opportunity for ensuring optimal child growth and development. Nutritional deficiencies during this period can lead to impaired cognitive development, compromised educational achievement, and low economic productivity. Improving infant and young child feeding (IYCF) practices in children aged 0–23 months is therefore critical to improved nutrition, health, and development. *Objective.* The aim of the study is to assess the prevalence of complementary feeding practice and its associated factors among mothers with children aged 6–23 months in Lasta District, Northeast Ethiopia, 2015. *Methods.* A community based cross-sectional study design was conducted among 476 mothers who had children aged 6–23 months in the study area. Simple random sampling technique was used to select the required sample. A face-to-face interview was done to collect data using structured questionnaire. Data were entered with EPI info version 3.5.1 and cleaning and analysis were done using SPSS version 16. Frequencies distribution and binary and multiple logistic regressions were done. *Results.* In this study only 56.5% of children aged 6–23 months received appropriate complementary feeding, considering timely introduction, minimum dietary diversity, and meal frequency. Exposure to public media [AOR = 2.50; 95% CI: 1.44, 4.35], occupation of mother [AOR = 9.50; 95% CI: 1.02, 14.25], mothers decision making role on how to use family income [AOR = 5.54; 95% CI: 1.19, 11.74], and use of postnatal care service [AOR = 5.98; 95% CI: 1.49, 13.96] were found to be independent predictors of complementary feeding practice. *Conclusion and Recommendation.* About 43.5% of mothers were not feeding their children complementary food appropriately, which would have negative implication on the health of infants and young children. There was a statistically significant association of inappropriate complementary feeding practices with mothers' occupation, postnatal care service, media exposure, and mothers' decision making role on how the money is used. Health professionals should focus on advising and counseling mothers on appropriate complementary feeding during prenatal, delivery, postnatal, and immunization services.

1. Introduction

An appropriate diet is a critical component for proper growth and development of children. The first two years of life are a critical window for ensuring optimal child growth and development [1, 2]. Nutritional deficiencies during this period can lead to impaired cognitive development, compromised educational achievement, and low economic productivity which become difficult to reverse later in life. Improving infant and young child feeding (IYCF) practices in children aged 0–23 months is therefore critical to improved nutrition, health, and development [3–5].

Scientific evidence indicates that various inappropriate complementary feeding practices such as untimely introduction of complementary food, improper feeding frequency, and low dietary diversity of complementary food have been shown to have numerous negative effects on children's health [6]. Appropriate complementary feeding entails introduction of complementary foods at 6 months with continued breastfeeding up to at least 2 years and beyond, feeding frequency for age, and consumption of a diverse diet [2, 5, 6]. For this study the following definitions were considered: introduction of solid, semisolid, or soft foods and proportion of infants aged six months who receive solid, semisolid, or soft foods during the previous day. Minimum dietary diversity was assessed by proportion of children of 6–23 months who receive four or more food groups during the previous day. Food groups used for tabulation of this indicator were cereals, legumes, dairy products (milk, yoghurt, and cheese), flesh foods (meat, fish, poultry, and liver/organ meats), eggs, vitamin A-rich fruits and vegetables, butter/oil, and sugar/honey. Minimum meal frequency was assessed by proportion of children aged 6–23 months who receive solid, semisolid, or soft food three times or more in the previous day. Complementary feeding practice was considered appropriate if the mother practices all the above three indicators, as recommended and inappropriate complementary feeding practice if at least one indicator was not fulfilled.

2. Methods

2.1. Study Area. Community based cross-sectional study design was used to determine complementary feeding practices of children aged 6–23 months in Lasta District, Amhara Region, Ethiopia. Lasta District is found in North Wollo zone 300 km away from Bahir Dar town which is the capital city of the region and the district has a total population size of 115,880 people of which 56,781 females (49%), 15,690 children of 0–59 months (13%), 5,852 <2 years (5%), 4165 6–23 months (district health office report 2015). The district has 24 health posts and 6 HCs. It is the fourth largest district in North Wollo zone and ranked among the most food insecure districts in the region (Lasta Woreda Health Office Data 2015). And the woreda has exposed for drought and degraded land. The main economic activities are small scale trading and farming (CSA, 2013). The area was chosen because most of the children were likely to be predisposed to suboptimal complementary feeding practices due to unknown factors that cause improper complementary feeding practices.

The district has 23 rural kebeles and of these 5 such as Yemrehanna-kristos, Bilballa, Geter Meda, Tilasefere, and Shimsha kebeles (21%) were selected randomly based on the rule of thumb for community based research. The lists of all study participants (mothers) were obtained from beneficiary folder of Food for Hungry Ethiopia (FHE) that provides food support for the area. Sample size was computed based on single population proportion formula assuming the prevalence (p) 0.10 which was taken from a previous community based study at Abyi Adi town, Tigray, Ethiopia [7]. A z-value of 1.96 was used at 95% confidence level and margin of error of 4% with 10% nonresponse rate and design effect of 2. Thus the total sample size was 476. Then the study participants from selected five kebeles were taken by considering proportional to size.

Seven diploma nurses and one BSC nurse were recruited in data collection and supervision, respectively. A structured and pretested questionnaire was used to collect the data. The questioner was prepared in English and translated to local language "Amharic" and back to English by two language

experts to check consistency. Pretest of the questionnaire was made on (5%) of the sample size in kebeles out of the main study area, two days' training for data collectors and the supervisor on how to approach the respondents and how to conduct interview based on the objective of the study. In addition the filled questionnaires were also checked daily by the supervisor for completeness and missing data to maintain the data quality. The collected data were coded and entered into Epi info version 3.5.1 and analyzed using SPSS version 16. Descriptive statics (frequency, mean, median, standard deviation, range, and percentage) was used for sociodemography and economic characteristics, maternal health care services of the population, knowledge, and complementary feeding practices. Bivariate and multivariable logistic regression was used in order to identify predictive variables and odds ratio (OR) with 95% confidence interval and p value was used as measure of the strength of association. Finally the variables which have significant association were identified on the basis of OR, 95% CI, and p value < 0.2 to identify eligible variables to fit into the final regression model and p value < 0.05 was used to identify predictor variables.

3. Results

3.1. Sociodemographic Characteristics of Study Participants. Among 476 sampled mothers, 470 participated in the study, making the response rate (98.7%). Biological mothers accounted for 471 (99%) whereas the remaining 5 (1%) were caregivers such as grandmothers and sisters. The median age of mothers/caregivers was 29 ± 6.7 years with age range between 15 and 70. Four hundred seventy two (99%) were Orthodox and four (1%) were Muslim by religion and four hundred sixty six (98%) belong to Amhara ethnic group and ten (2%) were Tigre. Concerning the educational status of the mothers, 126 (26%) had attended formal school. The majority of the mothers, 418 (88%), were married and 310 (65.1%) of mothers were farmers by occupation. More than three-fourths, 435 (91.4%), of mothers earned an average monthly income of less than or equal to 999 Ethiopian Birr (<47 USD). Husbands of 153 (32%) mothers had attended formal education. The median age of children was 16 months ± 5.7 with age range between 6 and 23 (Table 1).

3.2. Obstetrics and Health Service Related Variables. Almost all, 463 (97%), mothers had history of antenatal care follow-up at least once during their last pregnancy. About, 51% of mothers gave birth to their youngest child at health institution. Majority of the mothers (95%) had received postnatal care (PNC) at least once.

3.3. Complementary Feeding Knowledge and Practices. Approximately, 97% (462/476) of mothers had satisfactory knowledge and the remaining 1.6% (8/476) had poor knowledge about complementary feeding. However 56.5% of mothers had appropriate complementary feeding practice. Three hundred forty two (71.8%) mothers were inaccessible for complementary foods. Cereals (96.6%), legumes (93.3%), oil/butter (87.7%), and honey/sugar (79.6%) were the most commonly taken food item by the children in 24 hours

TABLE 1: Sociodemocratic, obstetric, and health related variables of mothers who had children aged 6–23 months ($n = 476$) in Lasta Woreda, Amhara, Northeast Ethiopia, April 2015 to October 2015.

Variable	Categories	Frequency	Percentage
Mothers' age	<20	46	9.7
	20–24	64	13.4
	25–29	125	26.3
	30–34	113	23.7
	≥35	128	26.9
Marital status	Married	419	88.0
	Single	16	3.4
	Divorced	35	7.4
	Widowed	6	1.3
Religion	Orthodox	472	99
	Muslim	4	1
Mothers' educational status	Illiterate	307	64.5
	Read and write	43	9.0
	1–4	29	6.1
	5–8	51	10.7
	9–12	43	9.0
	College/university	3	.6
Mothers' occupation	Government employed	9	1.9
	Private employed	4	.8
	Merchant	26	5.5
	Housewife	105	22.1
	Farmer	310	65.1
	Daily laborer	6	1.3
	Student	2	.4
	Housemaid	14	2.9
Monthly income (ETB)	≤999	435	91.4
	1000–2999	35	7.4
	3000–3999	4	.8
	≥4000	2	.4
Child's age in months	6–11	98	20.6
	12–17	129	27.1
	18–23	249	52.3
Number of children	1–3	473	99.4
	4–9	3	.6
ANC follow-up	Yes	456	95.5
	No	20	4.2
Place of delivery	Home	232	48.7
	Health institution	244	51.2
Postnatal care	Yes	454	95.4
	No	22	4.6

preceding the survey. However, the consumption of different food types in 24 hours preceding the survey was uniformly lower in 18–23 months age group, with the lowest rates reported for flesh foods (2.1%) (Table 2). In addition about 57.7% of mothers had introduced complementary feeding at the age of six months as per the recommended (Figure 1). And 60.7 mothers offered four or more food groups (the minimum recommended diversity) to their child and only

50.4 mothers fed their children ≥ three times a day (the recommended frequency) (Figure 2). The overall prevalence of appropriate complementary feeding practice combining the three mentioned indicators was 56.5%.

3.4. Factors Associated with Complementary Feeding. This section includes the results of multivariable analysis done between the independent variables (sociodemographic and

TABLE 2: Types of food given to children aged 6–23 months in the past 24 hours by age groups ($n = 476$) Lasta Woreda, Amhara, Northeast Ethiopia, April 2015 to October 2015.

| Food groups | Age of the child in months | | | | | |
| | 6–11 | | 12–17 | | 18–23 | |
	Yes (%)	No (%)	Yes (%)	No (%)	Yes (%)	No (%)
Cereals	94.9	5.1	96.9	3.1	97.2	2.8
Legumes	93.9	6.1	93.8	6.2	93.2	6.8
Milk/milk product	13.3	86.7	10.1	89.9	9.6	90.4
Meat/fish/chicken	5.1	94.9	3.9	96.1	2.1	98.0
Egg	52.0	48.0	41.1	58.9	34.9	65.1
Other fruits and vegetable	43.9	56.1	49.6	50.4	35.7	64.3
Honey/sugar	87.8	12.2	77.5	22.5	77.5	22.5
Butter/oil	89.8	10.2	91.5	8.5	84.7	15.3

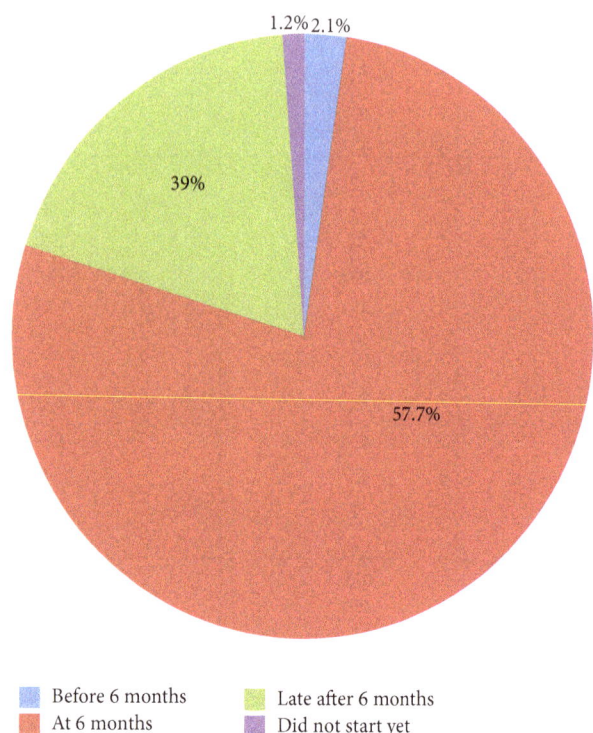

FIGURE 1: Time of starting complementary feeding for their children by study participants, Lasta District, Amhara region, Ethiopia, 2015.

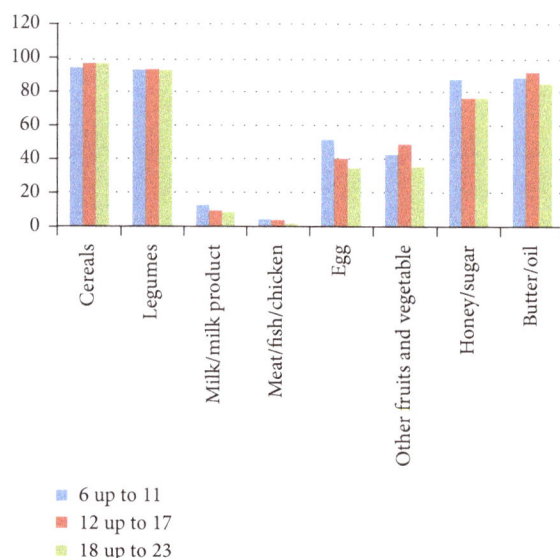

FIGURE 2: Varieties of foods used for complementary feeding by age groups, Lasta District, Amhara region, Ethiopia, 2015.

other variables) and the outcome variables of interest (complementary feeding practice). p value of <0.05 at 95% confidence level was taken as significant.

4. Discussion

The result of the study revealed that the prevalence of appropriate complementary feeding was 56.5% which is higher than research finding at Abyi Adi town, Tigray, Northern Ethiopia (10.75%) [7], Ethiopian National prevalence (4%) [5], Enemay district, Northwest Ethiopia (40.5%) [8], and India (17.5%) [2] and smaller than a study in Mekele (62.8%) [9], but it is consistent with a study done in Harar (54.4%) [10]. This relatively higher prevalence might be due to practices change with time, the presence of nutrition intervention program by nongovernmental organization in the study area, and the efforts of health extension workers, health professionals, and nutrition animators in the study area.

Findings of this study also showed that postnatal follow-up, occupation of mothers, exposure to public media (like radio, television), and mothers' decision making role on family income were predictors of complementary feeding practice. In this study mothers who had postnatal care follow-up were 5.9 times more likely to practice appropriate complementary feeding than those who did not follow the service [AOR = 5.98; 95% CI: 1.49, 13.96]. This might be due to the fact that health professionals have been educating and advising mothers on child nutrition (complementary feeding practice) during postnatal care. Postnatal care is a good platform for educating and advising mothers about feeding of children.

In South Asian countries, like in Bangladesh, India, Nepal, Pakistan, and Sri-Lanka, the most consistent determinants of complementary feeding practices across all countries including inadequate antenatal care, mode of delivery, and lack of postnatal contacts by health workers were among predictors of inappropriate feeding [11–17]. Another community based cross-sectional study conducted in Tigray at Abi-Adi town showed that mothers who followed postnatal care service were 2.8 times more likely to practice appropriate complementary feeding than those who did not follow the service [AOR = 2.86; 95% CI: 1.10, 7.46] [7]. And a study conducted at Enemay district, Northwest Ethiopia, found that maternal healthcare services (postnatal care) utilization was associated with optimal complementary feeding practice (OCFP) [8]. In line with this study another study conducted in Tanzania also showed that the main risk factor for inappropriate complementary feeding practice was lack of postnatal check-ups [18].

Profession of mothers was also another predictor for affecting the feeding practices of IYC (infant, young child). Housewife mothers were found to be about 9.5 times more likely to practice appropriate complementary feeding in comparison to government employees [AOR = 9.50; 95% CI: 1.02, 14.25] (Table 3). A study conducted in Addis Ababa found that employed mothers were more likely to introduce complementary foods before 6 months (AOR = 0.37) compared with mothers who stayed at home [11]. Similarly a study conducted at Enemay district supports this finding that mothers' occupation was significantly associated with complementary feeding practice [8]. Another study conducted in South West Ethiopia consistent with this study found that mothers who work as daily workers, farmers, merchant, and government employees were less likely to practice complementary feeding than housewife [19].

This study revealed that women whose husbands only decide on family income were more likely to have inappropriate complementary feeding practice than the women who are involved in decision making about how to use family income [AOR = 5.54; 95% CI: 1.19, 11.74] (Table 3). This might be due to the reason that mothers are more likely to purchase food items in the household and more responsible for care of children than fathers. In line with this finding a study done in Kenya also reported children belonging to families where mothers decide on how to use family income were more likely (chi square test; p value = 0.045) to have appropriate complementary feeding practice compared with children belonging to families where mainly husbands were deciding on family income (36.7%) [20].

This study also revealed that mothers who were exposed to public media were 2.5 times more likely to practice complementary feeding than mothers who were not [AOR = 2.50; 95% CI: 1.44, 4.35] (Table 3). This result is similar to another finding of the study done in Kenya which showed significant association between public media exposure and appropriate complementary feeding practice [20]. Another study conducted in Tanzania also indicated that one of the main risk factors for inappropriate complementary feeding

practices was limited access to mass media [18]. On the contrary community based studies conducted at Abyi Adi town, Tigray, Northern Ethiopia, and at Kamba woreda South West Ethiopia found that there is no significant association between media exposure and complementary feeding practice [7, 19]. The difference might be due to time difference of the study conducted.

This study did not find any statistically significant association between complementary feeding practice and sex of children, education of parents, income, child birth order, family size, maternal marital status, antenatal care, and place of delivery. The possible limitation of this study might be recall bias and social desirability bias as the data was based on self-report.

5. Conclusion and Recommendation

5.1. Conclusion

(i) Near half of mothers were not practicing appropriate complementary feeding practice, considering timely introduction, minimum dietary diversity, and frequency.

(ii) Mothers' occupation, postnatal care service utilization, media exposure, and mothers decision making role on family income were the independent predictors for appropriate complementary feeding practice.

(iii) Majority of mothers/caregivers were not using meat/fish/chicken and milk/milk products when they prepared complementary foods like porridge to their children.

5.2. Recommendations

For Mothers and Caregivers

(i) Mothers who work outside home had better to adopt workplace breastfeeding practices and breast milk expression in cup to feed the child when they spend long time outside their home due to different tasks.

(ii) Mothers should not miss meat/fish/chicken, milk/milk products, and vegetables diversification while preparing infants' and young children's porridge.

For Health Extension Workers and Health Professionals

(i) Health professionals should focus on advising and counseling mothers on appropriate complementary feeding during prenatal, delivery, postnatal, and immunization services.

For Government (Policy Makers)

(i) Developing motivational factors for mothers who practice complementary feeding appropriately could be promotion (advertising) of complementary feeding.

TABLE 3: Factors associated with inappropriate complementary feeding practice among mothers who had 6–23-month-old children at Lasta Woreda, Amharra, Northern Ethiopia, April to October 2015.

Variables (n = 476)	Appropriate N (%)	Inappropriate N (%)	COR (95% CI)	AOR (95% CI)
Sex of children				
Male	175 (75.4%)	57 (24.6)	1	1
Female	199 (81.6)	45 (18.4)	1.44 (.93, 2.24)	1.32 (.78, 2.22)
Child birth order				
1–3	273 (82.0)	60 (18.0)	1	1
4–6	97 (72.4)	37 (27.6)	5.69 (1.48, 21.81)	.27 (.13, .55)
7–10	4 (44.4)	5 (55.6)	3.28 (.83, 12.87)	.25 (.02, 2.60)
Public media exposure				
No	36 (35.3)	66 (64.7)	1	1
Yes	158 (42.2)	216 (57.8)	2.44 (1.53, 3.90)	2.50 (1.44, 4.35)**
Mothers decision making role on family income				
Mainly husband	29 (87.9)	4 (12.10)	1	1
Only husband	6 (60.0)	4 (40.0)	.20 (.04, 1.07)	5.54 (1.19, 11.74)*
Mainly wife	4 (40.0)	6 (60.0)	.09 (.02, .48)	.01 (.00, .14)
Only wife	32 (68.1)	15 (31.9)	.29 (.089, .99)	.20 (.02, 2.61)
Both jointly	303 (80.0)	73 (19.4)	.57 (.19, 1.68)	.15 (.03, .72)
ANC follow-up				
No	363 (80.1)	90 (19.9)	1	1
Yes	4 (40.0)	6 (60.0)	.29 (.10, .84)	.51 (.22, 1.20)
PNC follow-up				
No	90 (80.2)	12 (42.9)	1	1
Yes	364 (19.8)	10 (57.1)	.19 (.08, .45)	5.98 (1.49, 13.96)*
Mothers educational status				
Cannot read, write	242 (78.7)	65 (21.3)	1	1
Read & write	32 (74.4)	11 (25.6)	.79 (.37, 1.63)	.51 (.22, 1.22)
1–4	25 (86.2)	4 (13.8)	1.68 (.56, 4.99)	1.35 (.36, 5.01)
5–8	38 (74.5)	13 (25.5)	.79 (.39, 1.56)	.60 (.25, 1.46)
9–12	34 (79.1)	9 (20.9)	1.02 (0.46, 2.22)	1.33 (.41, 4.29)
College/university	3 (100.0)	0 (0)	4.34 (.00, . . .)	1.37 (.00, .00)
Mothers occupational status				
Government employed	7 (77.8)	2 (22.2)	1	1
Private employed	2 (50.0)	2 (50.0)	.29 (.02, 3.52)	.44 (.00, 7.45)
Merchant	18 (69.2)	8 (30.8)	.64 (.10, 3.80)	1.91 (.19, 8.84)
House wife	89 (84.8)	16 (15.2)	1.59 (.30, 8.35)	9.50 (1.02, 14.25)*
Farmer	242 (78.1)	68 (21.9)	1.02 (.20, 5.00)	3.56 (.42, 10.45)
Daily laborer	4 (66.7)	2 (33.3)	.57 (.06, 5.76)	1.90 (.08, 4.92)
Student	1 (50.0)	1 (50.0)	.27 (.01, 6.91)	.42 (.01, 7.00)
House maid	11 (78.6)	3 (21.4)	1.05 (.14, 7.93)	2.69 (.22, 3.68)
Maternal marital status				
Married	334 (79.9)	84 (20.1)	1	1
Single	11 (68.8)	5 (31.2)	0.55 (0.19, 1.63)	1.87 (.24, 13.73)
Divorced	24 (68.6)	11 (31.4)	0.55 (0.26, 1.16)	.92 (.11, 7.83)
Widowed	4 (66.7)	2 (33.3)	0.50 (0.09, 2.79)	.23 (.01, 4.29)
Family size				
1–4	176 (78.2)	49 (21.8)	1	1
5–8	195 (79.6)	50 (20.4)	1.09 (.68, 1.69)	1.79 (.85, 3.79)
9–11	3 (50.0)	3 (50.0)	.28 (.05, 1.42)	1.28 (.08, 2.79)

TABLE 3: Continued.

Variables ($n = 476$)	Appropriate N (%)	Inappropriate N (%)	COR (95% CI)	AOR (95% CI)
Place of delivery				
Health facility	200 (82.0)	44 (18.0)	1	1
Home	173 (74.9)	58 (25.1)	.66 (.42, 1.03)	.74 (.43, 1.29)

*p-value < 0.05, **p-value < 0.01, COR (Crude odds ratio) AOR (Adjusted odds ratio), CI (confidence interval)
Hosmer and Lemeshow's goodness-of-fit test was found to be chi-square of 8.147 with p-value of 0.232 hence the model was good because its p-value > (0.05).

(ii) Special emphasis should be given in empowering women to have a decision making role on family income using different strategies like public media.

(iii) Declaring six-month maternal leave after delivery for government employed mothers could be an alternative solution to improving complementary feeding practice.

(iv) It is better to assign nutrition professionals at health institution and woreda health office level.

(v) It is better to strengthen intersectorial involvement of organizations working on nutrition promotion to realize nutrition interventions.

For Researchers

(i) Further research should be conducted by using qualitative study design to understand deeply sociocultural and behavioral related factors toward complementary feeding to develop and implement better strategy on improving complementary feeding.

(ii) Researchers had better to use cohort study design in addition to cross-sectional one in assessing IYCF indicators.

Abbreviations

AOR: Adjusted odds ratio
COR: Crude odds ratio
FHE: Food for Hungry Ethiopia
IYCF: Infant and young child feeding
ORDA: Organization for Rehabilitation and Development in Amhara
DFAP: Development Food Aid Program
CSA: Central Statistical Agency.

Authors' Contributions

Menberu Molla, Tadese Ejigu, and Girma Nega have been involved in the conception, design, analysis, interpretation, report, and manuscript writing.

Acknowledgments

The authors would like to thank and sincerely appreciate study participant, data collectors, supervisors, and Lasta District authorities.

References

[1] WHO, "Indicators for assessing infant and young child feeding practices: part I," in *Proceedings of the Conclusions of a Consensus Meeting*, WHO, Washington, DC, USA, 2008.

[2] A. Aggarwal, S. Verma, M. M. A. Faridi, and Dayachand, "Complementary feeding—reasons for inappropriateness in timing, quantity and consistency," *The Indian Journal of Pediatrics*, vol. 75, no. 1, pp. 49–53, 2008.

[3] WHO, *Progress towards Developing Simple Indicators: Assessing Infant and Young Child Feeding*, WHO, Geneva, Switzerland, 2006.

[4] WHO, *Indicators for Assessing Infant and Young Child Feeding Practices: Part I. Conclusions of a Consensus Meeting Held in Washington D.C., USA*, WHO, 2008.

[5] Ethiopian Demographic Health Survey Report, 2011.

[6] K. K. Saha, E. A. Frongillo, D. S. Alam, S. E. Arifeen, L. Å. Persson, and K. M. Rasmussen, "Appropriate infant feeding practices result in better growth of infants and young children in rural Bangladesh," *American Journal of Clinical Nutrition*, vol. 87, no. 6, pp. 1852–1859, 2008.

[7] M. Ergib, S. Ashenafi, F. Semaw, and H. Fisha, "Magnitude and factors associated with complementary feeding among mothers having children 6–23 months of age in Northern Ethiopia," *Journal of Food and Nutrition Science*, vol. 2, no. 2, pp. 36–42, 2014.

[8] D. Gessese, H. Bolka, A. A. Abajobir, and D. Tegabu, "The practice of complementary feeding and associated factors among mothers of children 6–23 months of age in Enemay district, Northwest Ethiopia," *Nutrition and Food Science*, vol. 44, no. 3, pp. 230–240, 2014.

[9] A. Shumey, M. Demissie, and Y. Berhane, "Timely initiation of complementary feeding and associated factors among children aged 6 to 12 months in Northern Ethiopia: an institution-based cross-sectional study," *BMC Public Health*, vol. 13, no. 1, article 1050, 2013.

[10] A. Kume, "Infant and young child feeding practices among mothers living in Harar, Ethiopia," *Harar Bulletin of Health Sciences*, no. 4, pp. 66–78, 2012.

[11] S. Gebru, *Assessment of Breastfeeding Practice in Yeka Sub-City Addis Ababa, Ethiopia*, Community Health Department Medical Facility, Addis Ababa University, Addis Ababa, Ethiopia, 2007.

[12] I. Abukari, E. Kingsley, B. Penelope, P. Andrew, and J. Michel, "Determinants of inadequate complementary feeding practices among children aged 6–23 months in Ghana," *Journal of Public Health Nutrition*, vol. 18, no. 4, pp. 669–678, 2015.

[13] K. Jacob, *Determinants of complementary feeding practice and nutritional status of children 6–23 months of age [M.S. thesis]*, Kenyatta University, Nairobi, Kenya, 2013.

[14] M. E. Khan, F. Donnay, U. K. Tarigopula, and K. Aruldas, *Shaping Demand and Practices to Improve Family Health Outcomes: Findings from a Quantitative Survey*, Population Council, New Delhi, India, 2013.

[15] F. Saleh, F. Ara, M. A. Hoque, and M. S. Alam, "Complementary feeding practices among mothers in selected slums of dhaka city: a descriptive study," *Journal of Health, Population and Nutrition*, vol. 32, no. 1, pp. 89–96, 2014.

[16] H. Radwan, "Patterns and determinants of breastfeeding and complementary feeding practices of Emirati Mothers in the United Arab Emirates," *BMC Public Health*, vol. 13, no. 1, article 171, 2013.

[17] V. Khanal, K. Sauer, and Y. Zhao, "Exclusive breastfeeding practices in relation to social and health determinants: a comparison of the 2006 and 2011 Nepal Demographic and Health Surveys," *BMC Public Health*, vol. 13, no. 1, article 958, 2013.

[18] A. Kingsley, "Factors associated with inappropriate complementary feeding practices among children aged 6–23 months in Tanzania," *Maternal and Child Nutrition*, vol. 10, no. 4, pp. 545–561, 2012.

[19] E. Agedew, M. Demissie, and D. Misker, "Early initiation of complementary feeding and associated factors among 6 months to 2 years young children, in Kamba Woreda, South West Ethiopia: a community -based cross -sectional study," 2014.

[20] K. Jacob, *Determinants of complementary feeding practices and nutritional status of children 6–23 months old in Korogocho Slum, Nairobi County, Kenya [M.S. thesis]*, Kenyatta University, 2013.

11

Household Food Insecurity, Low Dietary Diversity, and Early Marriage Were Predictors for Undernutrition among Pregnant Women Residing in Gambella, Ethiopia

Mamo Nigatu (iD), **Tsegaye Tewelde Gebrehiwot** (iD), **and Desta Hiko Gemeda** (iD)

Department of Epidemiology, Institute of Health, Jimma University, Jimma, Ethiopia

Correspondence should be addressed to Mamo Nigatu; mamogebre14@gmail.com

Academic Editor: Ronald J. Prineas

Background. Maternal undernutrition affects the health of both mothers and children and, as a result, has broad impacts on economic and social development. *Objective.* The aim of this study was to assess magnitude of undernutrition and associated factors among pregnant women in Gambella town, 2014. *Methods.* Community based cross-sectional study was conducted on 338 randomly selected pregnant women from March to April 2014. Bivariate and multivariable logistic regressions were used for data analysis. *Result.* The prevalence of undernutrition among pregnant women in Gambella town was 28.6%. Pregnant women who were married before their age of eighteen, who were from food insecure households, and who had low dietary diversity score were nearly four (AOR = 3.9, 95% CI: 2.2–6.9), two (AOR = 2.3, 95% CI : 1.2–3.6), and two (AOR = 2.1, 95% CI: 1.3–4.16) times more likely to be undernourished as compared to their counterparts, respectively. *Conclusion.* Prevalence of undernutrition among pregnant women in Gambella town was unacceptably high. Stake holders should give due consideration to health education to delay age at first marriage and mainstreaming and strengthening nutritional activities that contribute to reduction of food insecurity and consumption of unbalanced nutrients.

1. Introduction

Nutrition is a fundamental pillar of human life, health, and development across the lifespan. From the earliest stage of fetal development, at birth through infancy, childhood, and adolescence, and into adulthood and old age, proper food and good nutrition are essential for survival, physical growth, mental development, performance and productivity, health, and well-being. It is an essential foundation of human and national development. For this reason everybody is expected to get adequate nutrition, especially woman of child bearing age [1, 2]. Pregnancy is one of the most critical and unique periods in woman's life cycle. A woman's body changes dramatically during pregnancy; hence there is a strong need to balance these changes with an adequate and nutritious diet [3].

Nutrients need typically an increase during pregnancy and lactation than during any other stage in woman's adult life. Additional nutrients are required during gestation for growth of the fetus as well as for the development of maternal tissues that support fetal development. The nutritional ingredients required for this rapid growth and development depend on the support from maternal diet [4, 5]. Proper dietary balance is necessary to ensure sufficient energy intake for adequate growth of the fetus without drawing on mother own tissues to maintain her pregnancy [6]. The common maternal nutritional problems during pregnancy include protein energy malnutrition, iron and folic acid deficiency, vitamin A deficiency, iodine deficiency, zinc deficiency, and vitamin B6 and vitamin B12 deficiency [4, 7].

Maternal undernutrition affects the health of both mother and children and, as a result, has broad impacts on economic and social development [7–10]. Undernourished pregnant woman has higher reproductive risks including death during or after child birth [6, 7, 11]. Many women suffer from combination of chronic energy deficiency, poor weight gain during pregnancy, anemia, and other micronutrient deficiency. These along with inadequate obstetric care contribute to high rates of maternal mortality and poor pregnancy outcomes [8, 12]. Maternal malnutrition in both the form of chronic energy and micronutrient deficiencies causes intrauterine growth retardation (IUGR), low birth weight, prematurity, infant and neonatal mortality, abortion, stillbirth, reduced physical activity, and poor cognitive development of the baby leading to poor educational capability and performance [2, 13–15].

Undernutrition's most damaging effect occurs during pregnancy and in the first two years of life, and the effect of this early damage on health, brain development, intelligence, educability, and reproductive is largely irreversible [6, 7, 9]. Maternal undernutrition has also intergenerational effect. Undernourished girls have a great likelihood of becoming undernourished mothers who in turn have a great chance of giving birth to low birth weight babies perpetuating an intergenerational cycle [4, 6].

Every day 800 women die during pregnancy or child birth and 8000 newborn babies die during their first month of life. Ninety-eight percent of newborn deaths and ninety-nine percent of maternal death occur in developing countries [16]. Many women in developing countries maintain pregnancies on dietary intake lower than those recommended by international agencies [17]. In a systematic review including sixty-two studies published from 1989 to 2011 Lee et al. reported that a large majority of pregnant women from Africa and Asia had taken lower energy and micronutrient than those recommended by Food and Agricultural Organization/World Health Organization (FAO/WHO). Lee et al. concluded that the problems of unbalanced macronutrient profiles and multiple micronutrient deficiencies are common among pregnant women in developing countries across the region of the world [18].

Studies have shown that cultural factors including lack of care for pregnant women, increased workloads, early marriage, and teenage marriage make the situation worse in Ethiopia [2, 7]. In order to identify, prioritize, and avert the devastating risk of malnutrition the government of Ethiopia has designed the national nutrition strategy (NNS) of which maternal nutrition during pregnancy is one of the priority areas [7].

In supporting the national nutrition strategy and other potential intervention programs, adequate evidence about undernutrition and its contextual determinants in children, pregnant, and lactating mothers are available in the highlands of Ethiopia [11, 19–22]. However, there is no evidence about the aforementioned problem in pregnant women in lowlands of the country like Gambella region as to the investigators knowledge. Gambella region is characterized by having hot climate condition, relative insecurity, diverse ethnicity, low sociodemographic and economic characteristics, pastoralist community, and common natural disasters like drought and flooding [23]. Therefore, this study was aimed at determining undernutrition and its contextual risk factors among pregnant mothers in Gambella town, a low land in Southwest Ethiopia.

2. Methods and Materials

2.1. Study Setting. Data were collected from March to April 2014 in Gambella town, Southwest Ethiopia. Gambella town is a separate district and the capital of the Gambella Region located at the confluence of the Baro River and its tributary the Jajjaba. The town has a latitude and longitude of 8°15'N 34°35'E and has an elevation of 526 meters above sea level having hot climatic condition. Gambella town is located 768 kilometers away from Addis Ababa, the capital city of Ethiopia in the southwest direction. The town harbors different ethnic groups. The majority of ethnic groups residing in the town are Nuire, Agnuhak, and Mejenger. However, there are also other ethnic groups including settlers from other highlands of the country. According to population projection for 2014, based on the 2007 Census report Gambella town has a total population of 51,696, of whom 18,232 were women [24]. The town had a total of 10,152 households with an average of 3.8 persons to a household.

2.1.1. Study Design. A community based cross-sectional study was utilized to address the magnitude of undernutrition and its contextual determinants among pregnant mothers.

2.1.2. Population. A sample of pregnant women who resided in Gambella town for at least six months was included in the study. Pregnant women who refuse to participate and are severely ill were excluded from the study.

2.1.3. Sampling. Sample size was calculated using single population proportion formula by considering proportion of pregnant women undernourished as 50% since there was no prior study in lowlands of Ethiopia, 5% margin of error, and 95% confidence level. In addition, correction formula was used due to small number of pregnant women ($N = 1,452$) in the town during the study period. Finally, by addition of 10% nonresponse rate, the expected sample size was 338 pregnant women.

A survey was done to identify pregnant women in Gambella town prior to the actual study. Every women of reproductive age group in all residential households was asked for self-report of current pregnancy status. Women who were pregnant as per their oral report were further asked to show proof of pregnancy, ANC card from health facilities. These women, who reported pregnancy but had no evidence from health facility, were further tested for pregnancy using urine test (HCT test) in the field. Finally, a total of 1,452 pregnant women were found in the town during the study period. Samples of 338 pregnant women were selected randomly using computer after entering the total pregnant women in to SPSS software using unique numbers.

2.1.4. Data Collection Procedure and Measurement. Variables included and measured in this study were sociodemographic variables which comprise age, marital status, educational status, husband's educational status, occupation, husband's occupation, and family size; socioeconomic variables which comprise household income and household food insecurity; sociocultural variables which include early marriage, history of teenage pregnancy, living in polygamy, and intrahousehold food distribution; individual and behavioral variables like knowledge about nutrition, health service contact, dietary practice, birth interval, number of children born to the women, and latrine possession.

Data on sociodemographic, socioeconomic, sociocultural, household food insecurity, and individual and behavioral factors was collected by face-to-face interview using pretested questionnaires adapted from related literatures and translated to Amharic language. Household food insecurity was assessed using Household Food Insecurity Access Scale (HFIAS) measurement consisting of nine items [9]. Each of the questions under HFIAS was asked with a recall period of four weeks (30 days) prior to the data collection period. The respondent was first asked an occurrence question, that is, whether the condition in the question happened at all in the past four weeks (yes or no). If the respondent answers "yes" to an occurrence question, a frequency-of-occurrence question was asked to determine whether the condition happened rarely (once or twice), sometimes (three to ten times), or often (more than ten times) in the past four weeks. A 24 hr dietary recall method was used to collect data on dietary intake.

Local languages speaking and fluent in Amharic diploma nurses were assigned as data collectors and verbally administered questionnaire to respondents. After conducting face-to-face interview, mid upper arm circumference of the respondents was measured on the left hand at the mid point between the tips of the shoulder and elbow to the nearest 0.1 cm by using nonstretchable mid upper arm circumference (MUAC) tape. MUAC was used to assess nutritional status of pregnant women [25]. Five trained diploma nurses were data collectors and two B.S. public health officers were assigned as supervisors. Data collectors and supervisors were given two-day training focusing on participant selection procedure, MUAC measurement, ethical procedure, and objective of the study. The responsibilities of data collectors were measuring the mid upper arm circumference of the respondent and filling the questionnaires. The supervisor provides all items necessary for data collection on each data collection day, checking filled questionnaire for completeness and consistency and solving problems during data collection. Before conducting the main study, pretesting was done on 17 pregnant women residing in Abobo town of Gambella region. Finally, data collection tool was refined based on the findings from the pretesting. Every day, all collected data was reviewed and checked for completeness and consistency by the supervisors.

2.2. Data Processing and Analysis. Data were checked and edited for completeness and consistency and partially coded manually. Data were entered into EpiData version 3.1 and exported to SPSS version 16 for statistical analysis. Descriptive statistics were computed to explore frequency distribution, central tendency, variability (dispersion), and distribution of outcome and explanatory variables. Bivariable logistic regression was done to identify candidate variables (p value = 0.2) for multivariable logistic regression analysis. To identify the independent predictors of undernutrition, multivariable logistic regression model was fitted using backward stepwise

method. Interaction between different variables was checked using Breslow-Day test of homogeneity of strata specific odds ratios. Multicollinearity between different predictor variables was also checked using variance inflation factor (VIF). In multivariable logistic regression, adjusted odds ratio with its 95% confidence interval was computed for variables maintained in the final model and statistical significance was declared by the confidence interval.

Individual dietary diversity score (IDDS) was calculated by summing a total of 14 food groups [(1) cereals; (2) vitamin A rich vegetables and tubers; (3) white roots and tubers; (4) dark green leafy vegetables; (5) other vegetables; (6) vitamin A rich fruits; (7) other fruits; (8) organ meat; (9) flesh meat; (10) eggs; (11) fish; (12) legumes, nuts, and seeds; (13) milk and milk products; and (14) oils and fats] consumed over reference period (24 hours before the data collection). For example, if one pregnant woman eats from each food group, her DDS will be 14 [26]. MUAC less than 21 cm in pregnant women was considered as undernutrition. Household food security is defined as a household which experiences none of the food insecurity (access) conditions or just experiences worry, but rarely, otherwise, food insecurity [26]. Dietary diversity score below six is said to be low dietary diversity score otherwise better.

2.2.1. Ethical Consideration. Ethical clearance letter was obtained from Institutional Review Board (IRB) of Jimma University. Permission letter to conduct the research was obtained from Gambella Regional Health Bureau. Prior to data collection, the participants were informed about the purpose of the study, their right to refuse participation and discontinue the interview or measurement, and their full right to say "no" (opt out), and it was clearly stated that their decision of "no" will not affect any of their right to health provisions intended for pregnant women. The interviewers discussed the issue of confidentiality and obtained verbal consent before the actual interviews were launched. For this purpose, a one page consent form was attached as cover page to each questionnaire. In addition, any identification information including the name of the participants was not written in the questionnaire. Undernourished pregnant women were linked to local nutritional programs in the area.

3. Results

3.1. Sociodemographic Characteristics. From the total 338 recruited pregnant women, twelve of them were refused to participate in the study, making the response rate 96.5%, and four were with incomplete data. Complete data were collected on 322 pregnant women.

Mean age of the participants was 26.7 with standard deviation of (SD ± 5.2) years. Majority (83.6%) of the participants were in the age range of 20 to 34 years. A tenth (10.2%), fifth (20.4%), and near to two-thirds (64.9%) of pregnant women were unmarried, illiterate, and housewives, respectively. The mean family size was 5.5 with the standard deviation of ±2.7 ranging from 2 to 15. One hundred thirty-seven (42.5%) were living in a family which had more than five members (Table 1).

TABLE 1: Sociodemographic characteristics of pregnant women in Gambella town, March-April 2014.

Socio demographic variables	Category	Number (%)	MUAC ≤ 21 cm	MUAC > 21 cm	Crude odds ratio (95% CI)	p value
Age in year	15–19	22 (6.8)	5 (22.7)	17 (77.3)	1.06 (0.36–3.15)	0.98
	20–24	90 (28.0)	29 (32.2)	61 (67.8)	1.71 (0.92–3.2)	0.092
	25–29	115 (35.7)	25 (21.7)	90 (78.3)	1	
	30–34	64 (19.9)	24 (37.5)	40 (62.5)	2.16 (1.1–4.23)	0.025
	≥35	31 (9.6)	9 (29.0)	22 (71.0)	1.47	0.396
	Total	322 (100)	92 (28.6)	230 (71.4)		
Ethnicity	Agnuak	89 (16.8)	35 (39.3)	54 (60.7)	1	
	Nuer	54 (27.6)	22 (40.7)	32 (59.3)	1.06 (0.53–2.11)	0.867
	Oromo	51 (15.8)	7 (13.7)	44 (86.3)	0.25 (0.10–0.61)	0.002
	Amhara	51 (15.8)	12 (23.5)	39 (76.5)	0.48 (0.22–1.03)	0.059
	Kambata	35 (10.9)	10 (28.6)	25 (71.4)	0.62 (0.26–1.14)	0.26
	Tigre	21 (6.5)	2 (9.5)	19 (90.5)	0.1 (0.036–0.74)	0.019
	Mejang	4 (1.2)	1 (25)	3 (75)	0.51 (0.05–5.14)	0.57
	Others	17 (5.3)	3 (17.6)	14 (82.4)	0.33 (0.089–1.24)	0.100
	Total	322 (100)	92 (28.6)	230 (71.4)		
Religion	Protestant	127 (39.4)	43 (33.9)	84 (66.1)	1	
	Orthodox	80 (24.8)	14 (17.5)	66 (82.5)	0.41 (0.21–0.82)	0.012
	Catholic	67 (20.8)	23 (34.3)	44 (65.7)	1.02 (0.55–1.91)	0.95
	Muslim	27 (8.4)	5 (18.5)	22 (81.5)	0.44 (0.16–1.25)	0.125
	Others	21 (6.8)	7 (33.3)	14 (66.7)	0.98 (0.37–2.6)	0.96
	Total	322 (100)	92 (28.6)	230 (71.4)		
Educational status	No formal education	65 (20.2)	23 (35.4)	42 (64.6)	1.91 (0.98–3.71)	0.057
	Primary education	136 (42.2)	42 (30.9)	94 (69.1)	1.56 (0.89–2.73)	0.123
	Secondary and above	121 (37.6)	27 (22.3)	94 (77.7)	1	
	Total	322 (100)	92 (28.6)	230 (71.4)		
Husband's educational status	No formal education	34 (10.6)	16 (47.1)	18 (52.9)	2.34 (1.13–4.85)	0.022
	Primary education	41 (12.7)	8 (19.5)	33 (80.5)	0.64 (0.28–1.45)	0.284
	Secondary and above	247 (76.7)	68 (27.5)	179 (72.5)	1	
	Total	322 (100)	92 (28.6)	230 (71.4)		
Marital status	Married	289 (89.8)	82 (28.4)	207 (71.6)	0.91 (0.42–2.00)	0.82
	Unmarried	33 (10.2)	10 (30.3)	23 (69.7)		
	Total	322 (100)	92 (28.6)	230 (71.4)		
occupation	Housewife	209 (64.9)	68 (32.5)	141 (67.5)	1.62 (0.83–3.14)	0.154
	Government employee	61 (18.9)	14 (23.0)	47 (77.0)	1	
	Merchant	25 (7.8)	5 (20.0)	20 (80.0)	0.84 (0.266–2.644)	0.77
	Others	27 (8.4)	5 (18.5)	22 (81.5)	0.76 (0.24–2.39)	0.64
	Total	322 (100)	92 (28.6)	230 (71.4)		
Husband's occupation	Government employee	189 (58.7)	54 (28.6)	135 (71.4)	1	
	Merchant	45 (14.0)	5 (11.1)	40 (88.9)	0.31 (0.12–0.834)	0.02
	Daily laborers	40 (12.4)	16 (40.0)	24 (60.0)	1.67 (0.82–3.38)	0.157
	Others	48 (14.9)	17 (35.4)	31 (64.6)	1.37 (0.70–2.68)	0.356
	Total	322 (100)	92 (28.6)	230 (71.4)		
Family size	>5	137 (42.5)	52 (38.0)	85 (62.0)	2.22 (1.36–3.63)	0.001
	≤5	185 (57.5)	40 (21.6)	145 (78.4)		
	Total	322 (100)	92 (28.6)	230 (71.4)		

Note. 1 = reference.

3.2. Prevalence of Undernutrition. The overall prevalence of undernutrition in lowland among pregnant women was 28.6%. Pregnant women who were in the age group of 30–34 years had higher prevalence (37.5%) of undernutrition compared to the other age groups. Pregnant women and their husbands who are illiterate had higher prevalence of undernutrition (35.4% and 47.1%) compared to their counterparts, who completed secondary education and above. Pregnant women who were married before the age of eighteen and conceived before the age of twenty had higher undernutrition prevalence (46.8% and 43.4%, resp.). Pregnant women who had meal frequency less than three and dietary diversity score (DDS) less than six had higher prevalence of undernutrition (45.8% and 41.5%, resp.) compared to pregnant women who had meal frequency greater than or equal to three and DDS greater than or equal to six (27.2% and 19.8%, resp.). Near to half (44.5%) of pregnant women living in food insecure households were undernourished whereas almost a fifth (16.8%) of pregnant women living in food secure households were undernourished (Tables 2 and 4).

3.3. Individual, Household, and Sociocultural Characteristics. The median age at first marriage was 18 ranging from 14 to 31 years. One hundred forty-one (43.8%) women were married before the age of eighteen. The mean age at first conception was 19.9 with the standard deviation of (SD $\pm$ 3.04) years ranging from 15 to 33 years of age. In two hundred forty-seven (76.7%) households, diets were shared equally even though the foods to be eaten were small during meal. In fifty-four (16.8%) households, foods were first given to husband and then shared among other family members. About one-third (33.2%) pregnant women said that they eat their diet after serving their husband and children (Table 2).

According to report from pregnant women, 41 to 44% of the households either are worried about not having enough food, are unable to eat preferred food, or ate few food types a month before commencement of data collection. One hundred fourteen (35.4%) households ate the foods they really do not want to eat while 28% of households ate a fewer meal a day during one month before data collection (Table 3).

From the total 322 pregnant women, 42.5% pregnant women were from food in secured households. Near to half (46.9%) of pregnant women had no better nutritional knowledge. The mean meal frequency per day was 3.43 meals with a minimum of two and maximum of six meals per day. Twenty-four (7.5%) pregnant women had eaten less than three meals a day. The mean dietary diversity score was 6 food groups out of 14 food groups with the standard deviation (SD) of $\pm$ 1.58 ranging from 2 to 13 food groups (Table 4). From the fourteen food groups, cereal food group was eaten by 100% of the pregnant women. From the cereal food group "teff" (58.4%) was the most consumed food followed by corn (54.7%), wheat (43.5%), and millet (36%). "Injera" (62.1%) and porridge (46%) were the most processed food eaten from cereal group (Supplementary Material (available here)).

3.4. Predictors for Undernutrition among Pregnant Women. The following candidate variables from bivariable logistic regression were considered to multivariable logistic

regression analysis: age, pregnant women and their husband's educational status, husband's occupation, family size, household's monthly income, household food insecurity, and dietary diversity. Similarly, nutritional knowledge, meal frequency, ANC visit, children size, latrine possession, and all sociocultural characterize of pregnant women were candidate variables to multivariable logistic regression analysis.

Multivariable logistic regression was fitted in order to identify independent predictors of undernutrition. Accordingly, early marriage, household food insecurity, and low dietary diversity score were independent predictors of undernutrition during pregnancy. Pregnant women who were married before the age of eighteen were nearly fourfold more likely to be undernourished compared to pregnant women who were married after the age of eighteen (AOR = 3.9, 95% CI: 2.2–6.9). Pregnant women who were from food insecure households were nearly two times more likely to be undernourished compared to pregnant women who were from food secure households (AOR = 2.3, 95% CI: 1.2–3.6). Pregnant women who had low dietary diversity score were two times more likely to be undernourished as compared to pregnant women who had better dietary diversity score (AOR = 2.1, 95% CI: 1.3–4.1) (Table 5).

4. Discussion

The current study tried to reveal the magnitude of undernutrition and its associated factors among pregnant women in Gambella, lowland of Ethiopia. Accordingly the project highlighted that near thirty percent of pregnant women in lowlands were undernourished and mainly influenced by household food insecurity, eating low dietary diversity and early marriage.

The magnitude of undernutrition among pregnant women in Gambella town was 28.6%. The result was almost similar to the result reported from Kenya which was 31.7% [27]. But magnitude of undernutrition reported in this study was far below the magnitude reported from Kersa Demographic Surveillance and Health Research Center (KDS-HRC) field site, Ethiopia, which was 47.3% [28], 71.1% in Southern Nations, Nationalities and peoples region (SNNPR) [29], and 34% in West Arsi Zone [22]. The big discrepancy observed may be due to different MUAC cut-off points used to determine undernutrition. However, the finding from this study was higher than other findings from highlands of Ethiopia 19.06% from eastern Ethiopia [21].

Early marriage was one of the sociocultural factors which independently associated with undernutrition during pregnancy. The median age at first marriage was 18 years. This is almost consistent with the EDHS 2011 report in which the median age at first marriage in Gambella region was 17.4 years. But, it was above the national median age at first marriage which was 16.5 years [30]. The difference may be due to disparity of age at first marriage among urban and rural women. From pregnant women who were married before the age of eighteen, 66 (46.8%) were undernourished whereas from those who married at their eighteen or more age, only 26 (14.4%) were undernourished. Pregnant women who were married before the age of eighteen were nearly fourfold more

TABLE 2: Sociocultural characteristics of pregnant women in Gambella town, March-April 2014 ($n = 332$).

Variables	Category	Frequency (%)	MUAC ≤ 21 cm	MUAC > 21 cm	Crude odds ratio (95% CI)	p value
Early marriage	Yes	141 (43.8)	66 (46.8)	75 (53.2)	5.3 (3.09–8.9)	0.001
	No	181 (56.2)	26 (14.4)	155 (85.6)		
History of teenage pregnancy	Yes	159 (49.4)	69 (43.4)	90 (56.6)	4.7 (2.7–8.02)	0.001
	No	163 (50.6)	23 (14.1)	140 (85.9)		
Living in polygamy	Yes	64 (19.9)	30 (46.9)	34 (53.1)	2.8 (1.6–4.9)	0.001
	No	258 (80.1)	62 (24.0)	196 (76.0)		
Measures taken when the food to be eaten was small	Shared equally	247 (76.7)	60 (24.3)	187 (75.7)	1	
	Given to children only	21 (6.5)	11 (52.4)	10 (47.6)	3.4 (1.4–8.5)	0.008
	First given to husband and shared	54 (16.8)	21 (38.9)	33 (61.1)	2.0 (1.1–3.7)	0.03
Allocation of the best portion of the food during meal	Shared equally	198 (61.5)	41 (20.7)	157 (79.3)	1	
	Give to husband	98 (30.4)	40 (40.8)	58 (59.2)	2.6 (1.6–4.5)	0.001
	Given to children	26 (8.1)	11 (42.3)	15 (57.7)	2.8 (1.2–6.6)	0.017
Time of dishing of mother's portion during meal	Along with husband	180 (55.9)	35 (19.4)	145 (80.6)	1	
	After husband	35 (10.9)	16 (45.7)	19 (54.3)	3.5 (1.6–7.5)	0.001
	After husband and children	107 (33.2)	41 (38.3)	66 (61.7)	2.6 (1.5–4.4)	0.001

Note. 1 = reference.

TABLE 3: Household food insecurity access scale (HFIAS) of pregnant women in Gambella town, 2014 ($n = 332$).

Household food insecurity access scale (HFIAS)	Frequency	Percentage
Worry about food		
Rarely	37	11.5
Sometimes	78	24.2
Often	25	7.8
No	182	56.5
Unable to eat preferred food		
Rarely	44	13.7
Sometimes	69	21.4
Often	22	6.8
No	187	58.1
Eat just a few kind of food		
Rarely	46	14.3
Sometimes	70	21.7
Often	17	5.3
No	189	58.7
Eat foods they really do not want to eat		
Rarely	40	12.4
Sometimes	64	19.9
Often	10	3.1
No	208	64.6
Eat a smaller meal		
Rarely	59	18.3
Sometimes	54	16.8
Often	7	2.2
No	202	62.7
Eat fewer meal in a day		
Rarely	69	21.4
Sometimes	20	6.2
Often	1	0.3
No	232	72
No food of any kind in household		
Rarely	9	2.8
Sometimes	2	0.6
No	311	96.6
Go to sleep hungry		
Rarely	6	1.9
Sometimes	1	0.3
No	315	97.8
Go a whole day and night without eating		
Rarely	2	0.6
No	320	99.4

likely to be undernourished compared to pregnant women who were married at or after the age of eighteen. This result is consistent with the study done in West Arsi, Ethiopia, in which pregnant women who married before the age of fifteen were sixteen times more likely undernourished compared to pregnant women who married between the ages of eighteen and nineteen years [22]. The 2012 USAID report on delaying age at marriage and reducing malnutrition of adolescent girls in India showed that early marriage was associated with early pregnancy and high fertility; close spacing of births, unwanted pregnancies, and pregnancy termination which cumulatively deteriorates nutritional status of adolescent girls [31].

Household food insecurity was also one of the socioeconomic factors which independently associated with undernutrition during pregnancy. Pregnant women who were from food insecure households were nearly two times more likely to be undernourished compared to pregnant women who were from food secured households. The result could be due to the fact that, in food insecure households, women pay a sacrificial role and are more vulnerable to be undernourished than other family members [7]. Pregnant women are particularly vulnerable to food insecurity and associated nutrient inadequacies for two major reasons. First, physiological vulnerability comes with childbearing. Maternal nutrient needs increase during pregnancy and breastfeeding, and when these needs are not met, mothers may experience wasting and fatigue. Second, women have a sociological vulnerability. Food security research indicates that, during periods of reduced food supply, women experience reduced intakes relative to men. Furthermore, mothers are likely to reduce their own intakes to secure those of infants and small children [32]. The Ethiopian national nutrition strategy also underpins that in food insecure households women and children are the most vulnerable groups and should be given special attention [7].

Low dietary diversity score was also independently associated with undernutrition. Pregnant women who had low DDS were two times more likely to be undernourished when they were compared with pregnant women who had better DDS. This is consistent with the result of survey done in Iran in which participants with scores $\geq$ six had greater body mass index, waist circumference, and waist-to hip ratio than in individuals with scores less than six [33]. The study is also similar to the community based study done in eastern Ethiopia in which pregnant women who improved their eating habits had a 53% lower risk of undernutrition than who did not [21]. The study done in Kenya also showed that pregnant women with better DDS had greater macro- and micronutrient intake when compared to pregnant women with low DDS [27].

This study had its own limitation; in that use of 24 hr dietary recall questionnaire may lend itself to over or underestimation of dietary intake as it is dependent on the respondents' ability to recall their dietary intake and persistence of the interviewer. The single 24 hr dietary recall method used in this study does not reflect seasonal variation of dietary intake. Similarly, household food insecurity and nutritional status during pregnancy may vary across seasons.

TABLE 4: Household, individual, and behavioral characteristics of pregnant women in Gambella town, 2014 ($n = 332$).

Variables	Category	Number (%)	MUAC ≤ 21 cm	MUAC > 21 cm	Crude odds ratio (95% CI)	p value
Nutritional knowledge	No	151 (46.9)	57 (37.7)	94 (62.3)	2.4 (1.4–3.9)	0.001
	Yes	171 (53.1)	35 (20.5)	136 (79.5)		
Meal frequency	≤3	24 (7.5)	11 (45.8)	13 (54.2)	2.3 (0.98–5.3)	0.057
	≥3	298 (92.5)	81 (27.2)	217 (72.8)		
Dietary diversity score	<6	130 (40.4)	54 (41.5)	76 (58.5)	3.9 (1.8–4.7)	0.001
	≥6	192 (59.6)	38 (19.8)	154 (80.2)		
ANC contact	Yes	240 (74.5)	64 (26.7)	176 (73.3)	0.7 (0.4–1.2)	0.197
	No	82 (25.5)	28 (34.1)	54 (65.9)	1	
	0	73 (22.7)	20 (27.4)	53 (72.6)		
Number of children	1–4	203 (63.0)	54 (26.4)	149 (73.4)	0.96 (0.5–1.8)	0.895
	≥5	46 (14.3)	18 (39.1)	28 (60.9)	1.7 (0.8–3.7)	0.183
Birth interval in year	≤3	206 (64.0)	61 (29.6)	145 (70.4)	1.6 (0.7–3.9)	0.283
	>3	34 (10.6)	7 (20.6)	27 (79.4)		
Latrine possession	No	88 (27.3)	39 (44.3)	49 (55.7)	2.7 (1.6–4.6)	0.001
	Yes	234 (72.7)	53 (22.6)	181 (77.4)		
Household food insecurity	Yes	137 (42.5)	61 (44.5)	76 (55.5)	4.0 (2.4–6.7)	0.001
	No	165 (57.5)	31 (16.8)	154 (83.2)	1	

Note. 1 = reference.

TABLE 5: Independent predictors of undernutrition among pregnant women in Gambella town, 2014 ($n = 332$).

Variables	Category	Number (%)	MUAC ≤ 21 cm	MUAC > 21 cm	Crude odds ratio (95% CI)	Adjusted odds ratio (95% CI)
Early marriage	Yes	141 (43.8)	66 (46.8)	75 (53.2)	5.3 (3.1–8.9)*	3.9 (2.2–6.9)*
	No	181 (56.2)	26 (14.4)	155 (85.6)		
Dietary diversity score	<6	130 (40.4)	54 (41.5)	76 (58.5)	3.9 (1.8–4.7)*	2.1 (1.2–3.6)*
	≥6	192 (59.6)	38 (19.8)	154 (80.2)		
Household food insecurity	Yes	137 (42.5)	61 (44.5)	76 (55.5)	4.0 (2.4–6.7)*	2.3 (1.3–4.1)*
	No	165 (57.5)	31 (16.8)	154 (83.2)		

*p value < 0.01.

5. Conclusions

This study found that the prevalence of undernutrition among pregnant women in Gambella town, lowland of Ethiopia, was within the range for highland area of Ethiopia, yet it is still unacceptably high. Household food insecurity, low dietary diversity score, and early marriage were independent predictors of undernutrition. Gambella region agricultural and rural development bureau should work in collaboration with other stakeholders to develop locally available crops to strengthen household food security and improve dietary diversity and quality. Responsible stake holders in the region should give due consideration to health education to delay age at first marriage. Further longitudinal study may be needed to fully understand household food insecurity and its relation to undernutrition across different seasons.

Acronyms

AOR: Adjusted odds ratio
cOR: Crude odds ratio
CSA: Central Statistical Agency
DDS: Dietary diversity score
EDHS: Ethiopian demographic and health survey
FAO: Food and Agriculture Organization
HCG: Human Chorionic Gonadotrophin
HFIAS: Household Food Insecurity Access Scale
IDDS: Individual diet diversity score
IUGR: Intrauterine Growth Restriction
JU: Jimma University
MDDS: Mean dietary diversity score
MOH: Ministry of Health
MUAC: Midupper arm circumference
OR: Odds ratio
PW: Pregnant woman
RDA: Recommended Daily Allowance
RDI: Reference Dietary Intake
SGA: Small for Gestational Age
SPSS: Statistical Package for Social Science
UNICEF: United Nation Children's Fund
USAID: United State Agency for International Development
WHO: World Health Organization.

Disclosure

Mamo Nigatu is a principal investigator.

Authors' Contributions

Mamo Nigatu, Tsegaye Tewolde, and Desta Hiko Gemeda made substantial contribution in conception, designing, data acquisition, statistical analysis, interpretation of the results, and drafting of the manuscript.

Acknowledgments

The authors are very grateful to Jimma University for financial support. They are also grateful to Gambella Regional Health Bureau for material support. Lastly, they would like to extend their thanks to research participants, data collectors, supervisors, and all friends who directly and indirectly supported them in preparing this scientific paper.

References

[1] WHO, *Nutrition for Health and Development*, Geneva, Switzerland, 2000, http://whqlibdoc.who.int/hq/.../WHO_NHD_00.6.p.

[2] T. Benson, *An assessment of the causes of malnutrition in Ethiopia A contribution to the formulation of a National Nutrition Strategy for Ethiopia*, Addis Abeba, Ethiopia, 2005.

[3] L. S. Brown, "Nutrition requirements during pregnancy," in *Nutrition Requirements During Pregnancy*, pp. 1–24, Jones and Bartlett Publishers, 1st edition, 2009.

[4] M. Melkie Edris, H. Tekle, Y. Fitaw, B. Gelaw, and Dagnew Engedaw. T. A., *Maternal Nutrition:For the Ethiopian Health Center Team*, Addis Abeba, Ethiopia, 2005.

[5] A. Bendich, *Nutrition and Health*, C. J. Lammi-Keefe, S. C. Couch, and EHP, Eds., Human Press, 2nd edition, 2008.

[6] Unicef, *Improving Child Nutrition*, New York, NY, USA, 2013, http://www.unicef.org/publications/index.htm.

[7] FMOH, National-Nutrition-Strategy.pdf., Addis Abeba, 2008.

[8] IYCN, *Guidance for Formative Research on Maternal Nutrition*, Washington, DC, USA, 2011.

[9] Worldbank, *Repositioning Nutrition as Central to Development*, Washington, DC, USA, 2006.

[10] R. E. Black, C. G. Victora, S. P. Walker et al., "Maternal and child undernutrition and overweight in low-income and middle-income countries," *The Lancet*, vol. 382, no. 9890, pp. 427–451, 2013.

[11] K. Haileslassie, A. Mulugeta, and M. Girma, "Feeding practices, nutritional status and associated factors of lactating women in Samre Woreda, South Eastern Zone of Tigray, Ethiopia," *Nutrition Journal* , p. 28, 2013.

[12] J. A. Opara, H. E. Adebola, N. S. Oguzor, S. A. Abere, and P. Harcourt, "Malnutrition during pregnancy among child bearing mothers in mbaitolu of south-eastern nigeria federal college of education (technical), omoku-rivers state , nigeria faculty of agriculture , rivers state university of science and technology," *Advances in Biological Research*, vol. 5, no. 2, pp. 111–115, 2011.

[13] D. Assefa, E. Wassie, M. Getahun, M. Berhaneselassie, and A. Melaku, *Harmful Traditional Practices*, Addis Abeba, Ethiopia, 2005.

[14] K. Abu-Saad and D. Fraser, "Maternal nutrition and birth outcomes," *Epidemiologic Reviews*, vol. 32, no. 1, pp. 5–25, 2010.

[15] F. Khoushabi and G. Saraswathi, "Association between maternal nutrition status and birth weight of neonates in selected hospitals in Mysore city, India," *Pakistan Journal of Nutrition*, vol. 9, no. 12, pp. 1124–1130, 2010.

[16] Savethechildren, Surviving the First Day, STATE OF THE WORLD'S MOTHERS, London; 2013, http://www.savethe-children.net.

[17] S. Huffman, E. Zehner, P. Harvey et al., *Essential Health Sector Actions to Improve Maternal Nutrition in Africa*, Washington, DC, USA, 2001, http://www.linkagesproject.org.

[18] S. E. Lee, S. A. Talegawkar, M. Merialdi, and L. E. Caulfield, "Dietary intakes of women during pregnancy in low- and middle-income countries," *Public Health Nutrition*, vol. 16, no. 8, pp. 1340–1353, 2013.

[19] F. H. Bitew and D. S. Telake, "Undernutrition among Women in Ethiopia. Bitew, Fikrewold H. and Daniel S. Telake. 2010. Undernutrition among Women in Ethiopia: Rural-Urban Disparity. DHS Working Papers No. 77," Tech. Rep. Report No.: 77, ICF Macro, Calverton, Md, USA, 2010.

[20] G. Woldemariam and G. Timotiows, *Determinants of the Nutritional Status of Mothers and Children in Ethiopia*, Calverton, Maryland, USA, 2002.

[21] H. Kedir, Y. Berhane, and A. Worku, "Magnitude and determinants of malnutrition among pregnant women in eastern Ethiopia: Evidence from rural, community-based setting," *Maternal & Child Nutrition*, vol. 12, no. 1, pp. 51–63, 2016.

[22] Y. Belete, B. Negga, and M. Firehiwot, "Under nutrition and associated factors among adolescent pregnant women in Shashemenne District , West Arsi Zone , Ethiopia: a community- based," *Journal of Nutrition & Food Sciences*, vol. 6, no. 1, pp. 1–7, 2016.

[23] A. Sewonet, *Breaking the Cycle of Conflict in Gambella Region*, Addis Abeba, Ethiopia, 2003.

[24] C. Statistical, *2007 Population and Housing Census of Administrative*, Addis Abeba, Ethiopia, 2012.

[25] FMOH, *Nutritin Blended Learning Module for the Health Extension Programme*, Health Education and Training in Africa, Addis Abeba, Ethiopia, 1st edition, 2004, Tom Heller and Lesley-Anne Long (Faculty of Health and Social Care at The Open University UK) http://www.moh.gov.et.

[26] FAO, *Guidelines for Measuring Household and Individual Dietary Diversity*, Rome, Italy, 2008.

[27] M. Lillian, *Dietary Diversity and Nutritional Status of Pregnant Women Aged 15-49 YearS Attending Kapenguria District Hospital West Pokot County*, Kenya, East Africa, 2013, https://www.lap-publishing.com/.../dietary-diversity-and-nutritional-statu.

[28] N. Assefa, Y. Berhane, and A. Worku, "Wealth status, mid upper arm circumference (MUAC) and Ante Natal Care (ANC) are determinants for low birth weight in Kersa, Ethiopia," *PLoS ONE*, vol. 7, no. 6, Article ID e39957, 2012.

[29] A. Sonko, "Assessment of dietary practice and anthropometric status of pregnant women in Aleta Chuko Woreda Southern Nations, Nationalities and People's™ Region /SNNPR/, Ethiopia: descriptive crosssectional study," *Journal of Epidemiology and Public Health Reviews*, vol. 1, no. 1, pp. 1–8, 2016.

[30] EDHS, *Ethiopia Demographic and Health Survey*, Addis Abeba, Ethiopia, 2011.

[31] USAID, *Delaying Age of Marriage and Reducing Anaemia Among Adolescent Girls in Jharkhand*, Mumbai, India, 2012, http://www.intrahealth.org/vistaar.

[32] USAID, *Maternal dietary diversity and the implications for children' s diets in the context of food security*, 2012, http://www.iycn.org.

[33] M. Vakili, P. Abedi, M. Sharifi, and M. Hosseini, "Dietary diversity and its related factors among adolescents: a survey in Ahvaz-Iran," *Global Journal of Health Science*, vol. 5, no. 2, pp. 181–186, 2013.

12

Households Sociodemographic Profile as Predictors of Health Insurance Uptake and Service Utilization: A Cross-Sectional Study in a Municipality of Ghana

Eric Badu [iD],[1,2] Peter Agyei-Baffour,[3] Isaac Ofori Acheampong,[4] Maxwell Preprah Opoku,[5] and Kwasi Addai-Donkor[6]

[1]Centre for Disability and Rehabilitation Studies, Kwame Nkrumah University of Science and Technology, Kumasi, Ghana
[2]The University of Newcastle, Callaghan, NSW, Australia
[3]Department of Health Policy, Management and Economics/School of Public Health, Kwame Nkrumah University of Science and Technology (KNUST), Kumasi, Ghana
[4]St. John of God Nursing Training College, Ministry of Health, Sefwi Asafo, Western Region, Ghana
[5]University of Tasmania, Hobart, TAS, Australia
[6]Ghana Health Service, Kwame Nkrumah University of Science and Technology, Kumasi, Ghana

Correspondence should be addressed to Eric Badu; badu3eric@gmail.com

Academic Editor: Carol J. Burns

Introduction. Attempts to use health insurance in Low and Middle Income Countries (LMICs) are recognized as a powerful tool in achieving Universal Health Coverage (UHC). However, continuous enrolment onto health insurance schemes and utilization of healthcare in these countries remain problematic due to varying factors. Empirical evidence on the influence of household sociodemographic factors on enrolment and subsequent utilization of healthcare is rare. This paper sought to examine how household profile influences the National Health Insurance Scheme (NHIS) status and use of healthcare in a municipality of Ghana. *Methods.* A cross-sectional design with quantitative methods was conducted among a total of 380 respondents, selected through a multistage cluster sampling. Data were collected using a semistructured questionnaire. Data were analysed using descriptive and multiple logistics regression at 95% CI using STATA 14. *Results.* Overall, 57.9% of respondents were males, and average age was 34 years. Households' profiles such as age, gender, education, marital status, ethnicity, and religion were key predictors of NHIS active membership. Compared with other age groups, 38–47 years (AOR 0.06) and 58 years and above (AOR = 0.01), widow, divorced families, Muslims, and minority ethnic groups were less likely to have NHIS active membership. However, females (AOR = 3.92), married couples (AOR = 48.9), and people educated at tertiary level consistently had their NHIS active. Proximate factors such as education, marital status, place of residence, and NHIS status were predictors of healthcare utilization. *Conclusion.* The study concludes that households' proximate factors influence the uptake of NHIS policy and subsequent utilization of healthcare. Vulnerable population such as elderly, minority ethnic, and religious groups were less likely to renew their NHIS policy. The NHIS policy should revise the exemption bracket to wholly cover vulnerable groups such as minority ethnic and religious groups and elderly people at retiring age of 60 years.

1. Introduction

The burden of out-of-pocket payment (OOP) for health services cannot be underestimated. Out-of-pocket payment for health services continues to dominate in the health system of most countries especially those in low and middle income settings [1, 2]. The global health statistics indicate that private health expenditure (PHE) in 2012 remained as high as 62.4% in low income countries and 66% in lower middle income countries (LMICs) compared with 40.7% in higher income countries [1]. Again, out-of-pocket payment out of total PHE for this same period remained as high as 77.6% for low income countries and 86.7% for LMICs compared with 38.5% in high income countries. The high proportion of PHE demonstrates that the large global population continues to face financial burden to health services due to OOP [1].

Consequently, the World Health Organization (WHO) in 2005 responded to this by tasking member states to ensure universal health financing through the removal of OOP for health services [3]. The use of prepayment system is recognized as effective means to remove financial burden to health services especially among the poor and vulnerable population. Prepayment measures involving the use of health insurance has the ability to achieve universal health financing. This system of payment is a common practice among countries in the developing world. Countries, such as UK, Germany, France, Italy, Canada, and Australia, have employed different forms of prepayment system for health services [4, 5]. There is evidence to support that most developed countries operate public and private health insurance as prepayment system of financing healthcare. In some settings, including Australia, Canada, Denmark, and Italy, the private health insurance operates as a complement to noncovered benefits and cost sharing as well as substitute for public insurance [5]. Across different settings, these insurance services are operated under guidance of central and regional government agencies [5].

Subsequently, countries in low and middle income settings are gradually closing the gap in addressing financial risk protection for the population. Several forms of prepayment systems including national health and private health insurance have been implemented in the last two decades [6–10]. There is again the emergence of social and community-based insurance scheme, which usually forms part of a social protection programmes and policies. Many countries in Africa including Ghana, Nigeria, Tanzania Rwanda, Kenya, and Senegal as well as those in Asia are practicing a variety of social and community health insurance schemes which mobilize resources from the public and private sectors to finance healthcare [2, 11–13]. This offers implementing countries the opportunity to expand financial access to the poorest populations. The use of varying types of health insurance is a strategy adopted by governments to establish compulsory schemes for public sector workers and establish equal scheme to cover workers in the informal sector simultaneously [14–16].

Ghana's response to universal health coverage (UHC) underscores the passage of the NHI bill into law in 2003 and subsequent operation in March 2005 [8, 17, 18]. The insurance was implemented to replace the previous "cash-and-carry" system which allowed patients to pay at the point of receiving care. Similar to other developing countries [7], the health insurance had a primary objective to make healthcare affordable and increase the general utilization of drugs and healthcare particularly among the most vulnerable groups including those in the deprived areas [19, 20]. There is evidence to support that the introduction of the insurance has increased out-patient utilization and subsequently increased out-patients per-capita [17, 19, 20]. Individuals who are insured against health risks are more likely to utilize outpatients care in public health facilities, especially in lower income communities [19, 21]. These individuals enrolled in NHIS have the greater chance of visiting clinics, obtain prescription, and seek formal healthcare [19, 22]. Pregnant women, in particular, have the likelihood of utilizing prenatal care, give birth in a health facility without facing financial barriers, and again have skilled attendants present at birth [11, 23–25]. The free maternal health policy [15] has contributed to the increased uptake of antenatal care among these pregnant women.

Notwithstanding this, most households in Ghana continue to experience unmet needs to health services due to OOP at the health facility [17, 26]. There has been inconsistency in the NHIS policy enrolment and renewal especially among households in rural and per-urban communities. The inability of these households to renew their subscription is attributed to varying factors at both health systems and individual levels. For instance, proximate factors such as unemployment [27], low level of income [28–30], limited education [27–29, 31], and individual's role within their families [27] discourage households from enrolling into the scheme. This apparently suggests that the health systems and sociodemographic factors of some households limit them from enrolling into the NHIS subscription, thereby preventing UHC. Subsequently, among the population who are able to register for the scheme, there has been inconsistency in renewal and utilization of healthcare. However, there is dearth of evidence that explores the influence of households' sociodemographic factors on NHIS active membership. This paper sought to examine how these factors influence active membership and subsequent utilization of health service among households in the Upper Denkyira East Municipality of Ghana. The evidence would inform NHIS policy decision, for instance, setting vulnerability exemption criteria for marginalized population.

Proximate Predictors of National Health Insurance Policy Uptake in Ghana. In Ghana, the sociodemographic information of households influences NHIS uptake. The sociodemographic information influences households' decision to enrol and renew their NHIS policy. These factors are mostly related to the social, economic, demographic, and health status of households [27–36]. Across different regional and geographic boundaries, social factor such as gender influences NHIS policy enrolment [27, 28, 30, 32, 34]. Past studies, for instance, have showed that females have more propensities to enrol and renew their NHIS policy compared with males [30, 31, 33]. Across different studies, females are 1.2–1.8 times [30, 33] and 1.4–1.9 times [31, 34] more likely to enrol and renew their NHIS policy subscription, respectively. The increased participation of females in the NHIS policy is mostly linked to their motherly role and vulnerability to healthcare. Similarly, married individuals in Ghana stand higher odds of enrolling and renewing their NHIS policy [34, 35]. Those in their reproductive age, for instance, are about 1.3 times (95% CI; 1.12, 1.73) more likely to enrol into the NHIS policy compared with singles [35]. The increased participation of this group in the NHIS is attributed to their perception towards the cost of seeking care. This population is more susceptible to the burden of OOP of care and subsequently influences their increased participation in the NHIS policy.

The religious affiliations of households have showed to influence their NHIS policy ownership. In some settings, including the Eastern and Central Regions of Ghana, previous studies have showed that households affiliated to some religion including Christianity, Islam, and Tradition were more likely to have NHIS active membership compared with those who were not affiliated to any religion [29, 31]. However, in a related study in the Upper West Region of Ghana, the increase in NHIS policy ownership according to religious affiliation varied based on gendered identity. For instance, males who were Muslims were more likely to have never enrol and to drop out of the NHIS policy compared with their Christian counterparts (OR = 2.6 and OR = 1.7, resp.). However, females who belonged to Muslim and Traditional religion were more likely to have enrolled (OR = 2.1 and OR = 1.6) compared to their Christian counterparts [25]. This difference could be attributed to the fact that the Upper West Region is a Muslim dominated setting.

Furthermore, the age of household members has been extensively demonstrated as a predictor of NHIS policy ownership [28–30, 33, 35]. In several studies, the odds of enrolling and renewing NHIS policy increase with the age of household [27–29, 31]. Among different age groups, previous evidence showed that the elderly people of 60–70 years and above stand at greater odds of enrolling and renewing their NHIS policy. Across different studies, the elderly people of about 60–70 years and above are about 1.8–4.2 times (mean = 2.45) more likely to enrol and renew their NHIS policy compared with those below this age category [29–33]. In the Eastern and Central regions of Ghana, for instance, the odds of enrolment into the NHIS among people in the richest quintile increase with the age; those aged 70 years and above were 13.6 times more likely to have NHIS active membership compared with the younger population [29]. The variation in NHIS policy ownership among different age categories further varies with vulnerability and gender identity. In some instances, vulnerable population including children and young women are more likely to own NHIS policy compared with other groups [30, 37]. However, previous evidence has showed that, among women in their reproductive ages, those in their 45–49 years were 0.64 times less likely to enrol in the NHIS scheme compared with those below 45 years [35]. The age, vulnerability, and gender disparity to the NHIS policy ownership are directly linked to various exemptions reserved for some people including children, pregnant women, and aged and marginalized groups [17, 19]. Also, the size of individual households predicts their NHIS policy ownership. The odds of enrolling and renewing NHIS policy decreases with household size [28, 32]. In a previous study, individuals with a larger household size, for instance, 12 and above (AOR = 0.33; 95% CI; 0.24, 0.45) were less likely to enrol in the NHIS scheme [32]. The burden of enrolling and renewing the NHIS policy could be challenging for individuals with a higher household size. This could be attributed to the increased charge or one-off payment for clients, especially if they are not well resourced.

In the Ghanaian setting, the ability of households to enrol and renew their NHIS policy is associated with the wealth quintiles mostly linked to income. It is previously reported that households with higher socioeconomic status have higher odds to enrol and renew their NHIS policy compared with those in poor socioeconomic standings [28–30]. The odds of enrolling and renewing NHIS policy among households in the highest socioeconomic status vary, ranging from about 1.6 to 4.1 times, higher than those in the lowest socioeconomic groups [27, 30]. This difference further varies by gender and age groups. In a previous study, for instance, the poorest males were 3.4 times less likely to enrol into the NHIS policy compared to their rich counterparts [25]. In the same instance, females in the poorest category were 3.8 times more likely to have never enrolled in the NHIS compared with those in the richest group [25]. Previous studies have again showed that, among women in their reproductive age, those in the richer (OR = 1.7; 95% CI; 1.2, 2.3) and richest wealth quintile (OR = 1.4; 95% 0.98, 2.11) were more likely to enrol in the NHIS policy [35]. Similarly, across different age groups, older people in the third (OR = 2.5; 95% CI; 1.0, 6.0) and fourth wealth quintile (OR = 3.8; 95% CI; 1.5, 9.4) were more likely to enrol in the NHIS policy compared to other groups [36]. This demonstrates that the variation in NHIS policy ownership among the poor and rich further differs according to different sociodemographic information such as gender and age.

Across different settings, the increase in the education level of households increases the odds of enrolling and renewing NHIS policy [27–29, 31]. It is previously reported that individuals educated at higher level, preferably tertiary, have higher odds of enrolling and renewing their NHIS policy. The increase in the odds of enrolling and renewing NHIS among households educated at tertiary level varies, ranging from about 2.1 to 5.9 times more higher than those with lower or no education [27, 28, 31]. Similarly, the increased odds of enrolling and renewing NHIS policy among educated households vary depending on the wealth quintiles. In a previous study, for instance, the odds of enrolling in the NHIS policy among clients educated at tertiary level increase from 29 for individuals in the first poorest quintile compared with 9.12 and 2.4 for the third and fourth quintile, respectively [29]. Again, the influences of educational attainment on NHIS policy ownership varies depending on the gender identify. Previous study on the Upper West Region of Ghana showed that males with primary or no education were more likely to have never enrolled (OR = 4.9 and OR = 6.9, resp.) and to drop out (OR = 4.8 and OR = 3.3, resp.) compared with university/college education [25]. Similarly, females with primary or no education had higher odds of never enrolled (OR = 12.8 and OR = 23.9, resp.) and drop out (OR = 1.6 and 2.06) compared with those educated at tertiary level [25].

Additionally, the health status of individuals influences their decision to continuously enrol and renew their NHIS policy. In previous studies, individuals with poor health status were about 1.13–1.9 times more likely to have NHIS active membership compared with those in good health [31, 34]. For instance, individuals with self-reported chronic conditions [30] and hospitalised [36] were about 1.9–2.2 times and 4.4 times, respectively, are more likely to enrol in NHIS scheme compared with those with no such conditions. The increased participation of people with chronic health condition especially the older population in the NHIS policy could be attributed to frequent healthcare needs. People who have poor health condition are at greater risk of experiencing health complications, which require immediate healthcare needs.

The responsible person to head a family influences their ability to enrol and renew their NHIS policy. Households headed by a male have showed to have increased odds (OR = 2.5; 95% CI; 1.2, 5.1) of enrolling and renewing their NHIS policy. The employment status of these household heads influences their economic ability to enrol and renew the NHIS policy. In instances where the individual household heads are engaged in a formal sector employment, they stand a higher propensity (OR = 3.7) to enrol and renew their NHIS policy [27].

2. Methods

2.1. Study Site. The study was conducted in the Upper Denkyira East Municipality. The Municipality covers a total land area of 1,700 square kilometers, which is about 17% of total land of Central Region, one of the four most deprived regions in Ghana. The municipality accommodates an estimated population of 79,793 people in 2013 [38]. Children under one year constitute 2,502 people whereas children under 5 years constitute 15,636 as of 2013. The municipality has 22 health facilities, including 17 public and 5 private facilities as of 2013 [38]. There were a total of 12 functional CHIP zones in the municipality in 2013 [38]. Social services such as schools and health facilities are located around the urban settings leaving the vast rural areas underserved and underdeveloped. The major economic activities are peasant farming and small scale alluvium mining along the basin of Ofin River. The municipality is known as one of the settings with poor health outcomes due to weakness in the municipal health systems and again ranked low on all poverty and economic indicators. The road network is poor with some portions unmotorable during the rainy season. There is also long distance to health centers and again high transport cost to service delivery centers. These weaknesses present unbearable challenges to the population in meeting their health service needs.

2.2. Study Design. The study used a cross-sectional design with quantitative methods of data collection. The design was used to collect data from all prospective respondents over three-month period (3 months, February, 2015–April, 2015). The cross-sectional design is relevant to measure the sociodemographic predictors of NHIS active membership and healthcare utilization. This was applicable as the researchers aimed to examine factors that influence active membership and service utilization. The quantitative data helped to make inferences about the situation of NHIS active membership within the municipality.

2.3. Sample Size and Sampling. The sample size was estimated using Cochran's [39, 40] sample size formula ($n_0 = (Z^2 * (p)(q))/d^2$), where z value = 1.96 or 95% confidence level, p = proportion of population enrolled in NHIS, d = degree

of freedom, and $q = 1 - p$). A proportion of 33% clients enrolled in the NHIS in the Upper Denkyira Municipality [38] was used to estimate the sample size. The formulae use a "z value" of 1.96 or 95% confidence, significance level of 0.05, and degree of freedom of 0.05. The first stage of the calculation arrived at 339.75, approximate of 340 respondents. The calculation further allowed a 10% nonresponse rate and design effects of 1.06 to arrive at 380 respondents.

The households for the study were identified through a multistage cluster and simple random sampling approaches. The first stage sampling identified communities in the Upper Denkyira Municipality. The communities sampled were Zongo, Dunkwa-Soro, Atechem, Mfuom, Kadadwen, and Compound [38]. The selected communities had a health center or clinic that accepts clients using NHIS. The second stage used simple random sampling to select households in each of the communities. In all, a maximum of 380 households were enrolled into the study. The researchers zoned the principal streets in each of the communities as initial point before moving from house to house. Numerical order of house numbers was used as a sampling frame. In each of the household visited, the study enrolled the head of the household as the respondent. All the heads of the households that were approached during the study were made to pick from a paper with an inscription "Yes" and "No" and all those who picked "Yes" and consented to participate (92%) were enrolled as respondents. This approach was repeated until the sample size of 380 households was reached. In all, less than 10% of prospective respondents answered "No." Again, in instances, where none of the household members met the inclusion criteria, the research team moved to the next household. Household in this context was operationally defined as individual or a group of people who live together in the same house or compound and share the same house-keeping arrangements [41] and depend on a common source of income for subsistence.

2.4. Data Collection. Data were obtained from respondents through administration of structured questions on face-to-face basis. Questions that were presented to the respondents were related to the sociodemographic information, current status of NHIS, and access and use of healthcare. The sociodemographic variables included gender, age, marital status, highest education, years of schooling, and religion. Questions on NHIS were related to the current status of clients on the scheme.

2.5. Data Analysis. The study used descriptive and inferential statistics to present results. The analysis first computed percentage distribution of the household profile of respondents. These frequencies and percentage distribution were grouped according to the type of variable-continuous and categorical. The continuous variables were age, monthly income, household size, and the number of dependents. The categorical variables were gender, education, marital status, occupation, place of residence, ethnic background, religion, NHIS status, and healthcare utilization. The analysis further used bivariate and multivariate logistics regression to examine the influence of sociodemographic factors on NHIS active membership. Odds ratio (OR) and adjusted odds ratio (AOR) were used to report the strength of influence of the sociodemographic factors on NHIS active membership. The main outcome variable for the analysis was the current NHIS status of respondents. Healthcare utilization was measured using individuals who had visited the health facility for care with the health insurance in the last twelve (12) months. The analysis was presented at 95% significance level at $\alpha = 0.01$, $\alpha = 0.03$, and $\alpha = 0.05$. The analyses set the reference group for both OR (odds ratio) and AOR (adjusted odds ratio) as 1.0. All statistical analyses were estimated using STATA version (14).

3. Results

3.1. Sociodemographic Characteristics of Respondents. A total of 380 respondents were recruited for the study. The average age of respondents was 34 years, and about 47.1% were between 18 and 27 years. Males (57.9%) dominated females in the study. More than a third (46.9%) of respondents had tertiary level education, whilst less than a fifth each had secondary, primary, and no formal education (Table 1). A little above half, 52.4%, were singles whilst more than one-third (36.5%) described their marital status as married.

More than a third of respondents (43.75%) were engaged in semiskilled employment, 36.9% as skilled workers, and 19.29% were not engaged in any employment. A little over a third, 34.4%, of respondents disclosed their places of residence as old town, 25.47% as peri-urban, and 18.16% as *Zongo* (literally means in Hausa dialect, "temporal abode," a suburb in a community where Muslims and other people from the savannah region live). As high as 7 in 10 and 6 in 10 said yes to use of NHIS and healthcare, respectively.

The median and average monthly income of respondents were GHC 200 (USD 52.35) (using 2016 exchange rate of GHC 3.82 = 1 USD equivalent) and GHC 412.94 (USD 108.12), respectively (Table 1). The mean household size was 5 persons per household. Average number of dependents was 3 persons and minimum and maximum was 1 and 12 persons, respectively. Most respondents, 80% and 53.9%, respectively, had Christian religious and Denkyira ethnic background.

3.2. The Influence of Sociodemographic Factors on NHIS Uptake. Table 2 presents the influence of sociodemographic factors on NHIS status. Sociodemographic factors such as age, monthly income, household size, gender, marital status, education, employment, place of resident, and religion influence the NHIS status of households in the crude odds ratio. The odds of renewing NHIS policy increased with the age of respondents. Households members within the age group of 28–37 years (OR = 3.15; 95% CI; 1.88, 5.29), 38–47 years (OR = 2.41; 95% CI; 1.37, 4.24), 48–57 years (OR = 3.13; 1.40, 6.93), and 58+ (OR = 3.0; 95% 1.27, 7.05) were more likely to renew their NHIS policy compared with those below 27 years. Similarly, females (95% CI 0.98, 2.61) and individuals who were married (OR = 4.27; 95% CI; 2.78, 6.54) were more likely to have their NHIS status active compared with males and singles, respectively.

TABLE 1: Sociodemographic characteristics of respondents.

Variable	Frequency	Percentage (%)
Continuous variable		
Age		
18–27	179	47.11
28–37	80	21.05
38–47	60	15.79
48–57	33	8.68
58+	28	7.37
Median; mean (SD); Min/Max	*28.5; 34 (13.96)*	
Monthly income (GHC)[1]		
>200	130	51.18
200–500	45	17.72
500–1000	64	25.20
1000–1500	9	3.54
1500+	6	2.36
Median; mean (SD); Min/Max	*200; 412.94 (417.55); 10/2000*	
Household size		
1–3	64	17.07
4–6	195	52.00
7–9	116	30.93
Mean (SD); Min/Max	*5.3 (1.93); 1/9*	
Number of dependents		
1–3	147	61.51
4–6	70	29.29
7–9	13	5.44
10+	9	3.77
Mean (SD); Min/Max	*3.4 (2.3); 1/12*	
Categorical variable		
Gender		
Male	219	57.94
Female	159	42.06
Education		
No formal education	49	12.93
Primary	59	15.57
Secondary	79	20.84
Tertiary	178	46.97
Other	14	3.69
Marital status		
Single	199	52.37
Married	139	36.58
Divorce	27	7.11
Widow	15	3.95
Occupation		
Skilled	136	36.96
Semiskilled	161	43.75
Unemployed	71	19.29
Place of residence		
Slum	22	5.33
Zongo	67	18.16
Old Town	127	34.42
Peri-Urban	94	25.47
New-Site	59	15.99
Ethnic background		
Denkyira	185	53.94
Other	158	46.06
Religion		
Christianity	296	80.00

TABLE 1: Continued.

Variable	Frequency	Percentage (%)
Islam	74	20.00
NHIS active		
Yes	277	74.26
No	96	25.74
Use of Healthcare		
Yes	215	63.61
No	123	36.39

[1]GHC 3.82 = USD 1, exchange rates from May 4, 2016.

The odds of enrolling and renewing NHIS subscription increased with the level of education. Individuals who had some educational credentials up to primary (OR = 2.22; 95% CI; 1.27, 3.87), secondary (OR = 2.71; 95% CI; 1.65, 4.47), and tertiary level (OR = 4.0; 95% CI; 2.76, 5.79) were more likely to have NHIS active membership compared with those with no education. Again, there was increase in the trends of the odds of using NHIS with the sector of employment. Individuals with public sector employment (OR = 4.5; 95% CI; 2.09, 9.68), Trading (OR = 3.0; 95% CI; 1.60, 5.61), and self-employment (OR = 4.70; 95% CI; 2.37, 9.30) were more likely to have active membership compared with those with no employment. Individuals who described their residency as *New sites and peri-urban* were 2.57 and 5.33 times, respectively, more likely to have their NHIS active compared with those who described their residence as *Slums*.

The income level of respondents increases the odds of enrolling and renewing NHIS policy. Individuals who earned above GHC 500–GHC 1000 (OR = 5.3; 95% CI; 2.69, 10.41) and 200–500 (OR = 2.63; 95% CI; 1.37, 5.17) were more likely to have their NHIS active compared with those who earned below GHC 200 (USD 52.37). Individuals who had more than 4–6 household size were 2.82 times more likely to have their NHIS status active compared with those who had less 1–3 household size. Individuals who mentioned their religious affiliation as Islam were 0.47 times (95% CI; 0.27, 0.80) less likely to have their NHIS status active.

Sociodemographic factors such as age, gender, marital status, education, ethnicity, and education consistently increased the odds of having active membership in the NHIS after the inclusion of other co-covariates. Individuals who were 38–47 years (AOR 0.06) and 58 years and above (AOR = 0.01) were, respectively, less likely to have their NHIS active after adjusting for other covariates. Consistently, being a female had a higher likelihood of having NHIS status as active AOR = 3.92 (95% CI; 1.21, 12.67) after accounting for the effect of other confounding variables. Different educational levels were consistently associated with active NHIS status after adjusting for other covariates. Respondents who were married consistently had higher odds (AOR = 48.9) of having their NHIS status active after adjusting for other covariates. Similar to the univariate analysis, the odds of having NHIS status active decreased with religious background; those with Islam religious background were less likely to have their NHIS active at AOR 0.12 (95% CI; 0.03, 0.52) compared with Christians after accounting for other covariates.

3.3. The Influence of Households' Profile on Healthcare Utilization. Table 3 presents the influence of households profile on healthcare utilization within the Upper Denkyira Municipality. Females were 1.16 times (95% CI; 0.14, 1.61) more likely to utilize healthcare compared with males. Respondents who had tertiary level education were 2.44 times (95% CI; 1.20, 4.97) more likely to use healthcare compared with those who reported no formal education. There was an increased odd of using healthcare with the marital status of respondents; those who reported as married as well as widow, respectively, were 1.47 times (95% CI; 1.00, 2.16) and 12.99 times (95% CI; 1.70, 99.37) more likely to use healthcare compared with those who were single. There was again increase in trends of the odds of using healthcare with employment; those who described their employment status as self-employed were 4.00 (95% CI; 2.06, 7.74) times more likely to use healthcare compared with those with no employment. The analysis further showed that the use of healthcare was associated with the monthly income of the respondents; those who earn more than GHC 200 (USD 52.37) and above were 2 times (95% CI; 1.09, 3.64) more likely to use healthcare compared with those who earn below GHC 200 (USD 52.37). Respondents who described their residency as peri-urban were 3.2 times more likely to use healthcare compared with those who lived in *Slums*.

Consistently, having tertiary level education had a higher likelihood of using healthcare AOR = 6.46 (95% CI; 0.89, 46.41) after accounting for the addition of other covariates like age, gender, and marital status. Also, respondents who were married and widowed consistently had higher odds (AOR = 10.32; AOR = 20.49) of using healthcare after adjusting for other covariates. Also, the place of residency of respondents was consistently associated with the use of healthcare after adjusting for the inclusion of other covariates.

4. Discussion

The study was conducted to examine households' profile that predicts NHIS active membership and subsequent utilization of healthcare in the Upper Denkyira East Municipality. The household profiles were categorized according to sociocultural, social class, economics, and spatial or geographical location.

The median and average ages of household members were 28.5 years and 34 years, respectively. The age characteristics demonstrate an active adult population in the study setting. This category of the population has the ability to contribute to the active labour force in both formal and informal sector. The trend of age distribution presents an inverse relationship between population growth and aging; an increase in the ages of the population presents a decreased population. The finding confirms similar trend of age distribution in the 2010 national population census [41]. The national population census presented an increased adult population with a decreasing aging population. Again, the study showed that more than 50% of households each constitute males and singles. The marital status of the population confirms the general characteristic of the Ghanaian population. In the recent population and housing census, singles were more dominant than married individuals [41]. However, the gender

Table 2: Logistic regression analysis of households' profile and NHIS uptake.

Variable	NHIS active membership					
	Model 1 OR	95% CI	p value	Model 2 AOR	95% CI	p value
Continuous variable						
Age						
18–27	1.00			1.00		
28–37	3.15	1.88, 5.29	**0.01**	0.47	0.06, 3.51	0.46
38–47	2.41	1.37, 4.24	**0.01**	0.06	0.00, 0.77	**0.05**
48–57	3.13	1.40, 6.93	**0.05**	0.24	0.02, 3.19	0.28
58+	3.00	1.27, 7.05	**0.01**	0.01	0.00, 0.25	**0.01**
Monthly income (GHC)[1]						
Below 200	1.0			1.00		
200–500	2.67	1.37, 5.17	**0.01**	0.96	0.17, 5.35	0.96
500–1000	5.3	2.69, 10.41	**0.01**	1.06	0.26, 4.36	0.92
1000–1500	3.5	0.72, 16.8	0.11	0.12	0.01, 1.47	
1500+	0.5	0.09, 2.72	0.42	0.23	0.02, 3.53	
Household size						
1–3	1.0			1.0		
4–6	2.82	2.04, 3.89	**0.01**	0.28	0.04, 1.64	0.16
7–9	3.07	2.00, 4.70	**0.01**	0.81	0.10, 6.35	0.84
Number of dependents						
1–3	1.0			1.0		
4–6	1.07	0.55, 2.10	0.84	3.83	0.93, 15.75	0.06
7–9	0.64	0.18, 2.24	0.48	2.84	0.17, 45.95	0.46
10+	2.54	0.31, 21.06	0.39	3.30	0.07, 155.4	0.54
Categorical variables						
Gender						
Male	1.0			1.0		
Female	3.86	0.98, 2.61	**0.00**	3.92	1.21, 12.67	**0.05**
Marital status						
Single	1.0			1.0		
Married	4.27	2.78, 6.54	**0.00**	48.9	4.46, 537	**0.01**
Divorce	2.0	0.89, 4.45	0.09	97.0	5.54, 1697	**0.01**
Widow	6.5	1.46, 28.80	0.14	2683	32.20, 2235	**0.01**
Education						
No formal education	1.0			1.0		
Primary	2.22	1.27, 3.87	**0.01**	9.87	1.52, 64.07	**0.05**
Secondary	2.71	1.65, 4.47	**0.00**	7.80	1.24, 49.10	**0.03**
Tertiary	4.0	2.76, 5.79	**0.00**	9.68	1.00, 92.92	**0.05**
Other	1.8	0.60, 5.37	0.29	15.31	0.58, 402.7	0.10
Occupation						
None	1.00			1.0		
Public sector	4.50	2.09, 9.68	**0.01**	1.85	0.14, 23.52	0.63
Farming	1.88	1.04, 3.38	**0.01**	0.69	0.05, 9.72	0.79
Trading	3.00	1.60, 5.61	**0.01**	1.38	0.09, 20.07	0.81
Apprenticeship	2.50	0.96, 6.44	0.06	2.66	0.09, 74.81	0.56
Self-employed	4.70	2.37, 9.30	**0.01**	1.77	0.08, 35.44	0.70
Other	3.31	1.89, 5.79	**0.01**	7.41	0.24, 220.6	0.24

TABLE 2: Continued.

Variable	NHIS active membership					
	Model 1 OR	95% CI	p value	Model 2 AOR	95% CI	p value
Place of residence						
Slum	1.00			1.0		
Zongo	2.67	1.55, 4.58	**0.01**	5.04	0.46, 55.38	0.18
Old Town	3.37	2.39, 5.88	**0.01**	3.57	0.41, 30.56	0.24
New site	2.57	1.63, 4.05	**0.01**	7.07	0.49, 102.1	0.15
Peri-urban	5.33	2.61, 10.86	**0.01**	1.92	0.16, 22.77	0.60
Other	1.5	0.42, 5.31	0.53	1		
Ethnic background						
Denkyira	1.00			1.0		
Other	0.69	0.41, 1.13	0.14	0.17	0.03, 0.78	**0.01**
Religion						
Christianity	1.0			1.0		
Islam	0.47	0.27, 0.80	**0.01**	0.12	0.03, 0.52	**0.01**

[1]GHC 3.82 = USD 1, exchange rates from May 4, 2016; OR = odds ratio; AOR = adjusted odds ratio; CI = confidence interval; Outcome measures: NHIS uptake; significance level: $\alpha = 0.01$, $\alpha = 0.03$, and $\alpha = 0.05$; OR and AOR for reference group were set as 1.0.

disparity contradicts the national dynamics. In the Ghanaian population, females generally have a higher ratio compared with men—1 : 6 according 2010 housing and population census [41].

The study showed that the median and average monthly incomes of households were GHC 200 (USD 52.35) and GHC 412.94 (USD 108.12), respectively. The average monthly income in particular was about 1.9 times higher than 2015 national monthly minimum wage of GHC 210 (USD 54.97) [42]. The rate suggests that households were relatively earning higher from their respective employment. This finding implies that the household members were relatively better-off when compared with the national standard. However, this may not translate to the actual standard of living among households in real terms. The households' welfare and standard of living could also be influenced by the size of individual household members. The average household size of 5 members could imply significant economic burden on the families especially when compared with the relative monthly income.

The study showed that 74% of household members were insured under the NHIS. This finding implies that most households were using the NHIS as their primary source of seeking healthcare. This number is about 2 times higher than the 2012 and 2013 national level active membership which stands at 37% and 38%, respectively. Again, the 74% insured clients were about 1.2 times higher than a similar study in Barekese district in the Ashanti Region of Ghana [28, 32]. The high rate of active policy membership may help to reduce the burden associated with out-of-pocket payment for healthcare. The discussion demonstrates that, across different districts of Ghana, active membership of NHIS differs. The variation in active policy ownership across different districts and regions could be attributed to varying factors, which may include individual sociodemographic factors.

The households profile such as age, gender, education, marital status, and ethnic and religious background influenced the NHIS active membership. These factors significantly influenced NHIS status, either likely increase or reduce active membership. The marital status of household members significantly influenced NHIS active membership. Married household members were more likely to have their NHIS active compared with singles. This finding could be attributed to the fact that married couples might fear the burden of out-of-pocket payment of healthcare particularly when there is a dependant. This finding confirms earlier studies in Ghana, which found that married individuals have higher odds of enrolling and renewing NHIS policy [34, 35]. This argument demonstrates that across different settings of Ghana, people who are married stand a higher chance of enrolling and renewing their NHIS policy. This demonstrates their continuous search for financial risk protection to healthcare.

In this study, females were more likely to have active NHIS policy. This finding could be attributed to the differences in health seeking behaviour between females and males. Females seem more responsive to sickness and will report promptly to health facilities than men who would usually wait till their condition deteriorates due to masculinity. Again, females are perceived as vulnerable especially during pregnancy and more prone to seeking care at the health facility. This may probably influence their decision to continually enrol and renew NHIS policy. This could also be linked to the free maternal health policy that grants exemption to payment of NHIS among pregnant women. This finding corroborate with previous studies across different settings of Ghana [30, 31, 33–35]. In a previous finding, females had increased odds of enrolling and renewing their NHIS policy compared with males. For instance, married women in their reproductive ages have demonstrated to be at greater odds in enrolling and renewing their NHIS policy [35]. The discussion has

TABLE 3: Logistic regression analysis of households' profile and healthcare utilization.

Variable	Use of healthcare with NHIS					
	Model 1 OR	95% CI	*p* value	Model 2 AOR	95% CI	*p* value
Continuous variable						
Age						
18–27	1.00			1.00		
28–37	0.64	0.34, 1.18	0.15	0.51	0.05, 4.95	0.56
38–47	0.39	0.18, 0.84	**0.05**	0.18	0.12, 2.73	0.22
48–57	0.84	0.31, 2.23	0.73	0.28	0.02, 2.86	0.34
58+	2.81	0.79, 9.95	0.10	12.53	0.31, 493.09	0.17
Monthly income (GHC)[1]						
Below 200	1.00			1.00		
200–500	2.00	1.09, 3.64	**0.01**	1.37	0.29, 8.49	0.39
500–1000	1.10	0.66, 1.82	0.70	0.39	0.07, 2.20	0.29
1000–1500	2.25	0.69, 7.30	0.17	1.01	0.04, 21.07	0.99
1500+	2.5	0.48, 12.88	0.27	1.00	-	
Household size						
1–3	1.00			1.00		
4–6	0.72	0.38, 1.37	0.38	1.20	0.31, 4.39	0.78
7–9	0.65	0.32, 1.32	0.24	0.23	0.04, 1.36	0.11
Number of dependents						
1–3	1.00			1.00		
4–6	0.82	0.43, 1.53	0.53	0.73	0.20, 2.64	0.63
7–9	1.40	0.34, 5.68	0.63	0,09	0.003, 2.92	0.18
10+	1.00	0.22, 4.38	1.00	2.85	0.03, 162.01	0.61
Gender						
Male	1.00			1.00		
Female	1.16	1.17, 2.35	**0.01**	0.48	0.14, 1.61	0.23
Education						
No formal education	1.00			1.00		
Primary	1.76	0.73, 4.27	0.19	1.00		
Secondary	1.82	0.82, 4.02	0.13	2.39	0.44, 12.80	0.30
Tertiary	2.44	1.20, 4.97	0.01	6.46	0.89, 46.41	**0.05**
Other	0.95	0.17, 5.28	0.95	4.92	0.63, 37.98	0.12
Marital status						
Single	1.00			1.00		
Married	1.47	1.00, 2.16	**0.05**	10.32	1.24, 85.94	**0.05**
Divorce	1.66	0.72, 3.80	0.22	6.89	0.86, 129.89	0.19
Widow	12.99	1.70, 99.37	**0.01**	20.49	0.63, 37.98	**0.05**
Occupation						
None	1.00			1.00		
Public sector	1.13	0.64, 1.98	0.66	0.42	0.04, 4.23	0.46
Farming	1.40	0.72, 2.71	0.32	1.20	0.09, 14.76	0.88
Trading	1.18	0.66, 2.08	0.56	0.47	0.03, 5.86	0.56
Apprenticeship	1.22	0.50, 2.94	0.65	3.24	0.18, 78.29	0.46
Self employed	4.00	2.06, 7.74	**0.01**	1.82	0.05, 65.81	0.74
Other	2.11	1.20, 3.69	**0.01**	1.00		

TABLE 3: Continued.

Variable	Use of healthcare with NHIS					
	Model 1 OR	95% CI	p value	Model 2 AOR	95% CI	p value
Place of residence						
Slum	1.00			1.00		
Zongo	1.65	0.61, 4.41	0.31	10.32	1.24, 85.94	**0.03**
Old town	1.61	0.67, 3.88	0.28	6.89	0.36, 129.89	**0.05**
Peri-urban	3.20	1.13, 9.07	**0.01**	20.49	0.57, 736.36	**0.05**
Other	2.75	0.24, 30.51	0.41	1.00		
Use NHIS [active]						
No	1.00			1.00		
Yes	1.67	0.95, 2.92	**0.05**	2.19	1.18, 4.07	**0.01**
Ethnic background						
Denkyira	1.00			1.00		
Other	0.75	0.45, 1.24	0.27	0.38	0.10, 1.46	0.16
Religion						
Christianity	1.00			1.00		
Islam	0.80	0.45, 1.45	0.466	1.18	0.23, 5.44	0.82

[1]GHC 3.82 = USD 1, exchange rates from May 4, 2016; OR = odds ratio; AOR = adjusted odds ratio; CI = confidence interval; outcome measures: use of healthcare; significance level: $\alpha = 0.01$ and $\alpha = 0.05$; OR and AOR for reference group were set as 1.0.

implication that, across different settings of Ghana, females especially those in their reproductive ages are more profound to enrol and renew their NHIS policy.

The age of individual household members influenced their decision to enrol and renew NHIS policy. The elderly people of age 58 years and above were less likely to have active membership to the NHIS though these groups frequently sought healthcare. This finding could be attributed to a number of factors including households financing sources for the scheme. For instance, the NHIS in Ghana has exemption for the aged 70 years and above. This exemption is an effort to cover the indigents otherwise classified as vulnerable including aged, children, pregnant women, and people with disabilities. However, the existing criteria peg exemption at 70 or more years and may have significant implication on payment sources for clients between 58 and 70 years. In Ghana, the compulsory retiring and retiring ages for the formal sector are 55 and 60 years, respectively. With the current exemption age pegged at 70 years and above, people who compulsorily retire from the public service may have to battle with the premium payment which invariably would restrict access to healthcare. Pension payments are so low that pensioners find it difficult to make ends meet let alone think about health expenditure. Individuals who are not resourced financially may not be able to enrol or renew their insurance policy. This is particularly true among elderly persons in the informal sector within the Upper Denkyira East Municipality who are predominantly peasant farmers with no regular pension scheme. This finding reinforces previous studies which suggest that the inability to pay for insurance premium constitutes the most frequently cited reason for limited enrolment [43, 44]. However, the finding generally contradicts previous studies that examined the influence of age on NHIS policy ownership. In previous studies, enrolment and renewal of NHIS policy increase with age. Elderly people of about 60–70 years and above have higher odds of enrolling and renewing into the scheme. Again, across people in the richest wealth quintile, the elderly population of 70 years and above have an increased odd of enrolling and renewing their NHIS. The differences in enrolment and renewal of NHIS among households in the current settings and those in previous studies could be attributed to the funding source to support enrolment.

The ethnic and religious affiliation of households plays a significant role in enrolling and renewing NHIS policy. The minority ethnic groups and Muslims were less likely to enrol and renew their NHIS policy. This finding could be explained by varying factors including limited funds, religious-cultural issues, and health seeking behaviour. This finding confirms previous evidence on the role of religion and ethnicity in determining enrolment and renewal of NHIS policy in Ghana. The role of religion in determining NHIS policy ownership varies according to geographical location and gendered identity. In the Upper West Region, previous finding showed that males who were Muslims were more likely to never enrol or drop out of their NHIS policy compared with Christians [25]. However, females who were Muslims had contrary exposure, where they were more likely to enrol and renew their NHIS policy compared with Christians [25]. Again, in some settings including Eastern and Central Regions of Ghana, individuals affiliated to a particular religion including Christianity, Muslim, and Tradition had higher odds of enrolling and renewing their NHIS policy [29, 31]. The variation in enrolment into the scheme according to religious affiliation could be attributed to religious-cultural beliefs and health seeking behaviour. The argument surrounding this generally demonstrates that there is variation in the enrolment and renewal of NHIS policy according to religious affiliation.

The study also found that the level of education consistently influenced households' decision to enrol and renew their NHIS policy. The odds of enrolling and renewing NHIS policy increased with the level of educational attainment. Individuals educated at secondary and tertiary level had higher odds of enrolling and renewing their NHIS policy. The finding implies that education plays a significant role in educating households about the important of enrolling and renewing NHIS policy. This finding confirms previous studies in Ghana [25, 27–29, 31] and other West Africa settings including Senegal and Mali [45]. Across these settings, individuals educated at the higher level, preferably secondary and tertiary education, were more profound to enrol and renew their NHIS policy [25, 27–29, 31]. However, individuals with low or no education are more likely to have never enrolled or possibly drop out of the scheme [25]. In some instances, the increased odds of enrolling and renewing NHIS policy further vary according to the wealth quintiles of the individuals. The increased policy enrolment among educated individuals could be linked to their basic understanding of the need to have financial risk protection. Again, in some instances, individuals that are educated at the higher level but fall within the lower wealth quintiles have higher odds of enrolling and renewing their NHIS policy compared with those in the wealthier quintile [29]. This demonstrates that, across different settings, education plays significant role in ensuring enrolment and renewal into NHIS policy. However, this could vary depending on the level and socioeconomic status of the individuals.

Limitation. The study was limited to only households in the Upper Denkyira East Municipality, without the perspectives of NHIS staff, health services providers, and health systems planners. Again, the study recruited a sample of 380 respondents across different communities to represent the entire municipality. In spite of these, the study employed several scientific scrutinies such as random sampling, pretesting of tools, informed consent processes, statistical analysis, and discussions of findings with relevant literature.

5. Conclusion

In this study, we examined the influence of households' profile on the use of NHIS and healthcare in the Upper Denkyira East Municipality. The factors influencing NHIS and use of healthcare were limited to only sociodemographic information compared with previous studies where management and health authorities' related factors are considered. Despite these, this study has provided insightful evidence to inform policy decision.

The study concludes that household's profile such as age, gender, income, education, and marital status influences individual's decision to renew their NHIS policy. Individuals who are married, females, and those with some educational credentials up to primary, secondary, and tertiary level were more likely to renew their NHIS policy. However, vulnerable population such as the elderly of 57–69 years and minority ethnic and religious groups including Muslims were less likely to renew their NHIS policy. The NHIS policy should revise

the exemption bracket to wholly cover vulnerable groups such as minority ethnic and religious groups and elderly people at retiring age of 60 years. This would help to remove out-of-pocket payment for healthcare for these vulnerable populations.

Disclosure

This is to certify that this paper is a finding from original work. The authors have duly acknowledged the work(s) of others they used in writing this article/manuscript and have duly cited all such work(s) in the text as well as in the list of the references and they have presented within quotes all the original sentences and phrases.

Authors' Contributions

Eric Badu wrote the first draft of the manuscript. Eric Badu, Peter Agyei-Baffour, Isaac Ofori Acheampong, Kwasi Addai-Donkor, and Maxwell Preprah Opoku performed the data analysis and interpretation of results. All authors reviewed and made inputs into the intellectual content and agreed on its submission for publication.

Acknowledgments

The authors wish to thank the Municipal NHIS Authorities and Health Directorate of Upper Denkyira East Municipal Assembly. They again wish to thank the Committee on

Human Research, Publications and Ethics, Kwame Nkrumah University of Science and Technology (KNUST), for approving the study protocol prior to its implementation. They are grateful to all the study participants for their support during the data collection.

References

[1] World Health Organization, *World Health Statistics 2015*, World Health Organization, 2015.

[2] S. Kwon, "Health care financing in Asia: Key issues and challenges," *Asia-Pacific Journal of Public Health*, vol. 23, no. 5, pp. 651–661, 2011.

[3] World Health Organization (WHO), *Book Health System Financing: The Path to Universal Coverage*, World Health Organization, 2010.

[4] S. Boyle, *Health Systems in Transition: United Kingdom (England)*, WHO Regional Office for Europe on behalf of the European Observatory on Health Systems and Policies, Copenhagen, Denmark.

[5] E. Mossialos, M. Wenzl, R. Osborn, and C. Anderson, *International Profiles of Health Care Systems*, The Commonwealth Fund, 2016.

[6] G. Carrin, M.-P. Waelkens, and B. Criel, "Community-based health insurance in developing countries: A study of its contribution to the performance of health financing systems," *Tropical Medicine & International Health*, vol. 10, no. 8, pp. 799–811, 2005.

[7] UNICEF, *National Health Insurance in Asia And Africa: Advancing Equitable Social Health Protection to Achieve Universal Health Coverage*, United Nations Children's Fund, New York, NY, USA, 2012.

[8] B. Garshong and J. Akazili, *Universal Health Coverage Assessment*, Global Network for Health Equity (GNHE), 2015.

[9] D. A. Adewole, M. Dairo, and O. Bolarinwa, "Awareness and Coverage of the National Health Insurance Scheme among Formal Sector Workers in Ilorin, Nigeria," *African Journal of Biomedical Research*, vol. 19, pp. 1–10, 2016.

[10] E. F. Adebayo, O. A. Uthman, C. S. Wiysonge, E. A. Stern, K. T. Lamont, and J. E. Ataguba, "A systematic review of factors that affect uptake of community-based health insurance in low-income and middle-income countries," *BMC Health Services Research*, vol. 15, no. 1, article no. 543, 2015.

[11] J. Mensah, J. R. Oppong, and C. M. Schmidt, "Ghana's national health insurance scheme in the context of the health MDGs: an empirical evaluation using propensity score matching," *Health Economics*, vol. 19, no. 1, pp. 95–106, 2010.

[12] N. J. Blanchet, G. Fink, and I. Osei-Akoto, "The effect of Ghana's National Health Insurance Scheme on health care utilisation," *Ghana Medical Journal*, vol. 46, no. 2, pp. 76–84, 2012.

[13] J. P. Jütting, "Do community-based health insurance schemes improve poor people's access to health care? Evidence from rural senegal," *World Development*, vol. 32, no. 2, pp. 273–288, 2004.

[14] A. Creese, S. Bennett, G. Schieber, and A. Maeda, "Rural risk-sharing strategies," *World Bank Discussion Papers*, pp. 163–182, 1997.

[15] D. M. Dror and C. Jacquier, "Micro-insurance: Extending Health Insurance to the Excluded," *International Social Security Review*, vol. 52, no. 1, pp. 71–97, 1999.

[16] B. Ekman, "Community-based health insurance in low-income countries: A systematic review of the evidence," *Health Policy and Planning*, vol. 19, no. 5, pp. 249–270, 2004.

[17] S. Witter and B. Garshong, "Something old or something new? Social health insurance in Ghana," *BMC International Health and Human Rights*, vol. 9, no. 1, article 20, 2009.

[18] J. Akazili, B. Garshong, M. Aikins, J. Gyapong, and D. McIntyre, "Progressivity of health care financing and incidence of service benefits in Ghana," *Health Policy and Planning*, vol. 27, no. 1, pp. i13–i22, 2012.

[19] National Health Insurance Authority, *National Health Insurance Authority*, NHIA, 2013.

[20] National Health Insurance Authority, *National Health Insurance Scheme*, National Health Insurance Authority, 2015.

[21] M. Jowett, A. Deolalikar, and P. Martinsson, "Health insurance and treatment seeking behaviour: Evidence from a low-income country," *Health Economics*, vol. 13, no. 9, pp. 845–857, 2004.

[22] E. K. Ansah, S. Narh-Bana, S. Asiamah et al., "Effect of removing direct payment for health care on utilisation and health outcomes in Ghanaian children: A randomised controlled trial," *PLoS Medicine*, vol. 6, no. 1, Article ID e1000007, pp. 0048–0058, 2009.

[23] C. M. Schmidt, J. H. Mensah, and J. R. Oppong, "Ghana's national health insurance scheme in the context of the health MDGs–an empirical evaluation using propensity score matching," *Ruhr Economic Paper*, 2009.

[24] J. Dixon, E. Y. Tenkorang, I. N. Luginaah, V. Z. Kuuire, and G. O. Boateng, "National health insurance scheme enrolment and antenatal care among women in ghana: is there any relationship?" *Tropical Medicine & International Health*, vol. 19, no. 1, pp. 98–106, 2014.

[25] J. Dixon, I. Luginaah, and P. Mkandawire, "The National Health Insurance Scheme in Ghana's Upper West Region: A gendered perspective of insurance acquisition in a resource-poor setting," *Social Science & Medicine*, vol. 122, pp. 103–112, 2014.

[26] A. S. Preker and G. Carrin, *Health Financing for Poor People: Resource Mobilization And Risk Sharing*, World Bank Publications, 2004.

[27] K. A. Alatinga and J. J. Williams, "Towards Universal Health Coverage: Exploring the Determinants of Household Enrolment into National Health Insurance in the Kassena Nankana District, Ghana," *Ghana Journal of Development Studies*, vol. 12, no. 1-2, p. 88, 2015.

[28] S. Manortey, J. Vanderslice, S. Alder et al., "Spatial analysis of factors associated with household subscription to the National Health Insurance Scheme in rural Ghana," *Journal of Public Health in Africa*, vol. 5, no. 1, pp. 1–8, 2014.

[29] C. Jehu-Appiah, G. Aryeetey, E. Spaan, T. de Hoop, I. Agyepong, and R. Baltussen, "Equity aspects of the national health insurance scheme in Ghana: who is enrolling, who is not and why?" *Social Science & Medicine*, vol. 72, no. 2, pp. 157–165, 2011.

[30] S. Chankova, S. Sulzbach, L. Hatt et al., *An Evaluation of The Effects of The National Health Insurance Scheme in Ghana*, Abt Associates Inc, Bethesda, MD, USA, 2009.

[31] C. Jehu-Appiah, G. Aryeetey, I. Agyepong, E. Spaan, and R. Baltussen, "Household perceptions and their implications for enrolment in the National Health Insurance Scheme in Ghana," *Health Policy and Planning*, vol. 27, no. 3, pp. 222–233, 2011.

[32] S. Manortey, S. Alder, B. Crookston, T. Dickerson, J. VanDerslice, and S. Benson, "Social deterministic factors to participation in the National Health Insurance Scheme in the context of

rural Ghanaian setting," *Journal of Public Health in Africa*, vol. 5, no. 1, pp. 1–18, 2014.

[33] S. Antwi, X. Zhao, E. K. Boadi, and E. O. Koranteng, "Socio-Economic Predictors of Health Insurance Claims: Evidence from Ghana," *International Journal of Economics and Finance*, vol. 6, no. 3, 2014.

[34] D. Boateng and D. Awunyor-Vitor, "Health insurance in Ghana: Evaluation of policy holders' perceptions and factors influencing policy renewal in the Volta region," *International Journal for Equity in Health*, vol. 12, no. 1, article no. 50, 2013.

[35] H. Amu and K. S. Dickson, "Health insurance subscription among women in reproductive age in Ghana: do socio-demographics matter?" *Health Economics Review (HER)*, vol. 6, article 24, 2016.

[36] D. Parmar, G. Williams, F. Dkhimi et al., "Enrolment of older people in social health protection programs in West Africa - Does social exclusion play a part?" *Social Science & Medicine*, vol. 119, pp. 36–44, 2014.

[37] S. Antwi, X. Zhao, and E. O. Koranteng, "Gender disparities in ghana national health insurance claims: an econometric analysis," *International Journal of Business and Social Research*, vol. 4, pp. 70–81, 2014.

[38] Upper Denkyira Municipal, *Municipal profile*, Ministry of Local Governance & Rural Development, 2013.

[39] W. G. Cochran, *Sampling Techniques*, John Wiley & Sons, 2007.

[40] L. Naing, T. Winn, and B. Rusli, "Practical issues in calculating the sample size for prevalence studies," *Archives of Orofacial Sciences*, vol. 1, pp. 9–14, 2006.

[41] Ghana Statistical Service [GSS], *2010 Population and Housing Census*, Ghana Statistical Services, 2012.

[42] "Government announces increment in minimum wage/salaries for public workers," http://www.ghana.gov.gh/index.php/media-center/news/2023-%09government-announces-increment-in-minimum-wage-salaries-for-public-workers.

[43] S. Sulzbach, B. Garshong, and G. Owusu-Banahene, "Evaluating the effects of the national health insurance act in ghana: baseline report," *Partners for Health Reformplus*, 2005.

[44] F. P. Diop, "Determinants of financial stability of mutual health organizations in the thies region of senegal: household survey component," *Partners for Health Reformplus*, 2006.

[45] S. Chankova, S. Sulzbach, and F. Diop, "Impact of mutual health organizations: evidence from West Africa," *Health Policy and Planning*, vol. 23, no. 4, pp. 264–276, 2008.

13

Views of First-Time Expectant Mothers on Breastfeeding: A Study in Three Health Facilities in Accra, Ghana

Freda Intiful, Claudia Osei, Rebecca Steele-Dadzie, Ruth Nyarko, and Matilda Asante

School of Biomedical and Allied Health Sciences, Department of Nutrition and Dietetics, University of Ghana, Accra, Ghana

Correspondence should be addressed to Freda Intiful; fdintiful@chs.edu.gh

Academic Editor: Carol J. Burns

The objective of this study was to evaluate the views of first-time expectant mothers on breastfeeding. A qualitative study approach using focus group discussions was used to solicit the views of 25 expectant first-time mothers. The results indicated the intention to breastfeed, though some were willing to opt for formula feeding when the need arises. Knowledge on breastfeeding issues was minimal among this group. Common sources of information on breastfeeding issues were obtained from home (relatives), hospital, and television. The need to support and provide adequate education on breastfeeding issues is critical among this category of women.

1. Introduction

The option to breastfeed or not is influenced by several factors including but not limited to cultural practices, health status of both mother and infant, nutrition knowledge, and support from family and other stakeholders. First-time expectant mothers may have several perceptions about breastfeeding based on what they have seen or heard from people about breastfeeding. Most of them may feel unskilled and therefore are unable to decide on feeding options while others may feel confident and therefore can decide on feeding options in the early stages of pregnancy [1].

In spite of the numerous established benefits of breastfeeding, feeding infants with baby formula has also gained a lot of recognition among first-time mothers. As a global public health strategy, the World Health Organization (WHO) recommends exclusive breastfeeding for the first six months as the gold standard for the feeding of infants during the first six months of life [2]. Some of the reported benefits of exclusive breastfeeding are its ability to reduce childhood morbidity and mortality [3–5]. Studies that were conducted in Denmark, Honduras, and New Zealand also demonstrated the effect of breastfeeding on intellectual and motor development of children [6–8]. The ability of breastfeeding to be protective against the development of chronic conditions

such as obesity and diabetes has been reported elsewhere. For example, it was reported that breastfed infants were more than 30% less likely to be obese later in life and also had about 33% increased risk of developing diabetes if not breastfed by the time of discharge from the hospital [9–11]. The economic benefits cannot be overemphasized especially in a developing economy like Ghana [12].

Many first-time expectant mothers may have the intention to breastfeed; however challenges during delivery may cause them to resort to other forms of feeding [13]. The decision to breastfeed could also be enhanced by the support they receive from family and other stakeholders [14].

In the most recent reports, Ghana has experienced reduced rates of exclusive breastfeeding from 63% in 2008 to 52% in 2013 [15, 16] (the 2013 Ghana Demographic Health Survey has the most current national data on exclusive breastfeeding rate in Ghana). Considering many benefits of breastfeeding to both mother and baby, it is crucial to address the barriers that prevent mothers from breastfeeding. If the first-time mother gets it right, then the likelihood of breastfeeding all subsequent children is high. Therefore, it is important to identify the barriers and beliefs in order to effectively address them. This qualitative study was conducted to evaluate the views of first-time expectant mothers on breastfeeding.

TABLE 1: Background characteristics of expectant mothers.

Characteristics	Frequency (*n*)	Percentage (%)
Age (mean age of participant 24.71 ± 6.18)		
≤25	12	48
26–40	11	44
>40	2	8
Religion		
Christian	21	84
Muslim	4	16
Marital status		
Married	15	60
Single	10	40
Employment status		
Employed	18	72
Unemployed	7	28
Educational level		
No education	4	16
Primary	3	12
Junior high school	4	16
Senior high school	9	36
Tertiary	5	20

2. Methodology

2.1. Study Site and Design. A qualitative study design involving focus group discussions was employed. The study was conducted in three health facilities (Kaneshie Polyclinic, Mamprobi Polyclinic, and Ussher Polyclinic). All three hospitals are located in the Accra Metropolis of the Greater Accra Region of Ghana. These three hospitals are located at areas with similar socioeconomic characterizations. The inhabitants of these areas mainly belong to the low and middle class. The main socioeconomic activity in these three areas is trading but there are those who also engage in white-collar jobs. Two major markets (Kaneshie Market Complex and Makola Market) are all situated within the catchment areas.

2.2. Participants. Twenty-five (25) first-time pregnant women participated in this study. They were made up of women between the ages of 18 and 46 years who had not delivered live babies or breastfed before. They were recruited from antenatal clinics at the various polyclinics. First-time pregnant women who came for antenatal for the first time were purposefully introduced to the researcher by the nurses. The researcher further explained the aim and procedures of the study to them. Those who consented to the study were recruited into the study.

2.3. Data Collection. A structured questionnaire was used to obtain information on the background of the expectant mothers. Three (3) different focus group discussions were held at the three (3) respective polyclinics. A facilitator moderated the discussions with the help of an assistant who took note of other relevant observations. The moderator used open ended questions to solicit views of expectant mothers on breastfeeding.

The discussions were held in Twi (a popular Akan dialect in Ghana) and recorded because most of the participants could not express themselves well in English. The discussions were then transcribed and translated verbatim into English. To reduce the effect to loss of meaning, the researcher moderated the translation process in collaboration with a translator to ensure that the intended meaning is maintained. Data were inputted into Microsoft word. Data were further coded manually by two of the researchers (FI and CO). Variations in coding were discussed and resolved. Agreed codes were categorized and developed into themes. These were further analyzed and discussed with reference to other relevant and current literatures.

2.4. Ethical Considerations. Ethical approval for this study was granted by the Ethics and Protocol Review Committee of the School of Biomedical and Allied Health Sciences, University of Ghana. The purpose and protocol of the study were explained to the participants and a written consent was obtained to ensure that participation was fully voluntary. Participants in the study were identified with pseudo names and therefore could not be linked with their comments.

3. Results

The mean age of the participants was 24.71 ± 6.18 years. Majority of the participants were Christians (84%). More than half (60%) of the participants were married. The employment rate among participants was 72%. Most of the participants had some form of education (Table 1).

The results from the focus group discussions were presented under the following themes; reactions of participants to the realization of being pregnant; feeding plan of first-time mothers; knowledge on breastfeeding; benefits of breastfeeding; views on formula feeding; other feeding options in case the mother cannot breastfeed; sources of information on breastfeeding; key people who may influence their breastfeeding; people and places for assistance during breastfeeding.

3.1. Reaction of Participants to the Realization of Being Pregnant.

The reactions of the participants to the news that they were expecting their first child were varied. Some were genuinely excited about their first child, others were not excited at all, and others, though were not planned, decided to accept their fate and cope with the situation. Here are some of the varied responses:

> I was very happy because I did not know that at my age God would remember me. [with so much passion] (46 year old woman)

> I was kind of disappointed because I was not prepared. (25 year old woman)

> I was happy. [shrugging her shoulders]. (18 year old woman)

3.2. Feeding Plan of First-Time Mothers.

Most of the respondents chose the option to breastfeed. Some however opted for formula feeding. One mother stated that

> I will breastfeed for the first four months and after that I will introduce porridges to the child because I think by 4 months the breastmilk will not satisfy the child, so I will add other foods to the breastmilk. (25 year old mother)

Another woman also indicated that she will rather feed her baby formula.

> I will give formula food to the baby. (18 year old woman)

3.3. Knowledge on Breastfeeding Issues.

Some of the respondents were familiar with the issues of breastfeeding. Others were not too conversant with the benefits of breastfeeding. Those who knew about the benefits of breastfeeding could explain in detail indicating that they had some education on breastfeeding. One woman commented that "breastmilk makes the child look nice and healthy and also strong." Others were also of the view that breastmilk improves the child's intelligence. In this regard a woman said that "breastmilk opens the mind of the child" (28 year old woman), literally meaning that the child becomes more intelligent. There was also the opinion to breastfeed no matter the circumstance. This was well expressed in the opinion of one woman:

> When you give birth to a child, you need to breastfeed the baby because it has all the necessary nutrients for the child to grow. Unless the child's

> mum is dead, the child would not be breastfed but so far as the mother is alive, the child should be breastfed. (25 year old woman)

3.4. Benefits of Breastfeeding.

When the women were asked about the benefits of breastfeeding to the mother and the baby, it appeared that they were more conversant with the benefits to the child than to the mother. The responses of the benefits included protection of the child from diseases, making the child strong, the ability of the mother to save some money, and also reducing the stress of having to visit the hospital periodically due to frequent illness of the baby. The following are some of the responses from the mothers:

> Well, what people have said and I have heard is that if you do not breastfeed, the breastmilk fills the breast and makes you uncomfortable and it is painful, so when you breastfeed, it helps you the mother feel comfortable. (32 year old woman)

> When you breastfeed, it helps you the mother save money and does not make your breast fill up and become painful. (26 year old woman)

> When you breastfeed the child, it makes the child more healthy than giving formula food, makes the child stronger and protects the child too from diseases. (23 year old woman)

> It helps prevent other health issues from arising and for your own good you have to breastfeed your child because it helps the child from getting health issues. It also saves you from the stress of going up and down to the hospital in case your child gets sick. (25 year woman)

3.5. Views on Formula Feeding.

There were varied views on formula feeding. Some expressed strong reservations with the use of formula to feed the newborn baby.

This is from the belief that the formula may not be safe because it is in a tin. Others also believed that the formula is full of chemicals therefore not appropriate for the baby. These were expressed in the sentiments of some of the women:

> Some of the children cannot tolerate formula food but with the natural foods they can eat it very well. Also with the formula foods, there are a lot of chemicals in it. So I would give the natural foods than the formula food. (34 year old woman)

> I think because it is a processed food it is not 100% safe. Also, because it is in a tin, it can rust as compared to breastmilk that we know is safe. (25 year old woman)

> As I said earlier on, these formula foods have chemicals in it and it is not healthy for your baby. So I would not give it at all. It also contains too much sugar from my sister's experience. (29 year old woman)

Some of the women were also of the view that circumstances such as the unavailability of the mother as a result of her work schedule could necessitate the introduction of formula. For example, one woman commented, *"It depends on the job you are doing. So maybe during the week, I will give formula food but on weekends, I will prepare both formula food and breastmilk and will give any of which the child prefers."* (24 year old woman)

Another woman also stated that *"I think it is good because if you are not around the child can still eat. Also, what you the mother is lacking in breastmilk, you can get it from formula foods."* (22 year old woman)

One other woman was strongly in support of formula feeding since she claims her friend used that option and found it to be very beneficial: *"It is good because I have a friend who gave her child formula food and the child is healthy, so formula food is good."* (19 year old woman)

3.6. Alternative Feeding Options When Mother Cannot Breastfeed. In the event of not being able to breastfeed, the women indicated various feeding options they would use. Feeding the child *"koko"* (fermented maize porridge) was the main choice for most of the women. Others could not give a definite answer as they had not thought about it before. Some also mentioned that they would give their baby formula food because it is close to the nature of breastmilk. The responses of the women allude to their preferences:

> *I will give my child porridge because formula foods are not good for the child's health, so instead I will give the child our local foods, mill it and put it down for the child to eat.* (29 year old mother)

> *I will give my child food that is close to the breastmilk or any light food.* (28 year old)

3.7. Source of Information and Key People Who Influence Breastfeeding. The women indicated that their main sources of information on breastfeeding were from the hospital, school, at home, and health talks on TV shows.

The women were asked key people they think would most likely influence their breastfeeding adherence. They were unanimous in stating that they would listen to their mothers and what is said in the hospital. Here is a response:

> *I would listen to my mother and the hospital.* (34 year old woman)

3.8. People and Places for Assistance during Breastfeeding. When they were further asked who they will go to for assistance when in challenges with regard to breastfeeding, most participants mentioned their mothers and the hospitals. Here are some responses:

> *From my mother, because she has given birth before and I am now about to.* (25 year old woman)

> *From the hospital because they can show you how to feed the baby well than the house.* (19 year old woman)

4. Discussion

This study aimed at providing more information to support the existing literature on breastfeeding. The qualitative nature of the study provides in-depth information concerning the views of expectant first-time mothers. The findings of this study will provide healthcare professionals, policy makers, and health program promoters information to help develop better support systems especially for expectant first-time mothers and know how to disseminate information to the mothers during their antenatal visits and the general public. This particular group was targeted because their views may be carried into the next phase of child care. In cases where these views become misconceptions, it may affect child care [17].

From this study, some expectant mothers expressed happiness on realization that they were pregnant while others were disappointed. Being happy about being pregnant is more likely to imply that they wanted the pregnancy. This is likely to impact on the decision of the expectant mother choosing to breastfeed as has been reported in another study in the US. The study observed that women with unwanted pregnancies were found less likely to breastfeed when compared to those who planned their pregnancies [18].

Breastfeeding is declining in Ghana. The challenge however is when it has to be done exclusively for the first six months. From the focus group discussions, it was realized that though they may opt to breastfeed their babies as advised during antenatal care sessions, the duration of the breastfeeding for the first six months was not certain. This can be attributed to the challenges they envisage that could hinder the ability to exclusively breastfeed. Some of these challenges are fuelled by perceptions and myths about breastfeeding. These myths and perceptions include the belief that breastmilk milk becomes polluted when the mother becomes pregnant while still lactating, colostrum being regarded as dirty, the fear of the lactating mother dying because of prolong breastfeeding, and the perception that breastmilk alone is not sufficient for the baby [19, 20]. Grandmothers, especially the mothers-in-law of breastfeeding women, are significant persons who can influence what to feed the newborn baby [21]. In addition the employment status of the breastfeeding mother can be a problem. For example among city dwelling professional Ghanaian women, exclusive breastfeeding rate was 10.3% in spite of the fact that 99% were aware of exclusive breastfeeding and 91% initiating breastfeeding within the first hour after birth [22]. Some cultural practices such as the giving of water, gripe water, and local herbs also prevent them from reaching the full six months of exclusivity [21].

Furthermore, the knowledge of the first-time mothers concerning breastfeeding had some gaps. Some of the expectant first-time mothers were conversant with some of the importance of breastfeeding to the baby. However, knowledge of the benefits of breastfeeding to the mother was minimal. This could be as a result of emphasis laid on the benefits of breastfeeding to the baby during educational sections to be more as compared to that of the mother. This calls for more thorough educational sections for women.

The views concerning formula feeding revealed that some mothers were not in favour of the use of formula foods as they deemed it unsafe and not healthy for their babies. During antenatal care sessions, the health professionals in charge such as the midwives and the nurses counsel the mothers on the advantages of breastfeeding over the use of formula. Concerns have also been raised about formula feeding that it may be contaminated with pathogens and chemicals and that it requires adequate hygiene in its preparation [23–25].

Research has shown that it is common for first-time mothers to have delayed lactogenesis [26]. However, the views of the expectant first-time mothers during the discussion reflected a level of nescience. This may be due to the fact that, during antenatal care, more emphasis is placed on the need to breastfeed the child leaving other areas unturned. It is imperative to get mothers equipped with the knowledge on what to do when they face challenges in breastfeeding. Support and education on what to do in cases of delayed lactogenesis may be minimal. This is evident in their responses as some opted to give porridges or food close to breastmilk. They may have an idea about what to do but not much education has been done concerning this. This brings to the fore the low level of support systems or groups to help mothers who want to exclusively breastfeed as has also been reported in the UK [27].

Regarding the source of information on breastfeeding, expectant first-time mothers had varied sources of information. This is indicative of the fact that education on breastfeeding was not only limited to the hospital. Similar findings were reported in an Australian study. Their main sources of information were from healthcare professionals, relatives/friends, television, and the Internet [28]. In this present study, key people who will be more likely to influence participants' breastfeeding were their mothers (i.e., grandmothers) and health professionals. These were the same people they would consult for assistance. In a systemative review of studies that investigated the role of grandmothers in both developing and developed countries, it became apparent that grandmothers had important influence on exclusive breastfeeding (Negin 2016). Support from healthcare professionals also strengthens the self-esteem of mothers, thereby encouraging them to exclusively breastfeed [29]. It is therefore crucial that these categories of people are well educated and equipped with the issues of breastfeeding so they can impact the mothers appropriately.

5. Conclusion

Breast feeding was the most preferred choice of feeding for the babies of the expectant mothers studied. The mothers were generally aware of the benefits of breastfeeding especially for their babies. There was a general disapproval for the use of formula to feed babies. The expectant mothers also indicated that they will solicit for help from their mothers (i.e., grandmothers) or health professionals when they are faced with challenges regarding breastfeeding.

It is recommended that further studies comprised of an educational component on breastfeeding and a subsequent evaluation analysis would be necessary to investigate how these views were put into action after they had delivered their babies. More detailed antenatal care sessions specific for expectant first-time mothers as well as strong support systems that encourage the education on breastfeeding should be done.

Acknowledgments

The authors wish to express their sincere thanks to all expectant mothers who volunteered to be part of this study and the staff of the antenatal clinics at the three polyclinics where the study was conducted.

References

[1] A. M. Stuebe and E. B. Schwarz, "The risks and benefits of infant feeding practices for women and their children," *Journal of Perinatology*, vol. 30, no. 3, pp. 155–162, 2010.

[2] *Global Strategy for Infant And Young Child Feeding*, WHO and UNICEF, Geneva, Switzerland, 2003.

[3] J. Clemens et al., "Early initiation of breastfeeding and the risk of infant diarrhea in rural Egypt," *Pediatrics*, vol. 104, no. 1, pp. e3–e3, 1999.

[4] M. Meremikwu, A. Asindi, and O. Antia-Obong, "The influence of breast feeding on the occurrence of dysentery, persistent diarrhoea and malnutrition among Nigerian children with diarrhoea," *West African journal of medicine*, vol. 16, no. 1, pp. 20–23, 1997.

[5] A. P. Betrán, M. De Onís, J. A. Lauer, and J. Villar, "Ecological study of effect of breast feeding on infant mortality in Latin America," *British Medical Journal*, vol. 323, no. 7308, p. 303, 2001.

[6] E. L. Mortensen et al., "The association between duration of breastfeeding and adult intelligence," *Jama*, vol. 287, no. 18, pp. 2365–2371, 2002.

[7] K. G. Dewey et al., "Effects of exclusive breastfeeding for four versus six months on maternal nutritional status and infant motor development: results of two randomized trials in Honduras," *The Journal of Nutrition*, vol. 131, no. 2, pp. 262–267, 2001.

[8] L. Horwood, B. Darlow, and N. Mogridge, "Breast milk feeding and cognitive ability at 7–8 years," *Archives of Disease in Childhood-Fetal and Neonatal Edition*, vol. 84, no. 1, pp. F23–F27, 2001.

[9] M. W. Gillman et al., "Risk of overweight among adolescents who were breastfed as infants," *Jama*, vol. 285, no. 19, pp. 2461–2467, 2001.

[10] M. L. Hediger et al., "Association between infant breastfeeding and overweight in young children," *Jama*, vol. 285, no. 19, pp. 2453–2460, 2001.

[11] M. E. Jones, A. J. Swerdlow, L. E. Gill, and M. J. Goldacre, "Pre-natal and early life risk factors for childhood onset diabetes mellitus: A record linkage study," *International Journal of Epidemiology*, vol. 27, no. 3, pp. 444–449, 1998.

[12] A. Kuma, "Economic and health benefits of breastfeeding: a review," *Food Science and Quality Management*, vol. 45, no. 39, 2015.

[13] J. Panczuk, S. Unger, D. O'Connor, and S. K. Lee, "Human donor milk for the vulnerable infant: A Canadian perspective," *International Breastfeeding Journal*, vol. 9, no. 1, article no. 4, 2014.

[14] M.-T. Tarkka, M. Paunonen, and P. Laippala, "What contributes to breastfeeding success after childbirth in a maternity ward in Finland?" *Women and Birth*, vol. 25, no. 3, pp. 175–181, 1998.

[15] G. S. S. GSS, "Ghana Demographic Health Survey 2008," in *Proceedings of the Ghana Health Service (GHS), and ICF International'08*, Demographic and Health, 2008.

[16] G. S. S. GSS, "Demographic Health Survey 2014," in *Proceedings of the Ghana Health Service (GHS), and ICF International*, Demographic and Health, 2015.

[17] A. Freund, *Expectations and experiences of first-time mothers [M.S. thesis]*, faculty of the University Graduate School in partial fulfillment of the requirements for the degree Master of Arts in the Department of Sociology, Indiana University, 2008.

[18] T. D. Dye, M. A. Wojtowycz, R. H. Aubry, J. Quade, and H. Kilburn, "Unintended pregnancy and breast-feeding behavior," *American Journal of Public Health*, vol. 87, no. 10, pp. 1709–1711, 1997.

[19] A. K.-A. Diji, V. Bam, E. Asante, A. Y. Lomotey, S. Yeboah, and H. A. Owusu, "Challenges and predictors of exclusive breastfeeding among mothers attending the child welfare clinic at a regional hospital in Ghana: A descriptive cross-sectional study," *International Breastfeeding Journal*, vol. 12, no. 1, article no. 13, 2017.

[20] A. Ayawine and K. A. Ae-Ngibise, "Determinants of exclusive breastfeeding: a study of two sub-districts in the Atwima Nwabiagya District of Ghana," *Pan African Medical Journal*, vol. 22, p. 248, 2015.

[21] R. A. Aborigo, C. A. Moyer, S. Rominski et al., "Infant nutrition in the first seven days of life in rural northern Ghana," *BMC Pregnancy and Childbirth*, vol. 12, article no. 76, 2012.

[22] E. J. Dun-Dery and A. K. Laar, "Exclusive breastfeeding among city-dwelling professional working mothers in Ghana," *International Breastfeeding Journal*, vol. 11, no. 1, article no. 23, 2016.

[23] K. D. Gribble and B. L. Hausman, "Milk sharing and formula feeding: Infant feeding risks in comparative perspective?" *Australasian Medical Journal*, vol. 5, no. 5, pp. 275–283, 2012.

[24] C. Siew et al., "Assessing a potential risk factor for enamel fluorosis: a preliminary evaluation of fluoride content in infant formulas," *The Journal of the American Dental Association*, vol. 140, no. 10, pp. 1228–1236, 2009.

[25] J. G. Schier, A. F. Wolkin, L. Valentin-Blasini et al., "Perchlorate exposure from infant formula and comparisons with the perchlorate reference dose," *Journal of Exposure Science and Environmental Epidemiology*, vol. 20, no. 3, pp. 281–287, 2010.

[26] L. A. Nommsen-Rivers, C. J. Chantry, J. M. Peerson, R. J. Cohen, and K. G. Dewey, "Delayed onset of lactogenesis among first-time mothers is related to maternal obesity and factors associated with ineffective breastfeeding," *American Journal of Clinical Nutrition*, vol. 92, no. 3, pp. 574–584, 2010.

[27] A. Grant, K. McEwan, S. Tedstone, G. Greene, L. Copeland et al., "Availability of breastfeeding peer support in the United Kingdom: A cross-sectional study," *Maternal and Child Nutrition*, 2017.

[28] R. Newby et al., "Antenatal information sources for maternal and infant diet," *Breastfeeding Review*, vol. 23, no. 2, p. 13, 2015.

[29] N. Alianmoghaddam, S. Phibbs, and C. Benn, "Resistance to breastfeeding: A Foucauldian analysis of breastfeeding support from health professionals," *Women Birth*, 2017.

14

Early Initiation of Antenatal Care and Factors Associated with Early Antenatal Care Initiation at Health Facilities in Southern Ethiopia

Mengesha Boko Geta[1] and Walelegn Worku Yallew[2]

[1]Kebado Primary Hospital, Hawassa, Ethiopia
[2]Institute of Public Health, College of Medicine and Health Sciences, University of Gondar, Gondar, Ethiopia

Correspondence should be addressed to Mengesha Boko Geta; mengeshaokkob@yahoo.com

Academic Editor: Jennifer L. Freeman

Antenatal care (ANC) is care given to pregnant mothers to timely identify and mitigate pregnancy related problems that can harm mother or fetus. Most of Ethiopian mothers present late for ANC. The aim of this paper was to assess determinants of early antenatal care initiation among pregnant women. Mothers attending Shebedino District Health Centers for ANC between January 12 and February 18, 2015, were invited to the study. Multistage sampling technique and structured questionnaire were used to collect data by trained data collectors. Univariate and bivariate analysis were conducted to study the association between explanatory and outcome variable. Out of 608 women, 132 [21.71%] had their first ANC within the recommended time [before or at 3 months]. Media access [AOR = 2.11 95% CI 1.00, 3.22], knowledge about the correct time of ANC booking [AOR = 4.49 95% CI 2.47, 6.16], and having been advised to book within 12 weeks [AOR = 4.14 95% CI 3.80, 5.21] were determinants of first-trimester booking. Health professionals and care providers should provide full information, advice, and appropriate care about early ANC for every eligible mother.

1. Introduction

The care that was given to the mother during pregnancy, during delivery, and after delivery is important for the well-being of the mother and the child. All pregnant ladies are recommended to go for their first antenatal check-up in the first trimester to identify and manage any medical complication as well as to screen them for any risk factors that may affect the progress and outcome of their pregnancy [1]. The first visit which is expected to screen and treat anemia and syphilis, screen for risk factors and medical conditions that can be best dealt with in early pregnancy, and initiate prophylaxis if required (e.g., for anemia and malaria) is recommended to be held by the end of fourth month [2]. ANC helps to ensure the well-being of the mother and fetus through early detection of risks in pregnancy, prevention of pregnancy, and labor complications and ensures the safe delivery of mother and child [3]. In Ethiopia, 34% of pregnant women attend antenatal care at least once and 19% of them attend four times

and only 11.2% attend early [4]. In Ethiopia, antennal care services increased in the past 15 years from 27 percent in 2000 to 62 percent in 2015. However, it needs further improvement to achieve [5–7].

Globally, approximately 515,000 women die from pregnancy related complications each year [8]. In developing world over 30 million women suffer each year from serious obstetric complications [9]. Inadequate access and underutilization of modern healthcare services are major reasons for poor health in the developing countries. This inequality in the health and well-being of women in the developing world is a growing concern [10]. Although services are given freely, a number of factors have been found to contribute to late initiation of ANC among pregnant women and these may vary between rural and urban areas [11].

Pregnant women should be offered screening for HIV infection early in ANC [12]. Low ANC coverage, few visits, and late attendance at first antenatal visit are common problems throughout Sub-Saharan Africa posing difficulty in accomplishing the WHO recommended ANC schedule [13].

Late ANC initiation may increase the total cost of caring for a pregnant woman [14]. A study conducted in Hadiya zone Southern Ethiopia revealed that, concerning time of initiating care, only 8.7% of the ANC attendants initiated care during the first trimester of pregnancy while 68.1% had the first visit during the third trimester [15]. Another study in Ethiopia showed that proper advice and information on timely booking from service providers and community level are very important for the effective utilization of the service [16].

Women in developing countries, particularly in Sub-Saharan Africa, tend to wait to start antenatal care until the second or third trimester [17]. The standard of care when evaluating a woman with a potentially complicated first-trimester pregnancy is to take a detailed history of the risk factors and ascertain the clinical course [18]. Educational status of the women and family income were independent factors for late initiation of ANC [19]. Pregnant mothers at younger age [20] register early for ANC compared to older age and younger women are more likely to accept modern health care as they are likely to have greater experience to modern medicine [21].

Women who have lower educational status, have good perception, and are urban residents are more likely to attend early for ANC compared to their counterparts [10, 22]. Parity [22] and late ANC initiation are also a factor for ANC utilization [23]. The aim of this study is to assess the magnitude and factors associated with early antenatal care initiation of mothers in health facilities.

2. Materials and Methods

Study was conducted in Shebedino district, which is one of 19 rural woredas of Sidama zone in Southern regions of Ethiopia, which is located 28 KM from capital city of southern regions, Hawassa, and organised by 32 rural and 3 urban kebeles for the purpose of administration. Source population was all mothers attending Shebedino district health facilities in Sidama zone. The study population was pregnant mothers attending Shebedino district health facilities for ANC services during study period with inclusion criteria of pregnant mothers attending those health facilities during study period for ANC services and exclusion criteria of pregnant mothers with some serious illness and labor. Five health centers were randomly selected by lottery method among 9 health centers in the woreda and 1 primary hospital. Multistage sampling technique was applied till the sample size was enough. Sample proportion or number of eligible pregnant mothers was calculated based on catchment population proportion using exit interview at every third mother.

The sample size was calculated using single population proportion based on the study conducted on timing of first ANC visit at Gondar Hospital, and a prevalence of 47.2% was taken to estimate the sample size [20]. Six hundred thirty mothers were included in the study with an assumption of 95% confidence interval, 5% margin of error, 10% nonresponse rate, and a design effect of 1.5.

A pretested questionnaire which consists of a sociodemographic characteristic, obstetric information, and decision-making status of women was used. The data collection was exit interview with pregnant mothers after service of ANC Department of Health Facilities. The data was collected by trained clinical nurses or midwifes who were selected from other catchments which are not selected for data collection. Data collectors were supervised by trained supervisors daily during data collection. Before data collection, ethical approval was taken from IRB of Addis Continental Institute of Public Health and informed consent and confidentiality were assured by data collectors to the participants.

Questionnaire was checked daily by the principal investigator for consistency. The selecting criteria of data collectors were ability to speak local language, interest to participate, and being well mannered and disciplined. Data was entered into EPI info version 3.5.1 and transferred to Statistical Package for Social Science (SPSS) version 20.0 software for analysis. Descriptive and summary statistics was carried out. P value 0.05 was considered statistical significance. Bivariate and multivariate logistic regression analyses were used to identify variables associated with early antenatal initiation.

3. Result

Out of 631 pregnant women who initiated to be included in this study, 608 [96.3%] have responded to the interview. The remaining 17 [2.7%] did not respond to the interview while 6 [1%] of them were unable to respond or they did not specify the gestational age when they started the ANC. The median age of respondents was 25 years ranging from 15 to 40 years (Table 1).

3.1. Obstetric History and Timing of First ANC Visits. Majority, 409 [67.3%], of respondents had parity one and above, while 184 [30.3%] have no parity and the remaining 15 [2.4%] of the respondents had history of parity greater than five (Table 2).

3.2. Knowledge and Perception of ANC Service Utilization and First Timing of ANC Visit. Majority, 596 [98.2%], of respondents perceived and rated that the importance of ANC for the health of the mother and fetus was highly important to the health of mother and fetus. Two-thirds, 410 [67.4%], of the respondents perceived that the correct time of ANC starting was after 12 weeks of gestation followed by 169 [27.8%] who perceived that the correct time of ANC starting was before 12 weeks of gestation. 26 [4.3%] respondents perceived that only one visit of ANC was enough, 76 [12.5%] perceived that two to three visits of ANC were necessary, 430 [70.8%] perceived that four to six visits of ANC were necessary, and 75 [12.4%] perceived that more than six ANC visits are necessary (Table 3).

3.3. Factors Associated with Timely ANC Initiation. Bivariate analysis showed that respondents who had media access (TV/radio) [OR = 1.485 95% CI 1.002, 2.202], who had perceived that the correct time of ANC booking is within 12 weeks of gestation [OR = 20.755 95% CI 12.816, 33.613],

TABLE 1: Sociodemographic characteristics of respondents by time of ANC booking in Shebedino district in 2015.

Variable	Description	Frequency	Percentage
Age in years: $n = 608$	15–19	66	10.8%
	20–24	247	40.6%
	25–29	195	32.0%
	30–34	65	10.7%
	35–39	28	4.6%
	40–45	7	1.1%
Ethnicity: $n = 608$	Sidama	548	90.1%
	Amahara	23	3.8%
	Guragie	18	2.9%
	Silte	5	0.8%
	Wolaita	14	2.3%
Religion: $n = 608$	Orthodox	37	6.0%
	Muslim	43	7.0%
	Protestant	510	83.8%
	Catholic	18	2.9%
Marital status: $n = 608$	Single [not married]	7	1.1%
	Married and live together	594	97.6%
	Cohabitation	5	0.8%
	Ever married but separated	2	0.3%
Educational level [completed]: $n = 608$	Illiterate [cannot read & write]	155	25.5%
	Illiterate [can read and write]	23	3.7%
	Primary [1–8]	333	54.7%
	Secondary [9–12]	63	10.7%
	Diploma and above	34	5.6%
Residence: $n = 608$	Urban	63	10.36%
	Rural	545	89.64%
Income per month: $n = 608$	<400.00 ETB	275	45.23%
	400.00-1000.00 ETB	235	38.65%
	>1000.00 ETB	98	16.12%
Media access (source of information) $n = 608$	Television	89	14.63%
	Radio	192	31.57%
	Village	284	46.70%
	None	43	7.07%

TABLE 2: Number of respondents by obstetric history and time of first ANC, Shebedino district in 2015.

Variable	Description	Frequency	Percentage
Parity $n = 608$	No parity	184	30.26%
	Parity 1–5	409	67.26%
	Parity >5	15	12.46%
Gravidity $n = 608$	No gravidity	170	27.96%
	One and above	438	72.04%
Abortion $n = 608$	Had no history of abortion	554	91.11%
	Had history of abortion	54	8.89%
Types of abortion $n = 54$	Had at least one spontaneous abortion	45	83.33%
	Had at least one induced abortion	9	16.67%
History of child death $n = 608$	Had history of child death	28	4.60%
	Had no history of child death	580	95.40%

who booked first ANC within the recommended time for the past pregnancy preceding the current [OR = 20.512 95% CI 12.671, 33.206], who received advise on early booking [OR = 17.885 95% CI 11.218, 28.513], who ever use ANC before current pregnancy [OR = 5.04 95% CI 2.85, 8.91], and who were prim gravid [OR = 1, 658 95% CI 1.100, 2.498] were positively associated and more likely to book first ANC within recommended time compared to their counterparts (Table 4).

Multivariate analysis showed that respondents with media access (who had TV/radio) [OR = 2.109 95% CI 1.001, 4.445], who perceived that the correct time of ANC booking is within 12 weeks of gestation [OR = 4.499 95% CI 4.470, 16.160], and who received advise on booking time within 12

TABLE 3: Knowledge and perception of ANC service utilization and timing of first ANC, Shebedino in district SNNPR, Ethiopia, in 2015.

Variable	Description	Frequency	Percentage
Perception of importance of ANC for health of mother n = 607	Highly important	596	98.18%
	Medium importance	4	0.65%
	Less important	7	1.15%
Perception of importance of care for the health of the fetus: n = 608	Highly important	598	98.35%
	Medium importance	2	0.32%
	Less important	8	1.32%
Perceptions on timing of first care: n = 608	Before and at 12 weeks of gestation	169	27.79%
	After 12 weeks of gestation	430	72.20%
Perceived number of ANC visits of pervious pregnancy n = 607	Only one ANC visit enough	27	4.44%
	2-3 ANC visits enough	76	12.52%
	4–6 ANC visits enough	430	70.84%
	>6 ANC visits enough	75	12.35%
Early antenatal booking is good for pregnancy of mother n = 608	I agree	599	98.51%
	I disagree	9	1.49%
Mother should go for antenatal booking before the third month of pregnancy n = 608	I agree	474	77.96%
	I disagree	134	22.04%
Antenatal follow up is good to monitor mother's and fetus' health n = 608	I agree	605	99.51%
	I disagree	3	0.49%

weeks [OR = 4.146 95% CI 5.806, 21.398] were also more likely to book ANC within the recommended time compared to corresponding counterparts and these factors were found positively associated (Table 4).

4. Discussion

In this study, only about 21.72% of respondents have started their ANC within the recommended time with 95% CI (18%, 25%) and the remaining 78.28% booked it lately with 95% CI (75%, 81%). The timing of first booking ranged from first month after last menstrual period to ninth month of gestation. The proportion of women who came for their first ANC within recommended time is lower than studies done in Gondar, Addis Ababa, and higher than studies conducted in Hadiya, Kembata zone, Yem special district, and EDHS 2011 [4, 13, 18–21]. Possible explanation for this might be those who have more proportion of early ANC due to better access and awareness regarding services while the lower proportion may be due to time variation in this study and the access and awareness improvement.

According to the result, mothers of age ≤ 25 years were found to be more likely to have early initiation of ANC when compared with others (COR = 1.309 95% CI 0.92, 2.458), but not significant. This idea was slightly supported by study done in Addis Ababa, Yem, Gondar, and Debrebrhan; this idea contradicts the study done in Tanzania (18–21, 8). This might be because younger mothers were more informed and convincible to seek appropriate prenatal care.

Respondents who had media access TV/radio initiated ANC within recommended time twice more likely when compared to those who had not (AOR = 2.109 95% CI 1.001, 4.445). This might be due to exposure to source of information, as result of the study indicated that prim gravid mothers start ANC timely 1.4 times more likely when

compared to multigravid mothers (AOR = 1.038 95% CI 1.02, 1.92). Another study conducted in Tanzania showed that higher gravidity is more likely to be predictor of late antenatal care initiation compared to early ANC initiation [8]. This could be because prim gravid mothers may be younger and educated and easily understand an advice to commence ANC early and different information.

Parity of respondents was found to be more likely predictor of timely booking of ANC (COR = 1.429 95% CI 0.951, 2.145), but not significant, and this finding was similar to that of study done in Debrebrhan and lower than the studies done in Gondar and Kembata Tembaro zone as parity was found as the most predictor for late utilization of ANC. The same studies revealed that pervious ANC utilization was also found to be a positive predictor for timely ANC booking [21, 22].

Perception of respondents concerning correct time of early initiation of ANC was highly associated with early initiation of ANC at recommended time and mothers who perceived right time to be in the first 12 weeks of gestation were nearly 4.5 times more likely to commence ANC timely than those who perceived right time beyond 12 weeks of gestation (AOR = 4.499 95% CI 2.470, 6.160) (P value = 0.000). This finding was supported by and higher than other findings of many studies conducted in different parts of our country [4, 14, 18, 20].

The finding of this study revealed that the maternal perception concerning the correct time to ANC booking was similar to that of study done in Gondar town. This in fact may be determinant factor for early ANC initiation at recommended time [22].

The result of the study indicates that respondents who received correct advice to book ANC during recommended time after amenorrhea used early ANC 4 times more likely than those not advised about correct time (AOR = 4.146 95% CI 3.806, 21.398) (P value = 0.001). The study conducted

TABLE 4: Association of factors with timely booking of first ANC, Shebedino district in 2015.

Variables	Time at first ANC visit		Crude OR [CI]	Adjusted OR [CI]
	Booked early	Booked late		
Age of mother				
Age ≥ 25	61 [19.48%]	252 [80.52%]	1.00	1.00
Age < 25	71 [24.06%]	224 [75.94%]	1.390 [0.93, 2.46]	0.88 [0.36, 2.15]
Place of residence				
Urban	13 [20.63%]	50 [79.36%]	0.93 [0.56, 2.04]	0.57 [0.20, 1.61]
Rural	119 [21.71%]	426 [78.29%]	1.00	1.00
Media access				
Had radio/TV	81 [26.04%]	230 [73.96%]	1.69 [1.02, 2.20]	2.11 [1.00, 4.44]**
Had no radio/TV	51 [17.17%]	246 [82.83%]	1.00	1.00
Educational level of mother				
Primary and below	109 [23.42%]	399 [76.58%]	1.00	1.00
Secondary and above	23 [23.00%]	77 [77.00%]	1.08 [0.63, 1.53]	1.64 [0.55, 4.89]
Educational level of husband				
Primary and below	98 [22.95%]	329 [77.05%]	1.00	1.00
Secondary and above	34 [18.78%]	147 [81.22%]	0.78 [0.49, 1.11]	0.41 [0.17, 1.00]
Occupation of mother				
Employed	10 [21.27%]	37 [78.73%]	0.97 [0.47, 1.47]	0.62 [0.18, 1.19]
Unemployed	122 [21.74%]	439 [78.26%]	1.00	1.00
Gravity				
Prim gravid	48 [28.23%]	122 [71.77%]	1.65 [1.10,2.19]	1.04 [1.02, 1.72]**
Two and above	84 [19.19%]	354 [80.81%]	1.00	1.00
Parity of mother				
No parity	48 [18.32%]	214 [81.68%]	1.00	1.00
Parity one and above	84 [24.27%]	262 [75.73%]	1.42 [0.95, 1.89]	0.14 [0.006, 3.46]
Perception on time of ANC initiation				
Perceived at and before 12 weeks	102 [53.96%]	87 [46.04%]	20.14 [12.81, 27.47]	4.49 [2.47, 6.16]***
Perceived after 12 weeks	22 [5.50%]	378 [94.50%]	1.00	1.00
Plan of pregnancy by mother				
Planned	102 [21.29%]	377 [78.71%]	0.89 [0.70, 1.08]	0.72 [0.26, 1.34]
Unplanned	30 [23.25%]	99 [76.75%]	1.00	1.00
Plan of pregnancy by husband				
Planned	109 [21.00%]	410 [79.00%]	0.76 [0.45, 1.07]	0.30 [0.09, 0.54]**
Unplanned	23 [25.84%]	66 [74.16%]	1.00	1.00
Advised when to start first ANC				
Advised to book before and at 3 months of gestation	93 [55.35%]	75 [44.65%]	17.80 [11.21, 24.39]	4.14 [3.80, 6.21]***
Advised to book after 3 months of gestation	19 [6.52%]	272 [93.48%]	1.00	1.00
Past experience of timing				
Book before and at 3 months of gestation	55 [31.97%]	117 [68.03%]	1.65 [1.10, 2.20]	2.50 [1.81, 3.45]***
Book after 3 months of gestation	19 [8.52%]	204 [91.48%]	1.00	1.00

Note. Significant at **$P \leq 0.05$ and ***$P \leq 0.001$.

at Addis Ababa also concluded that physical and financial accessibility alone cannot assure effective service utilization of ANC. The need for proper advice and information on timely booking from service providers and community level and/or health institution is very important for the effective

utilization of the service [16]. The current finding was also similar to that finding.

As revealed on the result of the study, occupation of the respondents had no effect on the early ANC initiation; this finding contradicts the study done in Kembata Tembaro

[21]. And others like educational level of mothers and their husbands, parity, and pregnancy plan by mothers and their husbands were not statistically significant findings.

5. Conclusion

Early time of initiation for ANC at recommended time is low. Perception of mothers on correct time of ANC initiation, advice on correct time of ANC initiation, past experience of early booking of ANC, and media access are the positive predictors or factors of early ANC initiation. Multigravid mothers start ANC more early than prim gravid mothers. Health professionals and care providers should provide full information and advice and appropriate care about early ANC for every eligible mother. Mass media worker should include early initiation of ANC. Care takers should consider the importance of past experience of early ANC and perceive appropriate time to start ANC.

Acknowledgments

The authors would like to thank their family, respondents, data collectors, and supervisors.

References

[1] A. M. Rosliza and H. J. Muhamad, "Knowledge, attitude and practice on ANC among orang asil women in JEMPOL, NEGERI SEMBILAN," *Malaysian Journal of Public Health Medicine*, vol. 11, no. 2, pp. 13–21, 2011.

[2] Population, Reproductive Health and the Global Effort to End Poverty, 2014.

[3] S. Babalola and A. Fatusi, "Determinants of use of maternal health services in Nigeria—looking beyond individual and household factors," *BMC Pregnancy and Childbirth*, vol. 9, article 43, 2009.

[4] Ethiopia Demographic and Health Survey, 2011.

[5] CSA, *Ethiopia Demographic and Health Survey 2015*, Central Statistical Agency (CSA), Addis Ababa, Ethiopia; ICF Macro, Calverton, Md, USA, 2016.

[6] CSA, *Ethiopia Demographic and Health Survey 2005*, Central Statistical Agency (CSA), Addis Ababa, Ethiopia; ICF Macro, Calverton, Md, USA, 2006.

[7] CSA, *Ethiopia Demographic and Health Survey 2000*, Central Statistical Agency (CSA), Addis Ababa, Ethiopia; ORC Macro; ICF Macro, Calverton, Md, USA, 2001.

[8] R. Carine and J. G. Wendy, "Maternal mortality: who, when, where, and why," *The Lancet*, vol. 368, no. 9542, pp. 1189–1200, 2006.

[9] WHO, *Make Every Mother and Child Count*, WHO, Geneva, Switzerland, 2005.

[10] B. Simkhada, E. R. Van Teijlingen, M. Porter, and P. Simkhada, "Factors affecting the utilization of antenatal care in developing countries: systematic review of the literature," *Journal of Advanced Nursing*, vol. 61, no. 3, pp. 244–260, 2008.

[11] I. Banda, C. Michelo, and A. Hazemba, "Factors associated with late antenatal care attendance in selected rural and urban communities of the copperbelt province of Zambia," *Medical Journal of Zambia*, vol. 39, no. 3, pp. 29–36, 2012.

[12] Centers for Disease Control and Prevention, "Revised recommendations for HIV screening of pregnant women," *MMWR Recommendations and Reports*, vol. 50, pp. 63–85, quiz CE1–19a2–CE6–19a2, 2001.

[13] W. Delva, E. Yard, S. Luchters et al., "A Safe Motherhood project in Kenya: assessment of antenatal attendance, service provision and implications for PMTCT," *Tropical Medicine & International Health*, vol. 15, no. 5, pp. 584–591, 2010.

[14] M. King, R. Mhlanga, and H. De Pinho, *The Context of Maternal and Child Health*, South African Health Review Health Systems Trust, Durban, South Africa, 2006.

[15] Z. Abosse, M. Woldie, and S. Ololo, "Factors influencing antenatal care service utilization in Hadiya zone," *Ethiopian Journal of Health Sciences*, vol. 20, no. 2, p. 78, 2010.

[16] TJ A, Why pregnant women delay to attend Prenatal care?, June 2008.

[17] W. Wang, S. Alva, S. Wang, and A. Fort, "Levels and trends in the use of maternal health services in developing countries," DHS Comparative Reports, ICF Macro, Calverton, Md, USA, 2011.

[18] K. T. Barnhart, B. Casanova, M. D. Sammel, K. Timbers, K. Chung, and J. L. Kulp, "Prediction of location of a symptomatic early gestation based solely on clinical presentation," *Obstetrics and Gynecology*, vol. 112, no. 6, pp. 1319–1326, 2008.

[19] T. W. Gudayu, S. M. Woldeyohannes, and A. A. Abdo, "Timing and factors associated with first antenatal care booking among pregnant mothers in Gondar Town; North West Ethiopia," *BMC Pregnancy and Childbirth*, vol. 14, article 287, 2014.

[20] T. Belayneh, M. Adefris, and G. Andargie, "Previous early antenatal service utilization improves timely booking: cross-sectional study at University of Gondar Hospital, Northwest Ethiopia," *Journal of Pregnancy*, vol. 2014, Article ID 132494, 7 pages, 2014.

[21] T. Tekelab and B. Berhanu, "Factors associated with late initiation of antenatal care among pregnant women attending antenatal clinic at public health centers in Kembata Tembaro zone, Southern Ethiopia," *Science, Technology and Arts Research Journal*, vol. 3, no. 1, pp. 108–115, 2014.

[22] D. Nigatu, A. Gebremariam, M. Abera, T. Setegn, and K. Deribe, "Factors associated with women's autonomy regarding maternal and child health care utilization in Bale zone: a community based cross-sectional study," *BMC Women's Health*, vol. 14, no. 1, article 79, 2014.

[23] A. Exavery, A. M. Kanté, A. Hingora, G. Mbaruku, S. Pemba, and J. F. Phillips, "How mistimed and unwanted pregnancies affect timing of antenatal care initiation in three districts in Tanzania," *BMC Pregnancy and Childbirth*, vol. 13, article 35, 2013.

15

Health-Related Quality of Life and Associated Factors among Women on Antiretroviral Therapy in Health Facilities of Jimma Town, Southwest Ethiopia

Yetnayet Abebe Weldsilase ⓘ,[1] Melaku Haile Likka,[2] Tolossa Wakayo,[1] and Mulusew Gerbaba ⓘ[1]

[1]Jimma University, Institute of Health Sciences, Department of Population and Family Health, Ethiopia
[2]Jimma University, Institute of Health Sciences, Department of Health Economics, Management and Policy, Ethiopia

Correspondence should be addressed to Yetnayet Abebe Weldsilase; mame.abebe@gmail.com

Academic Editor: Jennifer L. Freeman

Background. This study examined health-related quality of life and associated factors among HIV positive women receiving antiretroviral therapy in health facilities of Jimma town. *Methods.* A cross-sectional study was conducted, and consecutive sampling technique was employed to select 377 HIV positive women who were on antiretroviral therapy. Quality of life was measured using WHOQOL-BREF tool. Descriptive statistics, bivariate, and multivariable logistic regression analyses were performed. P values < 0.05 and adjusted odds ratio with 95% of confidence interval were used to determine statistical significance and report associations between the quality of life and independent variables. *Results.* Among the sampled participants, 344 were interviewed, yielding 91% of response rate. The mean ± standard deviation age of the respondents was 34.07 ± 8.76 years and 80.5% of them were urban dwellers. The proportion of women reporting good health-related quality of life was found to be 46.5%. Specific to each domain, the mean ± standard deviation of level of independence domain was the highest (14.08 ± 3.07) followed by physical (13.46 ± 2.95), social relationships (13.27 ± 3.91), psychological (12.97 ± 2.47), environmental (12.94 ± 3.25), and spiritual (12.39 ± 2.84) domains. Good social support (AOR: 4.99; 95% CI: [2.88, 8.34]), higher wealth status (AOR: 1.85; 95% CI: [1.02, 3.39]), and being on antiretroviral therapy for shorter duration (AOR: 1.85; 95% CI [1.14, 3.03]) were independently associated with better overall health-related quality of life among the participants. *Conclusions.* The study demonstrated high proportion of HIV positive women on ART had poor health-related quality of life which was affected by wealth index, social support, and duration on antiretroviral therapy.

1. Introduction

Over the past few decades, human immunodeficiency virus (HIV) has infected and killed millions of people globally, Sub-Saharan Africa (SSA) being most affected by the disease [1, 2]. Women, both globally and in least developed countries, bear higher burden of HIV infection than men due to various biological, social, and economic reasons. In Sub-Saharan region, gender aspect of the infection is more remarkable that women share the largest percent of the infected population. For instance, among young women aged 15–24, there are about 380,000 new HIV infections every year; and 15% of women living with HIV are aged 15–24, of whom 80% live in SSA [3, 4].

Ethiopia is one of the most affected SSA countries by HIV. In 2016, there were an estimated 718,500 people living with HIV in the country [5]. Like other SSA countries, women in Ethiopia are also disproportionately affected than men [3, 4]. In 2016, about two-thirds of the people living with HIV/AIDS (PLWHA) and newly infected individuals were women in this nation [5]. In addition, the social stigma and discrimination is higher against women than men [3].

In response to HIV pandemic, various interventions have been executed targeting improving diagnosis methods, treatment regimens, and strengthening HIV prevention and control programs [3, 6–8]. One of the interventions is the provision of antiretroviral therapy (ART) to the people who live with the infection [9, 10]. The treatment has resulted in decreased incidence of the disease and increased longevity of the people living with the infection [11, 12]. Antiretroviral therapy also improves health-related quality of life (HRQoL) of individuals receiving the treatment [13, 14]. However, the psychological and economic burden of the infection associated with its chronicity made the long-term HRQoL benefits of the treatment dubious [12, 15].

Health-related quality of life is a multidimensional and complex concept [16] and reflects subjective perceptions of individuals, their physical health, psychological state, level of independence, social relationships, personal beliefs, and relationship to salient features of their environment [17, 18]. Health-related quality of life is associated with physical, psychological, and social aspects which are obviously influenced by individuals' beliefs, expectations, and perceptions [19, 20].

There are evidence that HRQoL of PLWHA has significant role in ART retention, treatment adherence, and survival [21–24]. As a result, the issue is becoming increasingly important for policy makers, program implementers, and researchers. Studies across various areas indicate that HRQoL of PLWHA is affected by socioeconomic variables, presence of comorbidities, stage of the disease, psychological factors, perceived stigma, behavioral factors, and availability of social support [25–40]. Poor adherence to ART is also another factor for compromised HRQoL among PLWHA. The studies also indicate women with HIV/AIDS are of poorer QoL than their men counterparts though they are generally more adherent to ART and similar disease stages [19, 25, 41].

Though there is established evidence on gender character of HIV/AIDS related HRQoL, in Ethiopia there is dearth of studies on HRQoL of women on ART. Particularly in our study area there is no evidence examining perceived HRQoL among women receiving ART. Therefore, this study aimed to examine the status of HRQoL and associated factors of HRQoL among women attending ART clinics at health facilities in Jimma town, southwest Ethiopia.

2. Methods and Materials

2.1. Study Settings and Design. An institution based cross-sectional study was conducted among women on ART from health facilities in Jimma town from May to June 2016. Jimma town is located 346 kilometers southwest of Addis Ababa, the capital of Ethiopia. The town has two public hospitals (Jimma University Specialized Hospital (JUSH) and *Shenen-Gibe* Primary Hospital) and one health center (Jimma Town Health Center) which provide ART services.

2.2. Sampling and Data Collection Tool. During the study period, a total of 3,172 HIV positive women (2,437 at JUSH, 612 at Jimma Health Center, and 123 at *Shenen-Gibe* Primary Hospital) were receiving ART. A sample size of 377 women on ART was calculated by taking p = 50% (expected proportion of women on ART with good HRQoL), 5% margin of error, 95% confidence level, adjusting to finite population, and adding 10% expected nonresponse rate. The sample was proportionately allocated among the three health facilities based on their population size as 289, 73, and 15 to JUSH, Jimma Town Health Center, and *Shenen-Gibe* Primary Hospitals,

respectively. Finally, the required sample of study participants was selected consecutively till the required sample size was fulfilled. Women who were critically ill, less than 18 years of age, and pregnant during the data collection period are excluded.

The data were collected using pretested, structured questionnaire which comprises World Health Organization (WHO) Quality of Life HIV short form instrument (WHOQOL-HIV BREF) items, sociodemographics, wealth index, clinical, social support variables, and perceived stigma assessing questions.

WHOQOL-HIV BREF contains 31 items distributed into 6 domains: physical, social relationships, level of independence, and spirituality domains each with 4 items and psychological and environmental domains with 5 and 8 items, respectively. The individual items are rated on a 5-point Likert scale where 1 indicates low/negative perceptions and 5 indicates high/positive perceptions. The remaining two items measure overall perceived quality of life and general health perception of women living with HIV [20]. The items were contextualized to the study area and translated to the local language (*Amharic* and *Affan Oromo*).

Wealth index was assessed using a tool adopted from Ethiopian Demographic and Health Survey (EDHS) wealth index assessment questionnaire. Clinical variables were collected from patients' medical records. Social support variable was measured using a 19-item Medical Outcomes Study Social Support Survey (MOS-SSS) designed to measure participants' perception of the availability of functional support along 4 dimensions: emotional, affectionate, tangible, and positive social interaction dimensions. The items were rated on a five-point response format of availability ranging from "none of the time" (1) to "all of the time" (5). A total score was obtained by summing responses to all items (ranging 19–95), with higher scores reflecting greater available support. In addition, individuals scoring above the mean social support score were categorized as of "good social support", and those with below the mean were classified as "poor social support"[42].

Perceived stigma was measured by 23 questions adopted from Berger et al. that have been contextualized locally. The questions consist of four-point Likert scale (strongly disagree to strongly agree) questions focusing on perceived isolation, shame, guilt, and disclosure of the HIV status. The scores of perceived stigma range from 23 to 92. A person was said to perceive stigma if he/she scored above the mean, otherwise no perceived stigma [43].

2.3. Data Collection and Analysis. The questionnaires were administered through face-to-face interview by trained counseling nurses who were not affiliated to the health facilities in which the data were collected. Supervisors were also trained and deployed for checking each questionnaire for its completeness and cleaning at the end of each data collection day and overall data quality management. Furthermore, the data collection tool was tested prior to the actual data collection on 19 women on ART attending Agaro Hospital ART Clinic which is in a neighboring town of the study area.

Responses were coded, entered, and analyzed using Statistical Package for the Social Sciences (SPSS) version 21. The statistical analyses comprised three steps. First descriptive statistics (mean, standard deviation, median, range, frequency, and proportions) were computed to describe the participants' demographics and other characteristics. All domain scores in WHOQOL–HIVBREF were scaled in positive direction with higher score denoting good quality of life. Within each domain, the mean scores of the items were calculated and dichotomized into poor versus good. Then, bivariate analysis was carried out whereby those variables which had p-values < 0.25 in each of the six WHOQOL domains and overall HRQoL were considered candidates for multivariable logistic regression model. Finally, multivariate logistic regression model was fit, and the overall statistical significance of the model was reported using adjusted odds ratios (AOR) with its corresponding 95% confidence intervals. P value < 0.05 was considered statistically significant.

Ethical clearance was secured from Institutional Review Board of College of Health Sciences of Jimma University (Ref No. RPGC/167/2016). Verbal consent was obtained from the study participants before conducting the interview. The right of respondents not to participate in the interview or to withdraw at any time was also assured.

3. Results

3.1. Sociodemographic, Clinical, and Psychosocial Characteristics of Study Participants. Among the sampled 377 study participants, 344 were interviewed, yielding response rate of 91%. Majority of the study participants were from JUSH and urban residents, accounting for 76.8% and 80.2%, respectively. The mean ± standard deviation (SD) age of the respondents was 34.07 ± 8.76 years, nearly half of them being between ages of 29-39 years. Most (54.7%) of the participants were married and 60.5% of them completed elementary school education. About 47% of the respondents were self-employed. Forty percent (40%) of the respondents were Muslims and 44% Oromo by ethnicity (Table 1). The wealth index of the respondents showed that about one-third of the participants were in the second tertile.

The median time (in months) since the women had known their HIV status was 66 with range of 7-158. Regarding the functional status of the respondents, almost all of them were under working functional status category during the start of ART. About 62% of the respondents had CD4+ cells counts > 200 cells/mm^3 when they started receiving the treatment. However, this figure was observed to rise to 93% during the study periods. Almost all respondents were placed under the first-line ART drug regimen at the start of the treatment as well as during the time of data collection. At the beginning of the therapy, 45.3% of the participants were of WHO clinical stage 2 and during the study period, the proportion of this category was 91.3%. During the study period, more than 95% of the participants were not diagnosed with opportunistic infections. On average, the women were on ART for 57 months (Table 1).

The 19-item Likert scale social support tool was tested for reliability and it showed excellent internal consistency with Cronbach's α=0.960. Taking the mean as a cut-off point, majority of the respondents (61.3%) were categorized to have poor social support. It was also revealed that around half of the respondents perceived that they had been stigmatized (Table 1).

3.2. Health-Related Quality of Life of Women on Antiretroviral Therapy. As mentioned above, HRQoL of the participants was assessed using WHOQOLHIV-BREF tool. The tool's reliability was high (Cronbach's α=0.898). Internal consistency measures of each domain of the tool and other findings were presented in Table 2. Level of independence domain of HRQoL was the highest with mean ± SD of 14.08 ± 3.069. The mean score of overall HRQoL, composited from all the six domains, was 13.21 ± 2.19. The mean scores for each domain and the overall HRQoL were used as cut-off point to categorize the participants domains of HRQoL and overall HRQoL as poor (less than or equal to the mean score) or good (greater than the mean score). Accordingly, in all the domains, the participants' quality of life was found to be poor and 53.5% of the respondents had poor overall HRQoL (Table 2).

In addition to the six domains of HRQoL, the tool also measures general perceived quality of life (QoL) and health status. About 33% of the participants reported their general QoL as indifferent, whereas 23.6% said that it was poor or very poor. The remaining (43.3%) reported to be good or very good. Regarding satisfaction about their health, 50 (14.5%) of the respondents replied that they were dissatisfied or very dissatisfied, 137 (39.8%) neither satisfied nor dissatisfied, and 157 (45.6%) were satisfied or very satisfied.

3.3. Factors Affecting Overall Health-Related Quality of Life. In the multivariate analysis, higher wealth index, shorter duration since ART initiation, and good social support were found to have statistically significant associations with good overall HRQoL among the study participants. The third tertile (highest wealth index) was 1.85 times more likely to have good overall HRQoL than those who are in the second tertile of wealth index (AOR: 1.85; 95% CI: [1.02, 3.39]). But there was no statistically significant difference in overall HRQoL between women of the second and first wealth tertile. On the other hand, those who had been on ART for less than 57 months (5.5 years) were almost twice more likely to have better overall HRQoL (AOR: 1.85; 95% CI: [1.14, 3.03]) than those who had been more than 57 months on treatment. It was also shown that participants who reported to have good social support were about 5 times more likely to have good overall HRQoL in comparison with those who reported to have poor social support (AOR: 4.89; 95% CI: [2.88, 8.34]) (Table 3).

3.4. Factors Affecting Domains of Health-Related Quality of Life

3.4.1. Level of Independence Domain of Quality of Life. The multivariate analysis shows that only social support significantly associates with domain of level of independence. Those women who reported to have good social support were about

TABLE 1: Sociodemographic, clinical, and psychosocial characteristics of the study participant in, 2016 (n=344).

Descriptions		Frequency (%)
Sociodemographic variables		
Place of residence	Rural	68 (19.8)
	Urban	276 (80.2)
Age (years)	18-28	96 (28.0)
	29-39	165 (47.9)
	≥40	83 (24.1)
Marital Status	Single	71 (20.6)
	Married	188 (54.7)
	Others	85 (24.7)
Educational status	No education	41 (11.9)
	Elementary school	208 (60.5)
	Secondary school and above	95 (27.6)
Occupation	Employed	97 (28.2)
	Self-employee	161 (46.8)
	No job	86 (25.0)
Religion	Muslim	139 (40.4)
	Orthodox	131 (38.1)
	Others	74 (21.5)
Ethnicity	Oromo	151 (43.9)
	Dawro	55 (16.0)
	Amhara	84 (24.4)
	Others	54 (15.7)
Wealth index	1st tertile	114 (33.1)
	2nd tertile	117 (34.0)
	3rd tertile	111 (32.3)
Clinical Characteristics		
Time since they had known their HIV status	<66 months	173 (50.3)
	≥66 months	171 (49.7)
Functional status during start of ART	Working	259 (75.3)
	Ambulatory	70 (20.3)
	Bedridden	15 (4.3)
Current functional Status	Working	330 (95.9)
	Ambulatory	14 (4.1)
Opportunistic infection	No	327(95.0)
	Yes	17 (5.0)
CD4 count at start of ART	Below 200 cells/mm^3	129 (37.5)
	200 cells/mm^3 and above	215 (62.5)
Current CD4 count	Below 200 cells/mm^3	25 (7.3)
	200 cells/mm^3 and above	316 (92.7)
WHO clinical stage at start of ART	Stage 1	59 (17.2)
	Stage 2	156 (45.3)
	Stage 3	105 (30.5)
	Stage 4	24 (7.0)
Current WHO clinical stage	Stage 1	17 (4.9)
	Stage 2	314 (91.3)
	Stage 3	10 (2.9)
	Stage 4 or T1	3 (0.9)
ART regimen at start	1st line regimens	342 (99.4)
	2nd line regimens	2 (0.6)
Recent ART regimen	1st line regimens	341 (99.1)
	2nd line regimens	3 (0.9)

Public Health: Emerging Issues and Innovative Solutions

TABLE 1: Continued.

Descriptions		Frequency (%)
Duration on ART (in months)	<57	186 (54.1)
	≥ 57	158 (45.9)
Psychosocial Characteristic		
Social support	Poor social support	211 (61.3)
	Good social support	133 (38.7)
Perceived stigma	Low perceived stigma	171 (49.7)
	High perceived stigma	173 (50.3)

TABLE 2: HRQoL domains' mean score of women on ART in Jimma town health facilities, 2016 (n = 344).

QoL Domains (No. of items)	Cronbach's α	Mean	Std. Deviation	Domains of quality of life	
				Poor N (%)	Good N (%)
Physical (4)	0.703	13.4622	2.95324	195(56.7)	149(43.3)
Psychological (5)	0.698	12.9675	2.46975	194(56.4)	150(43.6)
Level of independence (4)	0.77	14.0843	3.06896	195(56.7)	149(43.3)
Social relationships (4)	0.813	13.2703	3.90852	188(54.7)	156(45.3)
Environmental (8)	0.794	12.9390	3.32528	172(50)	172(50)
Spiritual (4)	0.892	12.3895	2.83964	195(56.7)	149(43.3)
Overall HRQOL	0.898	13.2112	2.19448	184(53.5)	160(46.5)

TABLE 3: Factors associated with overall HRQoL among women on ART in health facilities, Jimma town, Ethiopia, 2016 (n=344).

Variables		Overall HRQoL	
		Crude OR [95% CI]	Adjusted OR [95% CI]
Age of the women in years	18-28	1.72 [1.03, 2.85]	1.18 [0.65, 2.16]
	29-39	1	1
	>39	1.92 [1.12, 3.28]	1.66 [0.89, 3.09]
Educational status	No education	1.74 [0.89, 3.42]	1.25 [0.57, 2.76]
	Primary school	1	1
	Secondary school & above	2.07 [1.26, 3.39]	1.49 [0.85, 2.63]
Social support	Poor s. support	1	1
	Good s. support	4.99 [3.12, 7.99]	4.99 [2.88, 8.34]*
Wealth index tertile	1st tertile	0.96 [0.57,1.66]	1.67 [0.72, 2.29]
	2nd tertile	1	1
	3rd tertile	1.65 [0.97,2.76]	1.85 [1.02, 3.39]*
Duration on ART	<57 months	1'	1
	≥57 months	0.67[0.44,1.03]	0.54 [0.33, 0.88]*

*Variable statistically significant at P< 0.05; AOR: adjusted odds ratio, COR: crude odds ratio; CI: confidence interval.

three times more likely to have better level of independence than those of poorer social support (AOR: 3.24; 95% CI: [1.98, 5.32]) (Table 4).

3.4.2. Physical Health Quality of Life Domain. Place of residence, educational status, and social support were found to have significant effects on physical health domain of QoL after controlling possible confounders. Women residing in urban area were 1.96 times more likely to have good physical

health QoL compared to their counterparts of rural resident (AOR: 1.96; 95% CI: [1.09, 3.57]). The study also revealed that women on ART who enrolled in secondary school or above were 1.98 times more likely to have good physical quality of life than those who were in the elementary school or had no education (AOR: 1.98; 95% CI: [1.17, 3.35]). It was also shown that those women who reported to have good social support were 1.78 times more likely to have good physical quality of life in comparison with those women who reported to have poor social support (AOR: 1.78; 95% CI: [1.10, 2.88]) (Table 4).

TABLE 4: Factors associated with domains of quality of life among women on ART in health facilities of Jimma Town, southwest Ethiopia, 2016 (n = 344).

Variables	Physical QoL		Psychological QoL		Level of Independence QoL		Social Relationship QoL		Environmental QoL		Spiritual QoL	
	COR [95% CI]	AOR [95% CI]	COR [95% CI]	AOR [95% CI]	COR [95% CI]	AOR [95% CI]	COR [95% CI]	AOR [95% CI]	COR [95% CI]	AOR [95% CI]	COR [95% CI]	AOR [95% CI]
Age (in years)												
18-28	1.59[0.96,2.65]	1.65[0.93, 2.95]			1.71[1.02, 2.84]	1.47[0.81, 2.68]						
29-39	1	1			1	1						
>39	1.47[0.86, 2.51]	0.97[0.53, 1.76]			1.62[0.95, 2.78]	1.08[0.58, 2.02]						
Place of residence												
Rural	1.36[0.79, 2.31]	0.51[0.28,0.92]*										
Urban	1	1										
Educational status												
No education	1.58[0.81, 3.11]	1.30[0.63, 2.68]	1.07[0.54, 2.11]	0.96[0.45,2.02]	1.41[0.72, 2.77]	1.25[,0.56, 2.78]	1.46[0.75, 2.85]	1.26[0.58, 2.75]				
Primary school	1	1	1	1	1	1	1	1				
Secondary School & above	2.10[1.28, 3.44]	1.98[1.17, 3.35]*	1.67[1.03, 2.73]	1.25[0.72, 2.20]	1.98 1.22, 3.23]	1.27[0.70, 2.29]	1.54[0.95, 2.52]	1.14[0.64, 2.04]				
Social support												
Poor s. support	1	1	1	1	1	1	1	1	1	1		
Good s. support	2.17[1.41, 2.94]	1.78[1.10, 2.88]*	3.38[2.15, 5.32]	3.38[2.05,5.56]*	3.98[2.51, 6.29]	3.24[1.98, 5.32]*	4.0[2.5, 6.25]	4.76[2.7, 8.33]*	4.69[2.92, 7.53]	4.85[2.83, 8.3]*		
Time since HIV diagnosed												
< 66 months					1.35[0.81, 2.23]	1.69[0.90,3.16]					0.65[0.39,1.10]	0.96[0.6,0.99]*
≥ 66 months					1	1					1	1

TABLE 4: Continued.

Variables	Physical QoL		Psychological QoL		Level of Independence QoL		Social Relationship QoL		Environmental QoL		Spiritual QoL	
	COR [95% CI]	AOR [95% CI]	COR [95% CI]	AOR [95% CI]	COR [95% CI]	AOR [95% CI]	COR [95% CI]	AOR [95% CI]	COR [95% CI]	AOR [95% CI]	COR [95% CI]	AOR [95% CI]
WHO Clinical Stage at the beginning of ART												
Stage 1							0.63[0.34,1.16]	0.70[0.35, 1.40]	0.61[0.33,1.13]	0.52[0.07,1.04]		
Stage 2							1	1	1	1		
Stage 3							0.96[0.58,1.57]	0.92[0.53,1.61]	1.32[0.80,2.16]	0.35[0.12,0.98]*		
Stage 4							2.27[0.92,5.62]	3.92[1.37,11.27]*	2.05[0.83,5.07]	0.46[0.16,1.33]		
Wealth index tertile												
1st tertile			1.19[0.70,2.02]	1.64[0.90,2.99]			0.67[0.39,1.13]	0.75[0.41,1.36]	1.11[0.66,1.85]	1.51[0.81,2.78]		
2nd tertile			1	1			1	1	1	1		
3rd tertile			2.18[1.28,3.70]	2.53[1.42,4.51]*			1.77[1.05,2.99]	1.96[1.09,3.52]*	1.90[1.12,3.22]	2.20[1.20,4.03]*		
Perceived stigma												
Low							1.79[1.18, 2.78]	2.13[1.3, 3.44]*				
High							1	1				
Duration on ART												
<57 months	1	1							1	1		
≥57 months	0.77[0.5, 1.19]	1.37[0.75, 2.49]							0.72[0.47,1.11]	0.57[0.35,0.93]*		
CD4 count during the beginning of ART												
<200 cells/mm³											0.49[0.32,0.78]	0.48[0.29,0.79]*
≥200 cells/mm³											1	1

* Variable statistically significant at P < 0.05; AOR: adjusted odds ratio, COR: crude odds ratio; CI: confidence interval.

3.4.3. Social Relationship Quality of Life Domain. Four variables (wealth index, WHO clinical stage during start of ART, social support, and perceived stigma) had significant associations with social relationship QoL after adjusting for confounders. Those women who were in clinical stage 4 were about four times more likely to have good social relationship QoL (AOR: 3.92; 95% CI: [1.37, 11.27]) than those who were in clinical stage 2. Respondents who perceived low stigma were two times more likely to have good social relationship QoL than those who had high perceived stigma (AOR: 2.13; 95% CI: [1.29, 3.44]). Similarly, respondents under third wealth tertile category were about twice more likely to have good social relationship QoL than those in other wealth index categories (AOR: 1.96; 95% CI: [1.09, 3.52]). It was also revealed that those women who reported that they get good social support were about 5 times more likely to have good social relationship QoL in comparison with those who received poorer social support (AOR: 4.76; 95% CI: [2.7, 8.33]) (Table 4).

3.4.4. Psychological Quality of Life Domain. In this domain, wealth index and social support had a significant association with psychological QoL. In the wealth index respondents belonging to third tertile were 2.53 times more likely to have better psychological QoL than those who are in the middle or first wealth tertiles (AOR: 2.53; 95% CI: [1.423, 4.505]). On the other hand, women who reported to have good social support were 3.38 times more likely to have better level of psychological QoL in comparison with those who reported that they receive poorer social support (AOR: 3.38; 95% CI: [2.05, 5.56]) (Table 4).

3.4.5. Environmental Quality of Life Domain. Among the variables assessed, WHO clinical stage during start of ART, social support, duration since ART initiation, and wealth index were found to be independent predictors of environmental QoL. Those women in clinical stage 2 were about three times more likely to have good environmental QoL than those women in clinical stage 3 (AOR: 2.86; 95% CI: [1.02, 8.33]). Similarly, respondents categorized under the third tertile of wealth index were twice more likely to have good environmental QoL than those women under the second tertile (AOR: 2.199; 95% CI: 1.20, 4.03]). Furthermore, respondents who reported to have good social support were about 5 times more likely to have good environmental QoL than those who have poor social support [AOR: 4.85; 95% CI: [2.83, 8.31]). The study also revealed that women who had been on ART for less than 57 months were more likely to have better environmental QoL than those for 57 months or more (AOR: 1.75; 95% CI: [1.07, 2.86]) (Table 4).

3.4.6. Spiritual Quality of Life Domain. CD4 count at the beginning of ART and time since they had been diagnosed for HIV had association with their spiritual QoL. Those women whose CD4 count at the start of ART was less than 200 cells/mm^3 were 52% less likely to have good spiritual QoL than those women whose CD4 count had been equal to or above 200 cells/mm^3 (AOR: 0.48; 95% CI: [0.29, 0.79]). In similar fashion, women that were diagnosed with HIV 5.5 years (66 months) prior to the study period were slightly more likely to have a better spiritual QoL than those who were diagnosed within 5.5 years during the study period (AOR: 0.96; 95% CI: [.60, .99]) (Table 4).

4. Discussion

This study revealed that majority of the women under study were from urban areas (80.2%), between the ages of 29 and 38 years (47.9%), and married (54.7%) and 60.5% of them attended elementary school. These sociodemographic characteristics are in line with the Ethiopian Demographic and Health Survey figures that indicate the burden of HIV/AIDS in the country with respect to the demographic and social status of PLWHA. According to the survey, female in urban areas and under the age group 29-30 years are more affected by HIV than the rural women and other age groups in Ethiopia [44].

In this study, it was shown that the overall HRQoL and each domain of QoL of women on ART in Jimma town health facilities were poor. This finding is consistent with other studies produced elsewhere in which HRQoL of people with HIV were documented to be poor [27, 30, 34, 39, 45, 46]. However, other studies came up with results which discord the current findings in relation to level of overall HRQoL [29, 47–52], in which the other studies show better overall HRQoL than the current findings. This difference is attributed to the socioeconomic differences across the study participants as most of these studies came from economically advanced countries. In addition, unlike the current study, others include both sexes as study population.

Level of independence domain was of the highest mean score among the six domains of HRQoL followed by physical health, social relationships, psychological, environmental, and spiritual QoL. These findings are not in line with those from other studies [25, 27, 41, 45, 53, 54]. The discrepancy may be attributed to the differences in the study areas and periods, and sociodemographic changes across the study populations.

This study also examined factors affecting the overall HRQoL and its domains among the study participants. The overall HRQoL of the participants was affected by wealth index, duration since ART initiation, and social support. Individuals with higher wealth index had better HRQoL. This evidence is also supported by studies from Nigeria and India in which higher income was associated with good QoL on the physical health, psychological health, level of independence, and spirituality/ personal beliefs domains [25, 29, 55, 56].

However, other sociodemographic variables assessed in this study such as age, place of residence, educational, marital, and employment status were not found to have statistically significant relation with overall HRQoL. Nevertheless, other studies indicated that employment and educational status were determined to be a positive factor for better overall HRQoL among PLWHA [34, 57–59]. The disagreement may be attributed to the differences in the study populations.

Clinical characteristics assessed in this study (current WHO clinical stage, ART regimen that the respondents were placed to, current CD4 cells count levels, and current functional status of the participants) had no statistically significant associations with neither overall HRQoL nor domains of QoL of PLWHA receiving ART in the study area. In contrast to this, several studies indicated that higher CD4 cell counts of PLWHA were associated with better HRQoL [21, 39, 60–64]. However, duration on ART was significantly associated with overall HRQoL of the participants, individuals with shorter duration on ART having better HRQoL. This might be due to the fact that HIV/ AIDS is one of the chronic illnesses affecting economic, psychological, and social aspects of patients. Improvement of QoL that resulted from the treatment may be outweighed by the negative impacts of chronicity of the disease. Furthermore, this finding is supported by a recent study carried out in Kenya in which it was reported that patients on ART for a relatively longer duration had had poorer HRQoL than those who had been on ART for lesser durations [46].

In this study, it was unveiled that better social support is a predictor for better HRQoL. This finding was concurrent with other studies across various countries [19, 25, 27, 29, 31, 32, 34, 36, 53, 65]. This is mainly because social support is crucial for adherence to ART drugs which in turn improves the patients' quality of lives [27, 29, 31, 32, 34, 36, 65] though adherence to the treatments and social support are not sufficient to ensure HRQoL.

Regarding the domains of HRQoL, among variables assessed, wealth index was found to be positively associated with psychological, social, and environmental domains of HRQoL but had no significant effect on physical, level of independence, and spiritual domains. This is supported by studies from other parts of the world in which women of better income had better physical HRQoL [32, 55]. Place of residence and educational status had significant associations with physical health domain. Women on ART who were more educated and residing in urban areas were more likely to have better physical heath than women who were less educated and living in rural areas. These associations may be attributed to the fact that better educational status and living in urban areas offer a better job opportunity, access to health care, and information. This finding is similar with the existing evidence [28, 29, 31, 32, 41, 65]. However, these variables as well as the remaining sociodemographic factors (age, religion, ethnicity, and marital status) had no significant effects on other domains of HRQoL. This result discords with other findings [12, 22, 66] in which the younger the patients, the better the various domains of HRQoL.

In this study, social support was found to positively affect five of the six domains of HRQoL. The finding is in line with those from other developing countries which documented that better social support positively affects physical health domain [28, 29, 31, 32, 34, 46, 67]. It is remarkable that social support is most important factor for improved QoL among women living with HIV in the study area.

Level of perceived stigma was found to affect only social relationship domain of the HRQoL in the current study setting. This is supported by longitudinal study conducted in developing countries that perceived HIV stigma has a significant negative and constant impact upon HRQoL for people with HIV infection [68]. Other studies also show

that the social relationship domain has negative impacts on HRQoL among PLWHA [69, 70].

Clinical variables (clinical stage when ART had been initiated, CD4 cell count during the start of ART, time since diagnosis of HIV by the participants, and duration since start of ART) had also significant associations with domains of HRQoL. WHO clinical stage of the women at the start of ART had positive relationship with social relationship domain and negative with environmental health domain. Women who had been at stage 4 (WHO Clinical Stage at the beginning of ART) were more likely to have better quality of social relationship domain than those in stage 2. This finding is in contrast with the findings in other studies in which lower clinical stages were associated with better QoL [65, 70].

On the other hand, women who had been in stage 2 were of better environmental health domain than that of stage 3. Women with less CD4 cells count during the start of the treatment were found to have poorer spiritual QoL. As CD4+ cells count increases in the body, the capability of protection from opportunistic infection also increases, which in turn leads to better QoL. Other studies conducted in India also showed that patients with higher CD4 count had better QoL [63, 69]. In contrast, a recent cohort study from Uganda revealed that there is no association between change in CD4 count and quality of life scores [27, 30]. However, amount of CD4 count during ART initiation or during the study period did not affect other domains of QoL in this study.

Time elapsed since the women had been diagnosed for HIV was found to be positively associated with spiritual domain. Living with the infection for longer time may lead to better adaptability and QoL. But this variable was associated with neither the other domains nor the overall HRQoL in this study. The other clinical variable which affected HRQoL of the respondents in the current study area was duration on ART. The longer they were on ART, the poorer environmental domain of QoL they had.

5. Limitations

As this study is cross-sectional, it cannot establish causality of the associations between the outcome variables and independent variables. Although variables which were presumed to have associated with HRQoL among PLWHA, such as alcohol use, smoking, and chewing khat, have been assessed, they cannot be analyzed because their observed frequencies were too low as the sample size is small.

6. Conclusion and Recommendations

This study demonstrated that the status of HRQoL among HIV positive women who were on ART treatment in Jimma town health facilities was poor. Along with this finding, wealth index, social support, and duration on ART were identified to affect HRQoL of the study participants in the study setting. The study also examined the proportion and associated factors of the six domains of HRQoL. Majority of the participants were found to have poor QoL in all the domains. These domains of QoL were affected by social support, place of residence, educational status, wealth index, duration since diagnosis, WHO clinical stage at start of ART, perceived stigma level, duration on ART, and CD4 count at start of the treatment.

We recommend branches of Ethiopian Ministry of Health and organizations concerned about welfare of PLWHA to enhance social support services delivered to women with HIV/AIDS to improve psychological, environmental, and overall HRQoL of the target group. In addition, strategies must be formulated and implemented to promote financial welfare of women with HIV/AIDS to enhance their quality of lives. We also recommend researchers to conduct further studies by applying stronger designs to establish causal relationship between health-related quality of lives of women on ART and factors identified to affect it, such as duration on ART treatment.

Abbreviations

AIDS:　Acquired Immuno-Deficiency Syndrome
AOR:　Adjusted odds ratio
ART:　Antiretroviral therapy
CI:　Confidence interval
COR:　Crude odds ratio
HIV:　Human Immunodeficiency Virus
HRQoL:　Health-related quality of life
PLWHA:　People living with HIV/AIDS
QoL:　Quality of life
SSA:　Sub-Saharan Africa
WHO:　World Health Organization.

Acknowledgments

We would like to thank Jimma University College of Health Sciences, for providing us with the opportunity to carry out this study. We would also like to thank all the data collectors and study participants for their participation and willingness to be involved in the study.

References

[1] United Nations Programme on HIV/AIDS (UNAIDS), *Global Report: UNAIDS Report on The Global AIDS Epidemic 2013*, UNAIDS, Geneva, Switzerland, 2013, Available from: http://www.unaids.org/en/resources/documents/2013/20130923_UNAIDS_Global_Report_2013.

[2] World Health Organization (WHO), *Global HIV/AIDS Response - Epidemic update and health sector progress towards Universal Access: Progress Report*, WHO, Geneva, Switzerland, 2011.

[3] World Health Organization, *Global Health Sector Response to HIV, 2000-2015: Focus on Innovations in Africa: Progress Report*, World Health Organization, Geneva, Switzerland, 2015.

[4] Federal HIV/AIDS Prevention and Control Office (FHAPCO), *Country Preogress Report on the HIV Response*, Federal Democratic Republic of Ethiopia, Addis Ababa, Ethiopia, 2014.

[5] The Ethiopian Public Health Institute, *HIV Related Estimates and Projectios for Ethiopia 2017*, The Ethiopian Public Health Institute, Ethiopia, 2017.

[6] World Health Organization, *Progress on Global Access to HIV Antiretroviral Therapy: a Report on "3 by 5" and Beyond*, WHO, Geneva, Switzerland, 2006, Available from: http://www.who.int/hiv/pub/2006progressreport/en.

[7] P. Iguot, D. Nanongo, and D. Odongo, *Accelerated Response to HIV and AIDS through Private-Public Capacity Building Partnerships: the Experience of TASO Uganda*, Uganda, 2008.

[8] President's Emergency Plan for AIDS Relief, *PEPFAR Funding: Fact Sheet*, President's Emergency Plan for AIDS Relief, Washington, DC, USA, 2015.

[9] World Health Organization, *Scaling up Antiretroviral Therapy in Resource-Limited Settings: Guidelines for A Public Health Approach*, WHO, Geneva, Switzerland, 2002, Available from: http://www.who.int/hiv/pub/prev_care/en/ScalingUp_E.pdf.

[10] World Health Organization, *Guideline on when to start antiretroviral therapy and on pre-exposure prophylaxis for HIV*, WHO, Geneva, Switzerland, 2015, http://www.who.int/hiv/pub/guidelines/earlyrelease-arv/en.

[11] S. Kasedde, C. Luo, C. McClure, and U. Chandan, "Reducing HIV and AIDS in adolescents: Opportunities and challenges," *Current HIV/AIDS Reports*, vol. 10, no. 2, pp. 159–168, 2013.

[12] J. Bor, A. J. Herbst, M.-L. Newell, and T. Bärnighausen, "Increases in adult life expectancy in rural South Africa: Valuing the scale-up of HIV treatment," *Science*, vol. 339, no. 6122, pp. 961–965, 2013.

[13] Federal HIV/AIDS Prevention and Control Office, Ministry of Health-Ethiopia, "Guide for Implementation of the Antiretroviral Therapy Programme in Ethiopia", Federal HIV/AIDS Prevention and Control Office, 2007.

[14] Federal Minstry of Health Ethiopia, *AIDS in Ethiopia 6th Report, 2006*, Federal Ministry of Health -Ethiopia, Addis Ababa, Ethiopia, 2006, http://www.etharc.org.

[15] S. G. Deeks, S. R. Lewin, and D. V. Havlir, "The end of AIDS: HIV infection as a chronic disease," *The Lancet*, vol. 382, no. 9903, pp. 1525–1533, 2013.

[16] R. W. Burgoyne and D. S. Saunders, "Quality of life among urban Canadian HIV/AIDS clinic outpatients," *International Journal of STD & AIDS*, vol. 12, no. 8, pp. 505–512, 2001.

[17] K. W. Smith, N. E. Avis, and S. F. Assmann, "Distinguishing between quality of life and health status in quality of life research: A meta-analysis," *Quality of Life Research*, vol. 8, no. 5, pp. 447–459, 1999.

[18] Department of Health and Human Sevices, *Healthy People 2020. Health-Related Quality of Life and Well-Being*, Department of Health and Human Sevices, Washington, DC, USA, 2013.

[19] O. O. Oguntibeju, "Quality of life of people living with HIV and AIDS and antiretroviral therapy," *HIV/AIDS—Research and Palliative Care*, vol. 4, pp. 117–124, 2012.

[20] Division of mental health and prevention of subsance abuse, *Measuring Quality of Life The World Health Organization Quality of Life Instruments (THE WHOQOL-100 and the WHOQOL-BREF)*, WHO, 1997.

[21] H. Jia, C. R. Uphold, S. Wu, G. J. Chen, and P. W. Duncan, "Predictors of changes in health-related quality of life among men with HIV infection in the HAART era," *AIDS Patient Care and STDs*, vol. 19, no. 6, pp. 395–405, 2005.

[22] A. Tomita, N. Garrett, L. Werner et al., "Health-related quality of life dynamics of HIV-positive South African women up to ART

initiation: Evidence from the CAPRISA 002 acute infection cohort study," *AIDS and Behavior*, vol. 18, no. 6, pp. 1114–1123, 2014.

[23] I. M. De Boer-van Der Kolk, M. A. G. Sprangers, J. M. Prins, C. Smit, F. De Wolf, and P. T. Nieuwkerk, "Health-related quality of life and survival among HIV-infected patients receiving highly active antiretroviral therapy: a study of patients in the AIDS therapy Evaluation in the Netherlands (ATHENA) cohort," *Clinical Infectious Diseases*, vol. 50, no. 2, pp. 255–263, 2010.

[24] S. B. Mannheimer, J. Matts, E. Telzak et al., "Quality of life in HIV-infected individuals receiving antiretroviral therapy is related to adherence," *AIDS Care*, vol. 17, no. 1, pp. 10–22, 2005.

[25] K. H. Basavaraj, M. A. Navya, and R. Rashmi, "Quality of life in HIV/AIDS," *Indian Journal of Sexually Transmitted Diseases and AIDS*, vol. 31, no. 2, pp. 75–80, 2010.

[26] K. A. McDonnell, A. C. Gielen, A. W. Wu, P. O'Campo, and R. Faden, "Measuring health related quality of life among women living with HIV," *Quality of Life Research*, vol. 9, no. 8, pp. 931–940, 2000.

[27] D. Mutabazi-Mwesigire, A. Katamba, F. Martin, J. Seeley, and A. W. Wu, "Factors that affect quality of life among people living with HIV attending an urban clinic in Uganda: A cohort study," *PLoS ONE*, vol. 10, no. 6, p. e0126810, 2015.

[28] E. Vigneshwaran, Y. Padmanabhareddy, N. Devanna, and G. Alvarez-Uria, "Gender differences in health related quality of life of people living with HIV/AIDS in the era of highly active antiretroviral therapy," *North American Journal of Medical Sciences*, vol. 5, no. 2, pp. 102–107, 2013.

[29] N. Wig, R. Lekshmi, H. Pal, V. Ahuja, C. M. Mittal, and S. K. Agarwal, "The impact of HIV/AIDS on the quality of life: A cross sectional study in North India," *Indian Journal of Medical Sciences*, vol. 60, no. 1, pp. 3–12, 2006.

[30] S. N. Mbalinda, N. Kiwanuka, D. K. Kaye, and L. E. Eriksson, "Reproductive health and lifestyle factors associated with health-related quality of life among perinatally HIV-infected adolescents in Uganda," *Health and Quality of Life Outcomes*, vol. 13, no. 1, article no. 170, 2015.

[31] M. Chokchai, B. E. M. K. Basamat, and N. Sutham, "People living with HIV/AIDS in the city of Bangkok: quality of life and related factors," *Journal of the Medical Association of Thailand*, vol. 95, no. 6, 2012.

[32] S. Yadav, "Perceived social support, hope, and quality of life of persons living with HIV/AIDS: a case study from Nepal," *Quality of Life Research*, vol. 19, no. 2, pp. 157–166, 2010.

[33] L. S. Briongos Figuero, P. Bachiller Luque, T. Palacios Martín, M. González Sagrado, and J. M. Eiros Bouza, "Assessment of factors influencing health-related quality of life in HIV-infected patients," *HIV Medicine*, vol. 12, no. 1, pp. 22–30, 2011.

[34] R. Patel, S. Kassaye, C. Gore-Felton et al., "Quality of life, psychosocial health, and antiretroviral therapy among HIV-positive women in Zimbabwe," *AIDS Care Psychological and Socio-medical Aspects of AIDS/HIV*, vol. 21, no. 12, pp. 1517–1527, 2009.

[35] M. K. Leow, K. Griva, R. Choo et al., "Determinants of Health-Related Quality of Life (HRQoL) in the Multiethnic Singapore Population – A National Cohort Study," *PLoS ONE*, vol. 8, no. 6, p. e67138, 2013.

[36] K. K. Pedersen, M. R. Eiersted, J. C. Gaardbo et al., "Lower self-reported quality of life in HIV-infected patients on cART and with low comorbidity compared with healthy controls," *Journal of Acquired Immune Deficiency Syndromes*, vol. 70, no. 1, pp. 16–22, 2015.

[37] K. Crothers, T. A. Griffith, K. A. McGinnis et al., "The impact of cigarette smoking on mortality, quality of life, and comorbid illness among HIV-positive veterans," *Journal of General Internal Medicine*, vol. 20, no. 12, pp. 1142–1145, 2005.

[38] P. T. Korthuis, L. C. Zephyrin, J. A. Fleishman et al., "Health-related quality of life in HIV-infected patients: The role of substance use," *AIDS Patient Care and STDs*, vol. 22, no. 11, pp. 859–867, 2008.

[39] L. N. Campos, C. C. César, and M. D. C. Guimarães, "Quality of life among HIV-infected patients in Brazil after initiation of treatment," *Clinics*, vol. 64, no. 9, pp. 867–875, 2009.

[40] C. Protopopescu, F. Marcellin, B. Spire et al., "Health-related quality of life in HIV-1-infected patients on HAART: A five-years longitudinal analysis accounting for dropout in the APROCO-COPILOTE cohort (ANRS CO-8)," *Quality of Life Research*, vol. 16, no. 4, pp. 577–591, 2007.

[41] A. Tesfay, A. Gebremariam, M. Gerbaba, and H. Abrha, "Gender Differences in Health Related Quality of Life among People Living with HIV on Highly Active Antiretroviral Therapy in Mekelle Town, Northern Ethiopia," *BioMed Research International*, vol. 2015, Article ID 516369, 9 pages, 2015.

[42] RAND Medical Outcomes Study, Social Support Survey Instrument, Available from: http://www.rand.org/health/surveys_tools/mos/socialsupport/surveyinstrumentinstrument.

[43] B. E. Berger, C. E. Ferrans, and F. R. Lashley, "Measuring stigma in people with HIV: psychometric assessment of the HIV stigma scale," *Research in Nursing & Health*, vol. 24, no. 6, pp. 518–529, 2001.

[44] Central Statistical Agency [Ethiopia] and ICF International, *Ethiopia Demographic and Health Survey 2011*, Central Statistical Agency and ICF International, Addis Ababa, Ethiopia and Calverton, Md, USA, 2012.

[45] M. H. Imam, M. R. Karim, C. Ferdous, and S. Akhter, "Health related quality of life among the people living with HIV," *Bangladesh Medical Research Council Bulletin*, vol. 37, no. 1, pp. 1–6, 2011.

[46] E. Mûnene and B. Ekman, "Does duration on antiretroviral therapy determine health-related quality of life in people living with HIV? A cross-sectional study in a regional referral hospital in Kenya," *Global Health Action*, vol. 7, no. 1, Article ID 23554, 2014.

[47] F. Razera, J. Ferreira, and R. R. Bonamigo, "Factors associated with health-related quality-of-life in HIV-infected Brazilians," *International Journal of STD & AIDS*, vol. 19, no. 8, pp. 519–523, 2008.

[48] B. Nirmal, K. Divya, V. Dorairaj, and K. Venkateswaran, "Quality of life in HIV/AIDS patients: A cross-sectional study in south India," *Indian Journal of Sexually Transmitted Diseases and AIDS*, vol. 29, no. 1, p. 15, 2008.

[49] M. Nojomi, K. Anbary, and M. Ranjbar, "Health-related quality of life in patients with HIV/AIDS," *Archives of Iranian Medicine*, vol. 11, no. 6, pp. 608–612, 2008.

[50] L. E. Eriksson, G. Nordström, T. Berglund, and E. Sandström, "The health-related quality of life in a Swedish sample of HIV-infected persons," *Journal of Advanced Nursing*, vol. 32, no. 5, pp. 1213–1223, 2000.

[51] K. Rüütel, H. Pisarev, H. Loit, and A. Uusküla, "Factors influencing quality of life of people living with HIV in Estonia: a cross-sectional survey," *Journal of the International AIDS Society*, vol. 12, no. 1, p. 13, 2009.

[52] S. Kovacevic, T. Vurusic, K. Duvancic, and M. Macek, "Quality of life of HIV infected persons in croatia," *Collegium Antropologicum*, vol. 30, Suppl 2, pp. 79–84, 2006.

[53] D. Haldar, P. Taraphdar, A. Dasgupta et al., "Socioeconomic consequences of HIV/AIDS in the family system," *Nigerian Medical Journal*, vol. 52, no. 4, pp. 250–253, 2011.

[54] M. L. Campsmith, A. K. Nakashima, and A. J. Davidson, "Self-reported health-related quality of life in persons with HIV infection: Results from a multi-site interview project," *Health and Quality of Life Outcomes*, vol. 1, article no. 12, 2003.

[55] A. O. L. Akinboro, S. O. M. Akinyemi, P. B. Olaitan et al., "Quality of life of Nigerians living with human immunodeficiency virus," *The Pan African Medical Journal*, vol. 18, p. 234, 2014.

[56] S. Bharat, P. Aggleton, and P. Tyrer, "India: HIV and AIDS-related discrimination, stigmatization and denial," *Joint United Nations Programme on HIV/AIDS, UNAIDS, Geneva, Switzerland*, 2001.

[57] A. L. Stangl, N. Wamai, J. Mermin, A. C. Awor, and R. E. Bunnell, "Trends and predictors of quality of life among HIV-infected adults taking highly active antiretroviral therapy in rural Uganda," *AIDS Care Psychological and Socio-medical Aspects of AIDS/HIV*, vol. 19, no. 5, pp. 626–636, 2007.

[58] A. C. Blalock, J. S. McDaniel, and E. W. Farber, "Effect of employment on quality of life and psychological functioning in patients with HIV/AIDS," *Psychosomatics*, vol. 43, no. 5, pp. 400–404, 2002.

[59] S. Rueda, J. Raboud, C. Mustard, A. Bayoumi, J. N. Lavis, and S. B. Rourke, "Employment status is associated with both physical and mental health quality of life in people living with HIV," *AIDS Care*, vol. 23, no. 4, 2011.

[60] R. Murri, M. Fantoni, C. Del Borgo et al., "Determinants of health-related quality of life in HIV-infected patients," *AIDS Care Psychological and Socio-medical Aspects of AIDS/HIV*, vol. 15, no. 4, pp. 581–590, 2003.

[61] S. A. Call, J. C. Klapow, K. E. Stewart et al., "Health-related quality of life and virologic outcomes in an HIV clinic," *Quality of Life Research*, vol. 9, no. 9, pp. 977–985, 2000.

[62] C. Armon and K. Lichtenstein, "The associations among coping, nadir CD4+ T-cell count, and non-HIV-related variables with health-related quality of life among an ambulatory HIV-positive patient population," *Quality of Life Research*, vol. 21, no. 6, pp. 993–1003, 2012.

[63] H. Jia, C. R. Uphold, Y. Zheng et al., "A further investigation of health-related quality of life over time among men with HIV infection in the HAART era," *Quality of Life Research*, vol. 16, no. 6, pp. 961–968, 2007.

[64] "WHO Guidelines," http://www.who.int/hiv/pub/guidelines/en/.

[65] M. Pereira and M. C. Canavarro, "Gender and age differences in quality of life and the impact of psychopathological symptoms among HIV-infected patients," *AIDS and Behavior*, vol. 15, no. 8, pp. 1857–1869, 2011.

[66] I. Ruiz Perez, J. Rodriguez Baño, M. A. Lopez Ruz et al., "Health-related quality of life of patients with HIV: Impact of sociodemographic, clinical and psychosocial factors," *Quality of Life Research*, vol. 14, no. 5, pp. 1301–1310, 2005.

[67] A. Charkhian, H. Fekrazad, H. Sajadi, M. Rahgozar, M. Haji Abdolbaghi, and S. Maddahi, "Relationship between health-related quality of life and social support in HIV-infected people in Tehran, Iran," *Iranian Journal of Public Health*, vol. 43, no. 1, pp. 100–106, 2014.

[68] M. Greeff, L. R. Uys, D. Wantland et al., "Perceived HIV stigma and life satisfaction among persons living with HIV infection in five African countries: A longitudinal study," *International Journal of Nursing Studies*, vol. 47, no. 4, pp. 475–486, 2010.

[69] T. Mahalakshmy, K. C. Premarajan, and A. Hamide, "Quality of life and its determinants in people living with human immunodeficiency virus infection in Puducherry, India," *Indian Journal of Community Medicine*, vol. 36, no. 3, pp. 203–207, 2011.

[70] A. P.-C. Fan, H.-C. C. Kuo, D. Y.-T. Kao, D. E. Morisky, and Y.-M. A. Chen, "Quality of life and needs assessment on people living with HIV and AIDS in Malawi," *AIDS Care Psychological and Socio-medical Aspects of AIDS/HIV*, vol. 23, no. 3, pp. 287–302, 2011.

16

Clinical Oral Health Recommended Care and Oral Health Self-Report, NHANES, 2013-2014

R. Constance Wiener⓪,[1] Nilanjana Dwibedi,[2] Chan Shen,[3]
Patricia A. Findley,[4] and Usha Sambamoorthi⓪[2]

[1]Department of Dental Practice and Rural Health, School of Dentistry, 104A Health Sciences Addition, P.O. Box 9415,
West Virginia University, Morgantown, WV 26506-9448, USA
[2]Department of Pharmaceutical Systems and Policy, West Virginia University School of Pharmacy,
Robert C. Byrd Health Sciences Center [North], P.O. Box 9510, Morgantown, WV 26506-9510, USA
[3]Departments of Health Services Research and Biostatistics, University of Texas MD Anderson Cancer Center,
1400 Pressler St., Houston, TX 77030, USA
[4]Rutgers University, School of Social Work, 536 George Street, New Brunswick, NJ 08901, USA

Correspondence should be addressed to R. Constance Wiener; rwiener2@hsc.wvu.edu

Academic Editor: Ronald J. Prineas

Purpose. The purpose of this study was to determine the concordance of self-reported responses to oral health questions versus clinically evaluated recommended need for oral healthcare by calibrated dentists to determine usefulness of the questions for epidemiological studies. We additionally examined other factors associated with concordant self-reports versus clinical evaluations. *Materials and Methods.* We used a cross-sectional study design with 4,205 participants, ages 30 years and above, who had complete oral health self-perception data and dental referral data in the NHANES 2013-14. Calibrated dentists completed clinical oral healthcare assessments. The assessments were dichotomized to (1) recommendation for immediate care and (2) routine oral health care. Self-reported oral health needs were measured with 6 items (an overall oral health self-perception question, oral pain within the previous year, impact on job/school, suspected periodontal disease, tooth appearance, and tooth mobility). The key item of interest was the overall oral health self-perception question. *Results.* Concordance with clinically evaluated recommended need for oral healthcare varied from 52.0% (oral pain) to 65.4% (overall oral health self-perception). Many subgroup differences were observed. *Conclusions.* The overall self-perception of oral health and the clinical evaluation of oral healthcare need were substantially concordant; other self-reported measures were moderately concordant. This is useful information and points to the need for a minimum set of measures that can provide actionable information and capture the need for clinical dental care.

1. Introduction

The World Dental Federation (FDI) policy-makers adopted a new definition of oral health in 2016. In addition to addressing well-being and the absence of disease or infirmity, they defined oral health as being multifaceted, *fundamental to health and quality of life*, and *subject to an individual's circumstances* [1]. The FDI policy-makers described oral health as involving speaking, smiling, tasting, touching, chewing, swallowing, and emoting [1]. The burden of poor oral health and its consequences have resulted in a call for

oral health to be included in all health policies [2]; a call derived from the voices of the people for overall better care, better health, and lower cost [3]. There are many known factors (social, psychosocial, economic, and cultural) that interact holistically with biological factors and have pivotal roles in *overall health* outcomes subject to an individual's circumstances [4]. Likewise, social, psychosocial, economic, and cultural factors also impact *self-perception* of health. However, in terms of clinical diagnoses and/or assessments, self-perception questions and clinical examinations may not have adequate agreement [5]. In a clinical setting, the discordance between patient's self-report of symptoms or lack thereof and a healthcare provider's clinically derived diagnosis/assessment is often resolved. However, on a population level, using data to learn about ways to improve quality requires measures (1) that are of importance, (2) that are efficient and do not involve a lot of time, (3) that measure what is intended, and (4) that are helpful in informing policy [3]. As such, to address a population's oral health needs for policy determination, it is important to know the agreement between questions involving oral health self-perceptions/self-report of needs versus clinically evaluated oral healthcare need so that the fewest and the best questions can be used in population research.

A number of researchers have examined oral health self-reports and oral health outcomes. For example, researchers found agreement between the self-reported number of missing teeth and the clinically determined number of missing teeth in adults, ages 70 years and above [6].

However, researchers also determined that self-reports of periodontal disease had good specificity but low sensitivity with clinical determinations among Veterans [7]. Among healthcare professionals, self-reports of periodontal surgery were associated with clinically determined periodontal disease measured in bone loss [8]. And, in a study in which researchers completed a full mouth clinical assessment for periodontal disease, the self-report of periodontal disease was in agreement with the clinical results [9]. In circumstances where only self-reports are available, valid correspondence with oral health needs is important to advance knowledge and to inform both treatment planning and policy development. Self-reported symptoms and health status matter. For example, since self-reported smokers were more than twice as likely to report poor oral health than nonsmokers and more likely to seek dental care symptomatically [10], report oral-facial pain [11], or report having higher dental needs [12], their dental treatment planning requires the consideration of their self-report.

However, there is a lack of consistency in epidemiological studies using self-reports with reference to oral health, due to the differences in which researchers ask oral health self-report questions, the end-points/outcomes for research that are considered, and the samples that are chosen. In summary, establishing which self-report questions have the best concordance with clinical evaluations has the potential to improve efficiency, improve reliability of epidemiological studies without the expense of clinical assessment, provide useful information for policy development, and ultimately improve oral healthcare without excessive measurement.

The purpose of this study was to determine the concordance of self-reported oral health questions versus the clinical evaluation of oral healthcare need by calibrated dentists to determine useful epidemiological questions. The determination of operant, valid questions about oral health is needed so that patient's behaviors/symptoms/conditions can be determined efficiently and diplomatically. Our focus is to provide data-driven evidence on the oral health questions that were relatively more concordant with the clinical determinations for the need of immediate or routine dental care. Tension exists for both the provider and patient when

required to collect *extraneous* data which wastes time, is not helpful, and does not improve health outcomes [3].

The present study received West Virginia University Institutional Review Board acknowledgement (protocol number 1606141771). The conceptual framework for this study was the Multidimensional Conceptual Model of Oral Health in which clinical oral health need is identified as oral tissue damage [13]. In the model, tissue damage and oral disease (oral pain and discomfort, oral functional limits, and oral disadvantage) are factors for self-rated oral health.

2. Methods

2.1. Data Source. The data source for the present study was National Health and Nutrition Examination Surveys (NHANES) 2013-14 [14], which is available to researchers from the NHANES website. The Centers for Disease Control and Prevention researchers for the NHANES used stratified, multistage probability sampling designs for the surveys. The NHANES participants were civilians who were noninstitutionalized and who lived in the U.S., including Washington, DC. The researchers for the NHANES oversampled smaller subgroups to increase estimate accuracy.

Data for the full mouth periodontal examination were collected in a mobile examination center by calibrated licensed dentists who used #5 reflecting mirrors, Hu Friedy PCP-2 (Hu Friedy, Chicago, IL) periodontal probes with markings of 2-4mm; 6-mm, and 10-12 mm parallel to the tooth's long axis for the periodontal examination, and #23 dental explorers for the dental examination [14]. A reference examiner conducted 20-25 examination replications per year to verify calibration. The examiners reported if there was a need for a participant to seek dental care, or if the participant needed to continue routine care. Participants for the periodontal examination in the NHANES, 2013-14 were ages 30 years and above. Participants for the dental examination in the NHANES, 2013-2014 were ages 1 year and above.

The participants in the NHANES, 2013-2014, also responded to interview questions involving the status of their teeth and gingiva, demographic information, and questions regarding health and nutrition. Details of the NHANES study are available at the NHANES website, https://wwwn.cdc.gov/nchs/nhanes/Default.aspx[14].

Eligibility for this study's data set included complete data for the dentists' oral health recommendations and responses from questions about oral health self-perception and oral pain in adults aged 30 years and above. The final sample size consisted of 4,205 adults.

2.2. Multidimensional Measures of Self-Reported Oral Health. We used six self-reported oral health measures: overall oral health self-perception; oral pain; impact on work/school; suspected periodontal disease; tooth appearance; and tooth mobility. The key oral health self-perception question was as follows: Overall, how would (you/survey participant [SP]) rate the health of (your/his/her) teeth and gums?" The possible responses were "Excellent, Very Good, Good, Fair, and Poor." [14] The responses to these questions were dichotomized to Excellent/Very Good/Good and Fair/Poor.

The question about oral pain was as follows: "How often during the last year (have you/ has SP) had painful aching anywhere in (your/his/her) mouth?" The impact on work/school question was as follows: "How often during the last year (have you/has SP) had difficulty doing (your/his/her) usual jobs or attending school because of problems with (your/his/her) teeth, mouth or dentures? The possible responses were "Very Often, Fairly Often, Occasionally, Hardly Ever, or Never." [15] The responses for these questions were dichotomized to (1) Very often/Fairly often; and (2) Occasionally and Hardly Ever/Never.

The periodontal question was as follows: "People with gum disease might have swollen gums, receding gums, sore or infected gums or loose teeth" followed by asking "(Do you/Does SP) think (you/s/he) might have gum disease?" The tooth appearance question was as follows: "During the past three months, (have you/has SP) noticed a tooth that doesn't look right?" [15] And the tooth mobility question was the mobile tooth question: the possible responses to these questions were yes or no.

The "How often during, suspected periodontal disease, appearance of a tooth or teeth not looking right during the previous three months, and a loose tooth/teeth not due to injury" were also used [14].

2.3. Concordance/Discordance between Self-Reports and Recommended Oral Health Care. We grouped adults into two groups: (1) the concordant group (self-reported responses which were in agreement with the clinical evaluation of oral healthcare need such that a self-report of concern/need and clinical evaluation of immediate need agreed *or* a self-report of no concerns/needs and clinical evaluation of routine care agreed); and (2) the discordant group (self-reported responses and clinical evaluation of oral healthcare need were not in agreement).

2.4. Outcomes. The primary outcome was the concordance of the overall oral health self-perception question with the clinical evaluation of oral healthcare need. We determined the percentage of agreement between the self-perception of fair or poor care and the clinical evaluation of oral healthcare need.

We were also interested in the specificity of the overall health self-perception question versus clinical evaluation of oral healthcare need. We determined the percentage of agreement between the self-perception of excellent/very good/good and the clinical evaluation of routine care.

2.5. Statistical Analyses. Due to the complex nature of NHANES, SAS® version 9.4 (SAS Institute, Inc., Cary, NC) was used with the supplied weights in the data set. The analyses also accounted for stratification, primary sampling unit values, and eligibility. We used chi-square tests to assess the statistical significance of unadjusted associations. We also performed logistic regressions on concordance between clinical evaluation of recommended care and self-reported oral health measures after controlling for sex, race/ethnicity, age, education, federal poverty level, insurance coverage, obesity, alcohol use, smoking status, physical activity, presence

of chronic conditions (cancer, cardiovascular disease, and diabetes), general health status, and dental visits.

The level of statistical significance for alpha was set at 0.05. Strength of concordance was set at 0-20% as poor; 21-20% as slight; 41-60% as moderate, 61-80% as substantial; and 81-100% as almost perfect, based upon similar guidelines for the Kappa coefficient by Landis and Koch [16].

3. Results

In Table 1, we report the weighted percentages for the clinical evaluation of oral healthcare need versus the self-reported responses to questions about oral health status (overall oral health self-perception, oral pain, impact on work/school, suspected periodontal disease, tooth appearance which "does not looking right", and tooth mobility). The percentages in the columns are for immediate or routine oral healthcare need for each self-reported response. Each response to the questions about oral health status was statistically significant, that is, more people who reported fair/poor oral health self-perception were more likely to have a clinical determination of needing immediate care; more people reporting pain were more likely to have a clinical determination of needing immediate care; more people who reported that there was an impact on work/school due to an oral condition were more likely to have a clinical determination of needing immediate care; more people reporting a suspected periodontal disease were more likely to have a clinical determination of needing immediate care; and more people who reported that a tooth's appearance did not look right were more likely to have a clinical determination of needing immediate care.

Table 2 has the concordance of the self-reported oral healthcare measures with the clinical evaluation of oral healthcare need in which the concordant group was in agreement with the self-report of a need with a clinical evaluation of oral healthcare need, *or was in* agreement with the self-report of no need with a clinical evaluation of routine oral healthcare; and the discordant group was in disagreement with the clinical evaluation of oral healthcare need. Clinical evaluation of oral healthcare need and the self-report for overall oral health self-perception had the highest concordance at 65.4%. The lowest concordance was with oral pain (aching anywhere in the mouth during the last year) at 52.0%.

The bivariate associations of concordant self-reported oral health with clinical evaluation of oral healthcare need are in Table 3. There were significant differences in concordance when considering sex, race/ethnicity, education, federal poverty level, insurance coverage, and diabetes for both overall oral health self-perception and oral pain. There were also significant differences in concordance when considering body mass index, smoking, cardiovascular disease, self-reported general health, and dental visit for the relationship with oral pain.

The adjusted odds ratios (AOR) and 95% confidence intervals (CI) from logistic regressions on concordance are in Table 4. Overall, females were more likely to have concordance than males. Non-Hispanic White individuals were more likely to have concordance than racial minorities. Participants with insurance, who were not obese, or who

TABLE 1: Oral health and recommended care versus variables of interest. Adults aged 30 years or older in National Health Examination and Nutrition Survey 2013-2014.

	Immediate Care		Routine Care		Chi-sq	Prob	Sig
	N	wt %	N	wt %			
ALL	**2,411**	**50.2**	**1,794**	**49.8**			
Overall oral health self-perception							***
Fair/Poor	1,089	79.3	253	39.6	368.373	< .001	
Ex/Vg/Good	1,322	20.7	1,541	60.4			
Oral Pain[1]							***
Yes	221	66.6	83	49.1	27.625	< .001	
No	2,190	33.4	1,711	50.9			
Impact on work/school							***
Yes	295	66.6	106	48.7	39.768	< .001	
No	2,116	33.4	1,688	51.3			
Suspected periodontal disease[2]							***
Yes	558	67.3	208	46.7	63.326	< .001	
No	1,853	32.7	1,586	53.3			
Tooth appearance does not look right							***
Does not look right	*581*	*82.3*	99	45.7	184.747	< .001	
Looks right	*1,830*	*17.7*	1,695	54.3			
Tooth mobility[3]							***
Mobile	*527*	*71.9*	181	46.8	106.808	< .001	
No mobility	*1,884*	*28.1*	1,613	53.2			

Note: based on 4,205 participants, who were 30 years and older and who had no missing data for the dentists' oral health recommendations and responses from questions about oral health self-perception and oral pain. Ex/Vg/Good, Excellent/Very Good/Good. [1] Aching anywhere in the mouth during the last year. [2] If participant thought he or she "might have gum disease" (NHANES, 2017). [3] Participant was asked if "any teeth [were] becoming loose without an injury" (NHANES, 2017).

TABLE 2: Concordance of self-reported oral health measures and oral health recommended care. National Health and Nutrition Examination Surveys 2013-2014.

Total	N 4,205	Wt %
Overall oral health self-perception		
Concordant	2,630	65.4
Discordant	1,575	34.6
Oral pain[1]		
Concordant	1,932	52.0
Discordant	2,273	48.0
Impact on work/school		
Concordant	1,983	52.6
Discordant	2,222	47.4
Suspected periodontal disease[2]		
Concordant	2,144	55.6
Discordant	2,061	44.4
Tooth appearance "does not look right" within the previous 3 months		
Concordant	2,276	57.8
Discordant	1,929	42.2
Tooth mobility.[3]		
Concordant	2,140	55.7
Discordant	2,065	44.3

Note: based on 4,205 participants, who were 30 years and older and who had no missing data for the dentists' oral health recommendations and responses from questions about oral health self-perception and oral pain. [1] Aching anywhere in the mouth during the last year. [2] If participant thought he or she "might have gum disease" (NHANES, 2017). [3] Participant was asked if "any teeth [were] becoming loose without an injury" (NHANES, 2017).

TABLE 3: Weighted % of concordance between clinical oral health recommended care and self-reported oral health measures adults aged 30 years or older in National Health and Examination Nutrition Survey, 2013-14.

	Overall Oral health self-perception	Oral Pain[1]	Impact on Job or school	Suspected Periodontal Disease	Tooth Appearance "does not look right"	Tooth mobility[3]
ALL	65.4	52.0	52.6	55.6	57.8	55.7
Sex	***	***	***	***	***	***
Female	69.2	57.1	57.8	59.8	62.4	60.4
Male	61.4	46.5	47.0	51.2	52.9	50.8
Race/Ethnicity	***	***	***	***	***	***
Non-Hispanic White	68.0	57.0	56.9	60.4	61.5	60.4
Non-Hispanic Black	57.5	40.0	42.1	45.0	49.5	45.8
Hispanic	61.9	39.3	42.3	43.4	50.8	43.9
Other	58.6	44.2	45.3	48.0	48.1	46.7
Age groups		*			*	
30 - 44 years	67.4	54.4	55.8	56.0	60.7	57.0
45 - 54 Years	68.7	51.8	52.0	56.4	59.8	57.2
55 - 64 Years	64.4	47.6	48.5	55.1	53.2	52.2
65, or older	65.5	55.9	54.9	57.0	59.4	61.1
Education	***	***	***	***	***	***
Less than high school	67.2	41.2	42.2	46.2	52.1	44.0
High school graduate	61.1	41.6	43.3	50.6	51.2	50.7
Some College	64.7	50.3	51.4	54.3	55.8	53.6
College	68.2	65.1	64.3	64.3	66.7	66.2
Federal Poverty Level	*	***	***	***	***	***
0 - < 1.25	63.3	38.4	39.4	45.4	52.4	44.4
1.25 to < 2.00	62.6	44.1	44.5	50.7	53.6	48.7
2.00 - < 4.00	62.9	48.1	50.7	52.7	54.0	54.3
4.00 and above	69.1	64.6	63.6	65.3	65.5	65.3
Missing	67.2	52.5	52.4	52.9	55.1	54.4
Insurance coverage	**	***	***	***	***	***
Yes	66.4	55.7	55.9	58.8	60.4	59.2
No	59.7	35.5	34.0	37.9	43.6	36.7
Obesity		***	***		*	*
No	66.7	55.4	55.7	57.0	60.0	58.3
Yes	63.5	47.2	48.2	53.5	54.8	52.0
Alcohol use		***	***	***	***	***
Non-Drinker	64.2	51.9	54.6	55.9	57.2	54.5
Moderate use	68.3	58.7	59.3	61.6	63.2	62.1
Heavy use	62.1	42.8	41.8	46.4	50.2	48.5
Missing	63.7	46.0	46.1	51.3	54.4	49.9
Smoking		***	***	***	***	***
Current	66.1	40.0	40.3	42.1	49.7	43.2
Former	63.1	51.9	51.3	57.1	57.3	56.0
Never	66.4	56.1	57.3	59.5	60.8	59.8
Physical activity				*	*	*
Yes	65.8	52.7	53.3	56.6	58.8	56.6
No	64.3	50.1	50.6	53.0	55.2	53.2

TABLE 3: Continued.

	Overall Oral health self-perception	Oral Pain[1]	Impact on Job or school	Suspected Periodontal Disease	Tooth Appearance "does not look right"	Tooth mobility[3]
Cancer			*			*
Yes	68.3	56.3	58.1	58.8	59.6	60.3
No	65.0	51.3	51.7	55.1	57.6	55.0
Cardiovascular disease		*				
Yes	65.4	52.5	53.8	59.2	59.6	53.3
No	65.5	52.0	52.5	55.2	57.7	56.0
Diabetes	*	***	***		*	**
Yes	60.4	43.4	42.7	52.2	51.0	48.6
No	66.4	33.6	54.4	56.3	59.1	57.1
General health		***	***	*	**	***
Excellent/very good	65.9	59.6	59.1	59.3	61.7	62.8
Good	63.1	48.6	50.0	54.1	54.6	52.5
Fair/poor	69.1	44.3	44.7	52.1	56.6	48.7
Missing	65.5	49.5	53.1	53.0	57.6	53.8
Dental visit		***	***	***	***	***
1 year or less	65.7	59.3	59.7	60.2	61.2	62.6
More than 1 year	64.9	39.1	39.9	47.6	51.8	43.6

Note: based on 4,205 participants, who were 30 years and older and who had no missing data for the dentists' oral health recommendations and responses from questions about oral health self-perception and oral pain. Asterisks represent significant group differences in concordance versus discordance based on Rao-Scott Chi-square tests.[1]Aching anywhere in the mouth during the last year.[2]If participant thought he or she "might have gum disease" (NHANES, 2017).[3]Participant was asked if "any teeth [were] becoming loose without an injury" (NHANES, 2017). *** $p < .001$; ** $.001 \leq p < .01$; * $.01 \leq p < .05$.

were never-smokers were more likely to be concordant. Reported fair/poor *general health was* associated with high concordance between clinical oral health recommended care and oral health self-perception.

4. Discussion

When using multidimensional measures of self-reported oral health, we found that the greatest concordance with clinical evaluation of oral healthcare need was with the question for overall oral health self-perception. Clinical evaluation of oral healthcare need and the self-report for overall oral health self-perception had a substantial concordance at 65.4%. The question may be a useful tool in oral health epidemiological studies, similar to the usefulness of the overall self-rated *general* health question in systemic epidemiology [17–19].

Another noteworthy finding is the moderate concordance of the *appearance* of teeth with clinically evaluated oral healthcare need. Although we do not know whether participants were self-conscious of the *color, or shape* rather considering than carious/periodontal condition of their tooth/teeth when they answered the question, the literature does include "pressures to conform" as a factor influencing body image and self-awareness [20]. The media present images of the perfect smile and ultra-white teeth with which to compare one's teeth. Reports in the media include the obsession of many people with ultra-white teeth [21], and those cultural influences may be affecting the participants' responses to this particular question.

Although not a focus of this study, additional analysis indicated that the specificity of the overall oral health self-perception question was 60.4%; and, the specificities of the other measures were between 50.9% and 53.3%. These findings have implications for referral patterns. Future research is needed to explore the reasons behind the low specificity. Additionally, when these measures are used in epidemiological research, caution is necessary in interpreting results associated with these oral health questions.

The subgroup analyses also included variations in concordance between the clinical evaluation of oral healthcare need and self-reports. Some subgroups were consistently concordant (example: female, racial minorities) on all of the measures; other groups were not. These findings suggest that when researchers use the self-reported measures on some subpopulations (smokers, middle-aged adults), the self-reported measures may not be as reliable in indicating clinical need.

4.1. Similar Studies. There is a lack of recent, similar studies with which to compare this study due to the differences in which the questions for self-report are asked, the endpoints/outcomes considered, and populations chosen for the research. For example, in a study of black women (median age 38 years), there were similar self-report questions; however, only periodontal disease status and intensity (and not all other clinical evaluations of oral healthcare needs) were considered [22]. Similarly, in another study, there was moderate agreement with the women's self-report of the removal

TABLE 4: Adjusted odds ratios (AORs) and 95% confidence intervals (CIs) from logistic regressions on concordance between recommended care and self-reported oral health measures. Adults Aged 30 and older in National Health and Examination Nutrition Survey, 2013-14.

	Overall Oral Health Self-Perception	Oral Pain[1]	Impact on job or school	Suspected Periodontal Disease[2]	Tooth appearance "does not look right"	Tooth mobility[3]
	AOR [95%CI]	AOR [95%CI]	AOR [95%CI]	AOR [95%CI]	AOR [95%CI]	AOR [95%CI]
Sex						
Female	1.46*** [1.28, 1.67]	1.57*** [1.33, 1.84]	1.58*** [1.28, 1.95]	1.45** [1.12, 1.86]	1.54*** [1.29, 1.82]	1.59*** [1.35, 1.87]
Male (ref)						
Race/ethnicity						
Non-Hispanic Black	0.56*** [0.43, 0.72]	0.51*** [0.40, 0.66]	0.59*** [0.46, 0.77]	0.54*** [0.44, 0.66]	0.60*** [0.49, 0.75]	0.59*** [0.50, 0.70]
Hispanic	0.66* [0.46, 0.94]	0.54*** [0.40, 0.66]	0.61*** [0.46, 0.77]	0.52*** [0.38, 0.73]	0.63** [0.47, 0.85]	0.57*** [0.45, 0.71]
Other	0.52*** [0.35, 0.78]	0.47*** [0.34, 0.65]	0.52*** [0.36, 0.75]	0.50*** [0.35, 0.73]	0.47*** [0.33, 0.67]	0.47*** [0.35, 0.61]
Non-Hispanic White (ref)						
Age in years						
30 - 44 years (Ref)						
45 - 54 years	0.99 [0.80, 1.22]	0.76* [0.60, 0.97]	0.73 [0.53, 1.00]	0.92 [0.73, 1.16]	0.83 [0.66, 1.05]	0.85 [0.64, 1.14]
55- 64 years	0.80 [0.57, 1.14]	0.56*** [0.40, 0.77]	0.57** [0.38, 0.84]	0.78 [0.56, 1.09]	0.58*** [0.41, 0.82]	0.62* [0.40, 0.97]
65, or older	0.81 [0.54, 1.22]	0.74 [0.54, 1.02]	0.69 [0.45, 1.08]	0.78 [0.57, 1.05]	0.72 [0.49, 1.04]	0.83 [0.61, 1.12]
Insurance coverage						
Yes (ref)						
No	0.71** [0.57, 0.89]	0.51*** [0.40, 0.64]	0.55*** [0.44, 0.70]	0.54*** [0.44, 0.66]	0.58*** [0.49, 0.69]	0.55*** [0.46, 0.65]
Self-reported General Health						
Fair/poor	1.51*** [1.22, 1.86]	0.97 [0.72, 1.31]	0.98 [0.76, 1.27]	1.17 [0.99, 1.39]	1.26 [0.91, 1.74]	0.98 [0.77, 1.26]
Excellent/very good/good (ref)						
Physical Activity						
No	0.96 [0.79, 1.17]	1.02 [0.86, 1.21]	0.98 [0.76, 1.26]	0.84 [0.69, 1.02]	0.86 [0.74, 1.01]	0.95 [0.83, 1.08]
Yes (ref)						
Obese						
Obese	0.74** [0.61, 0.90]	0.62*** [0.51, 0.76]	0.65*** [0.52, 0.81]	0.78 [0.60, 1.01]	0.67*** [0.55, 0.82]	0.67** [0.52, 0.87]
No (Ref)						
Smoking status						
Current smoker	0.93 [0.67, 1.29]	0.57*** [0.43, 0.77]	0.56*** [0.39, 0.80]	0.46*** [0.31, 0.67]	0.65** [0.47, 0.88]	0.56 [0.67, 1.18]
Former smoker	0.88 [0.64, 1.21]	0.85 [0.64, 1.14]	0.85 [0.60, 1.20]	0.86 [0.67, 1.09]	0.90 [0.64, 1.27]	0.89 [0.67, 1.18]
Never smoker (ref)						

TABLE 4: Continued.

	Overall Oral Health Self-Perception	Oral Pain[1]	Impact on job or school	Suspected Periodontal Disease[2]	Tooth appearance "does not look right"	Tooth mobility[3]
	AOR	AOR	AOR	AOR	AOR	AOR
	[95%CI]	[95%CI]	[95%CI]	[95%CI]	[95%CI]	[95%CI]
Dental visit						
More than 1 year	0.97	0.48***	0.50***	0.70***	0.73***	0.51***
	[0.73, 1.29]	[0.40, 0.57]	[0.42, 0.59]	[0.60, 0.82]	[0.61, 0.87]	[0.41, 0.65]
1 year or less (ref)						

Note: based on 4,205 participants, who were 30 years and older and who had no missing data for the dentists' oral health recommendations and responses from questions about oral health self-perception and oral pain. Asterisks represent significant group differences in concordance compared to the reference group based on logistic regressions. [1]Aching anywhere in the mouth during the last year.[2]If participant thought he or she "might have gum disease" (NHANES, 2017).[3]Participant was asked if "any teeth [were] becoming loose without an injury" (NHANES, 2017).*** p < .001; ** .001 ≤ p < .01; * .01 ≤ p < .05.

of periodontally involved teeth and (clinically determined) severe periodontitis (Kappa=0.25; 95%CI, 0.17, 0.31); however, the study's focus was periodontal disease and not overall oral health [23].

4.2. Study Strengths. This current study has several strengths. The researchers used a large, current, nationally representative study for the data source. Several self-report questions were included in the research. The dental examiners who conducted the research to establish the NHANES 2013-2014 data source were calibrated, licensed dentists who determined if a dental need existed or if routine care should be maintained. "Overall oral health need" was used in this study. This is consistent with the 2016 FDI World Dental Federation members' emphasis upon the new definition for oral health; that is, oral health is multifaceted such that speech, sensing (smell, taste, and touch), and muscle action (chewing, swallowing, and emoting) can occur with confidence and without pain/discomfort/disease of the craniofacial complex [24]. Included in the definition are the influences of physical and mental well-being (recognized as a continuum influenced by individual and cultural values/attitudes); biopsychosocial attributes of life leading to quality life; and change (circumstantial, perceptual, experiential, etc.) [24].

4.3. Study Limitations. There are challenges to the use of broad questions concerning oral health in research. Measures need to be valid and consistently used by researchers. In a study in New Zealand and Australia, Locker's single question for global oral health rating [25] was slightly altered and validated with caries, tooth loss, periodontal disease, and the short form of the Oral Health Impact Profile (OHIP-14) in adults, ages 35-44 years [26]. Altered questions make comparisons difficult. Additionally, the FDI definition suggests that age, sex, and culture will influence oral health self-perception. Self-perception questions are less involved than clinical oral evaluations; however, they must be considered proxies that vary by population and questions posed. A consensus-based set of measures for oral healthcare is being developed with patient perception as a major feature; therefore, having the

appropriate measures may improve research and quality of care [27].

In addition to the limitations imposed by definition variability, there are other limitations. One includes the nature of the observational study design's purpose to establish association rather than causation. Studies in which self-report is used also have the potential for social desirability bias and therefore misclassifications. Although many covariates were used in this study, there is also the potential for having missed an important confounding factor.

4.4. Clinical Considerations. The ultimate goal of oral health research is to provide the information for oral healthcare practitioners to learn the evidence-based practices to provide the best preventive and restorative care for their patients, to improve oral healthcare quality, and eliminate redundancy and waste. To maximize these effects, research studies need good study designs with more uniform/standardized questions and terminologies which accurately reflect the patient presentation. Having useful questions to direct the conversation not only is more efficient, but also is more respectful and considerate of the patient's time and circumstances.

5. Conclusion

The overall self-perception of oral health and the clinical evaluation of oral healthcare need were substantially concordant; other self-reported measures were moderately concordant. This is useful information and points to the need for a minimum set of measures that can provide actionable information and capture the need for clinical dental care.

Disclosure

The content is solely the responsibility of the authors and does not necessarily represent the official views of the National Institutes of Health.

Authors' Contributions

All authors contributed to the conception and design of the research. R. Constance Wiener and Usha Sambamoorthi conducted the statistical analyses. R. Constance Wiener wrote the first draft. All authors contributed to the manuscript and approved the final version.

Acknowledgments

Research reported in this publication was supported by the National Institute of General Medical Sciences of the National Institutes of Health under Award no. U54GM104942, WVCTSI.

References

[1] J. Y. Lee, R. G. Watt, D. M. Williams, and W. V. Giannobile, "A New Definition for Oral Health," *Journal of Dental Research*, vol. 96, no. 2, pp. 125–127, 2016.

[2] M. Glick and D. M. Meyer, "Defining oral health," *The Journal of the American Dental Association*, vol. 145, no. 6, pp. 519-520, 2014.

[3] D. M. Berwick, "Era 3 for medicine and health care," *Journal of the American Medical Association*, vol. 315, no. 13, pp. 1329-1330, 2016.

[4] K. S. Reddy, D. Doshi, S. Kulkarni, B. S. Reddy, and M. P. Reddy, "Correlation of sense of coherence with oral health behaviors, socioeconomic status, and periodontal status," *Journal of Indian Society of Periodontology*, vol. 20, no. 4, pp. 453–459, 2016.

[5] A. R. D. Nascimento, F. B. D. Andrade, and C. C. César, "Factors associated with agreement between self-perception and clinical evaluation of dental treatment needs in adults in Brazil and Minas Gerais," *Cadernos de Saúde Pública*, vol. 32, no. 10, p. e00039115, 2016.

[6] C. W. Douglass, J. Berlin, and S. Tennstedt, "The Validity of Self-reported Oral Health Status in the Elderly," *Journal of Public Health Dentistry*, vol. 51, no. 4, pp. 220–222, 1991.

[7] W. Pitiphat, R. I. Garcia, C. W. Douglass, and K. J. Joshipura, "Validation of self-reported oral health measures.," *Journal of Public Health Dentistry*, vol. 62, no. 2, pp. 122–128, 2002.

[8] K. J. Joshipura, W. Pitiphat, and C. W. Douglass, "Validation of self-reported periodontal measures among health professionals.," *Journal of Public Health Dentistry*, vol. 62, no. 2, pp. 115–121, 2002.

[9] P. I. Eke, B. A. Dye, L. Wei et al., "Self-reported measures for surveillance of periodontitis," *Journal of Dental Research*, vol. 92, no. 11, pp. 1041–1047, 2013.

[10] J. Csikar, J. Kang, C. Wyborn, T. A. Dyer, Z. Marshman, and J. Godson, "The self-reported oral health status and dental attendance of smokers and non-smokers in England," *PLoS ONE*, vol. 11, no. 2, Article ID e0148700, 2016.

[11] W. J. Millar and D. Locker, "Smoking and oral health status," *Journal of the Canadian Dental Association*, vol. 73, no. 2, pp. 155-155, 2007.

[12] B. A. Dye, N. M. Morin, and V. Robison, "The relationship between cigarette smoking and perceived dental treatment needs in the United States, 1988-1994," *The Journal of the American Dental Association*, vol. 137, no. 2, pp. 224–234, 2006.

[13] G. H. Gilbert, R. P. Duncan, M. W. Heft, T. A. Dolan, and W. B. Vogel, "Multidimensionality of Oral Health in Dentate Adults," *Medical Care*, vol. 36, no. 7, pp. 988–1001, 1998.

[14] Centers for Disease Control and Prevention and National Center for Health Statistics, *National Health and Nutrition Examination Survey Data Hyattsville*, Department of Health and Human Services Centers for Disease Control and Prevention, 2013-2014.

[15] Centers for Disease Control and Prevention and National Center for Health Statistics, *National Health and Nutrition Examination Survey Questionnaire (or Examination Protocol, or Laboratory Protocol)*, Department of Health and Human Services Centers for Disease Control and Prevention, 2013-2014.

[16] J. R. Landis and G. G. Koch, "The measurement of observer agreement for categorical data," *Biometrics*, vol. 33, no. 1, pp. 159–174, 1977.

[17] J. Schnittker and V. Bacak, "The increasing predictive validity of self-rated health," *PLoS ONE*, vol. 9, no. 1, Article ID e84933, 2014.

[18] D. S. Brown, W. W. Thompson, M. M. Zack, S. E. Arnold, and J. P. Barile, "Associations between health-related quality of life and mortality in older adults," *Prevention science : the official journal of the Society for Prevention Research*, vol. 16, no. 1, pp. 21–30, 2015.

[19] E. R. Berchick and S. M. Lynch, "Regional variation in the predictive validity of self-rated health for mortality," *SSM - Population Health*, vol. 3, pp. 275–282, 2017.

[20] U. Kenny, M.-P. O'Malley-Keighran, M. Molcho, and C. Kelly, "Peer Influences on Adolescent Body Image: Friends or Foes?" *Journal of Adolescent Research*, vol. 32, no. 6, pp. 768–799, 2017.

[21] M. Crain, "The Crimson White," 2017, http://www.cw.ua.edu/article/2016/03/non-goals-how-social-media-affects-body-image.

[22] B. Heaton, N. B. Gordon, R. I. Garcia et al., "A clinical validation of self-reported periodontitis among participants in the black women's health study," *Journal of Periodontology*, vol. 88, no. 6, pp. 582–592, 2017.

[23] M. J. La Monte, K. M. Hovey, A. E. Millen, R. J. Genco, and J. Wactawski-Wende, "Accuracy of self-reported periodontal disease in the Women's Health Initiative Observational study," *Journal of Periodontology*, vol. 85, no. 8, pp. 1006–1018, 2014.

[24] FDI World Dental Federation, FDI unveils new universally applicable definition of "oral health, 2016.

[25] D. Locker, *Oral Health Indicators and Determinants for Population Health Surveys. A Report for Health Canada*, University of Toronto, Toronto, Canada, 2001.

[26] W. M. Thomson, G. C. Mejia, J. M. Broadbent, and R. Poulton, "Construct validity of locker's global oral health item," *Journal of Dental Research*, vol. 91, no. 11, pp. 1038–1042, 2012.

[27] F. Baâdoudi, A. Trescher, D. Duijster et al., "A Consensus-Based Set of Measures for Oral Health Care," *Journal of Dental Research*, vol. 96, no. 8, pp. 881–887, 2017.

17

Improving Completeness of Inpatient Medical Records in Menelik II Referral Hospital, Addis Ababa, Ethiopia

Kasu Tola,[1] Haftom Abebe,[1] Yemane Gebremariam,[1] and Birhanu Jikamo[2]

[1]*Mekelle University College of Health Sciences School of Public Health, Mekelle, Ethiopia*
[2]*Hawassa University College of Medicine and Health Sciences School of Public and Environmental Health, Hawassa, Ethiopia*

Correspondence should be addressed to Kasu Tola; kasu.tola@yahoo.com

Academic Editor: Ronald J. Prineas

Introduction. The incompleteness of medical records is a significant problem that affects the quality of health care services in many hospitals of Ethiopia. Improving the completeness of patient's records is an important step towards improving the quality of healthcare. *Methods.* Pre- and postintervention study was conducted to assess improvement of inpatient medical record completeness in Menelik II Referral Hospital from September 2015 to April 2016. Simple random sampling technique was used. Data was collected using data extraction checklist and independent sample t-test was used to compare statistical difference that exists between pre- and postintervention outcomes at confidence interval of 95% and P value less than 0.05 was considered statistically significant. *Result.* The overall inpatient medical record completeness was found to be 84% after intervention. An enhancement of completeness and reporting of inpatient medical record completeness increased significantly from the baseline 73% to 84% during postintervention evaluation at P value < 0.05. *Conclusion and Recommendation.* The finding of this project suggests that a simple set of interventions comprising inpatient medical record format and training healthcare provider showed a significant improvement in inpatient medical record completeness. The Quality Officer and Chief Executive Officer of the study hospital are recommended to design and launch intervention programs to improve medical record completeness.

1. Introduction

Medical record completeness is a key performance indicator that is related with delivery of healthcare services in the hospital [1]. At hospital level, statistics collected from medical records are used to review the incidence and type of diseases treated and different procedures performed. At hospital level statistics derived from the daily bed census and medical records are used to assess the utilization of services and enable the hospital to make appropriate financial and administrative plans and to conduct vital research [2].

Patient medical record review is the most applied technique to investigate adverse events in hospitals. The determination with which information is recorded may influence the visibility of adverse events. Poor quality of the information in patient medical records may be a cause or a consequence of poor quality of care and associated with higher rates of adverse events [3]. Better quality of healthcare data in patient medical records can affect clinical and administrative decision making in health economics and patient safety [4].

Adverse events occur in an estimate of 2.9 to 3.7 percent of acute care hospitalizations in the United States of America (USA) and it is estimated that between 44,000 and 98,000 patients die in hospitals each year as a result of medical error explained as the failure of planed action to be completed as intended [5].

Despite the importance of medical records to high quality and efficient care management of patients' medical records, especially in developing countries like Ethiopia, it has not been a priority, generally inadequately supported and poorly managed. The study done in a rural hospital in Ethiopia shows that only 45.7% of medical records were complete [6].

A facility based cross-sectional study was conducted in Ayder Referral Hospital and six-month data have been assessed and showed that 36.7% was inaccurate [7].

The study done in a Dalefage Primary Hospital, West Afar, Ethiopia, showed that an enhancement of completeness and reporting of inpatient medical record completeness improved significantly from the baseline 0% to 73.6% during postintervention evaluation [8].

In Menelik II Referral Hospital baseline assessments were collected and inpatient medical record completeness showed 73% which is low against the standard in which medical record completeness is expected to be 100%. In line with this there is a gap of study on medical record completeness particularly inpatient medical records. Knowledge gap and shortage of medical record format were accepted as root cause for existence of incomplete inpatient medical records.

Objective of the study is to improve the completeness of inpatient medical records from 73% to 93% at the end of April 30, 2016, at Menelik II Referral Hospital.

A patient medical record provides two important functions; the first helps to support direct patient care by assisting physician on clinical decision making and provides communication. The second provides a legal record of care given and helps as a source of data to support clinical audit, research, resource allocation, monitoring and evaluation, epidemiology, and service planning [9–11].

Improving medical record completeness services is an important step towards improving the quality of healthcare. It can also provide valuable information to help measure progress and effectiveness. The medical record has become an important legal document; good medical records are essential not only for the present and future care of the patient but also as a legal document to protect the patient and the hospitals from litigation [1, 2].

Medical record is a very important document that is used to communicate and document critical information among health professionals. The incompleteness of medical records compromises the quality of care of patient's and results in different medical errors and patient dissatisfaction. To alleviate the problem the medical record completeness is part of national key performance indicators to monitor the magnitude of the problem and intervene according to the necessity.

2. Methodology

2.1. Setting/Study Area. The study was conducted at Menelik II Referral Hospital, governmental hospital found in capital city of Ethiopia in Addis Ababa. Menelik II Referral Hospital has various professionals that included 59 physicians, 203 nurses, 123 other health professionals, and 250 administrative staff, making a total of 635 staff. The study was conducted from September 2015 to April 2016.

2.2. Study Design. Pre- and postintervention study was conducted at inpatient departments of Menelik II Referral Hospital.

2.3. Population. All inpatient medical records of patients treated and discharged from Menelik II Referral Hospital were sourced for review medical records after implementing

the best intervention. Baseline data were collected in September 2015 and postintervention data was collected in May 2016 and schedule for intervention was carried out in January, February, March, and April 2016.

2.4. Sample Size Determination. The sample size calculation for comparing proportions was used to make a valid statistical computation and conclusion; the following sample size calculation for comparing two proportions was made [12]:

$$n = \frac{(Z\alpha/2 + Z\beta)^2 P(1-P)}{(P-Po)^2}, \quad (1)$$

where n is sample size and $P = (Po + P1)/2$, $Po = 73\% = 0.73$ (baseline data surveys were collected and analysis was done which gives 73% of inpatient medical record as being completed in Menelik II Referral Hospital). $P1 = 93\% = 0.93$ (planned proportion after the best intervention implemented in Menelik II Referral Hospital is expected to be 93% because of shortage of resources and time to accomplish the tasks). $P = Po + P1/2 = 0.83$ (average population proportion that is between preintervention and postintervention proportion); $Z\alpha/2$ with 95% confidence interval equal to 1.96, power = 80%, and $Z\beta = 0.84$.

$$n = \frac{(1.96 + 0.84)^2 \, 0.83 \, (1 - 0.83)}{(0.83 - 0.73)^2}, \quad (2)$$

$$n = 111.$$

2.5. Sampling Technique and Procedures. Simple random sampling technique was used during the study period which means that for preintervention, September 2015, the total discharged patients were 605 and among these 50 medical records were sampled and for postintervention, May 2016, the total discharged patients were 582 and among these 111 medical records were sampled, respectively, using lottery methods. The above sample size was taken based on Ethiopian Federal Ministry of Health Hospital performance and monitoring improvement reports [13].

2.6. Intervention

2.6.1. Training for Inpatient Healthcare Worker (Physician and Nurse). Training for physician and nursing staff consists of the following:

(i) Awareness and sensitization creation on the importance of medical records.

(ii) Medical record as part of hospital reform.

(iii) Medical record as part of hospital key performance indicator for quality of care.

2.6.2. Avail Medical Record Format. During intervention implementation the main focus was to provide training for inpatient healthcare worker (physician and nurses) for one day for 122 nurses and 67 physicians totally for 189 healthcare providers on inpatient medical record completeness as well hospital reform by providing onsite training to solve lack of awareness and knowledge gap on the overall hospital reform.

2.7. Evaluation. The type of evaluation that was conducted is the cycle of problem solving, PDSA cycle of continuous quality improvement.

Process indicators

(i) Availability of necessary formats

(ii) Trained healthcare provider (Physician and Nurse)

Outcome indicators

(i) Score of completeness of inpatient medical records after intervention.

2.8. Data Collection Procedure and Quality Control. The training was given to two nurses for one day. These trained data collectors used data extraction checklist and collect information from medical charts. To maintain data quality, training was given to data collectors and supervision was carried out by principal investigator on daily basis to check completeness and consistency so as to ensure quality of data, during the data collection procedures.

2.9. Operational Definition

Medical Record. They are papers that document the care and treatment a patient received.

Completeness of Medical Record. It is the presence of all the necessary information of patients based on the standard formats attached at the annex and all entries are dated and signed.

Inpatient Medical Record. It is the official record of patient that contains information of admitted patients to general ward.

2.10. Data Entry and Analysis Procedure. After data is collected, it was coded and entered into Epi data of version 3.1 and was exported to SPSS for windows version 22 for cleaning, editing, and analysis, and t-test was used to compare statistical difference that exists between preintervention and postintervention. P value less than 0.05 was considered statistically significant. Ethical clearance was obtained from Mekelle University College of Health Science, School of Public Health, as the study was conducted as part of Master's thesis for the first author and prior to commencement of the study. Official letter of permission from the school was submitted to Menelik II Referral Hospital administration in order to conduct the project. Following this, searching and obtaining of the selected samples' medical record was processed with assigned person. Finally, strict care for the patients' medical records and the confidentiality of records that could identify study participants was protected.

3. Result

The completeness of medical records was assessed in terms of physician note, physician order sheet, nursing care plan, medication administration sheet, and discharge summary. Accordingly, the result showed that physician note format was attached for 111 (100%) and completed for 103 (92.8%), physician order sheet was attached for 111 (100%) and completed for 107 (96.4%), nursing care plan was attached for 109 (98.2%) and completed for 85 (76.6%), medication administration format was attached for 103 (92.8%) and completed for 78 (70.3%), and at last discharge summary was attached for 107 (96.4%) and completed for 93 (83.8%) (Figure 1).

There are prepared standardized formats and three of them were completed by physician (inpatient physician notes, physician order sheet, and discharge summary) and two of them completed by nurses (nursing care plan and medication administration sheet). An enhancement of completeness and reporting of inpatient medical record completeness improved significantly from the baseline 73% before intervention to 84% after intervention (P value < 0.05, Table 1).

Since calculated t-value exceeds the critical value, the null hypothesis has been rejected and the alternative hypothesis has been accepted, implying that intervention done has brought a significant change.

4. Discussion

The result of the study showed that the intervention done has increased the overall inpatient medical record completeness by 11% from 73% to 84% (P value < 0.05). When compared with study done in Netherland the nursing record was unavailable in 1% of the patient records and the medication administration list in 21% of the reviewed patient records but relatively similar to the study in which medication administration list is incomplete for 29.7% [3].

When compared with aspects of medication administration sheet the study done in England shows that the medication history in the hospital medical record is often incomplete, as 26% of used medication is not recorded. Similarly in this study medication administration sheet is incomplete for 29.7% of the medical records [14].

Aspects of discharge summary in this study: 16.2% of inpatient medical record is incomplete in comparison with study done in Canada which shows discharge summaries were assessed for completeness and accuracy. Most items were completely reported with given items missing in 5% of summaries. However there is improvement of completeness of discharge summary as compared to preintervention but low as compared to study done in Canada. The reason for this observation might be that the country gives due attention for medical records for better health information and decision making [15].

The study done in a rural hospital in Ethiopia shows that the proportion of medical records that were complete increased significantly (6.5% preintervention and 45.7% postintervention, P < 0.01); in line with this, in our study there is also significant improvement in inpatient medical record completeness which implies giving due attention to

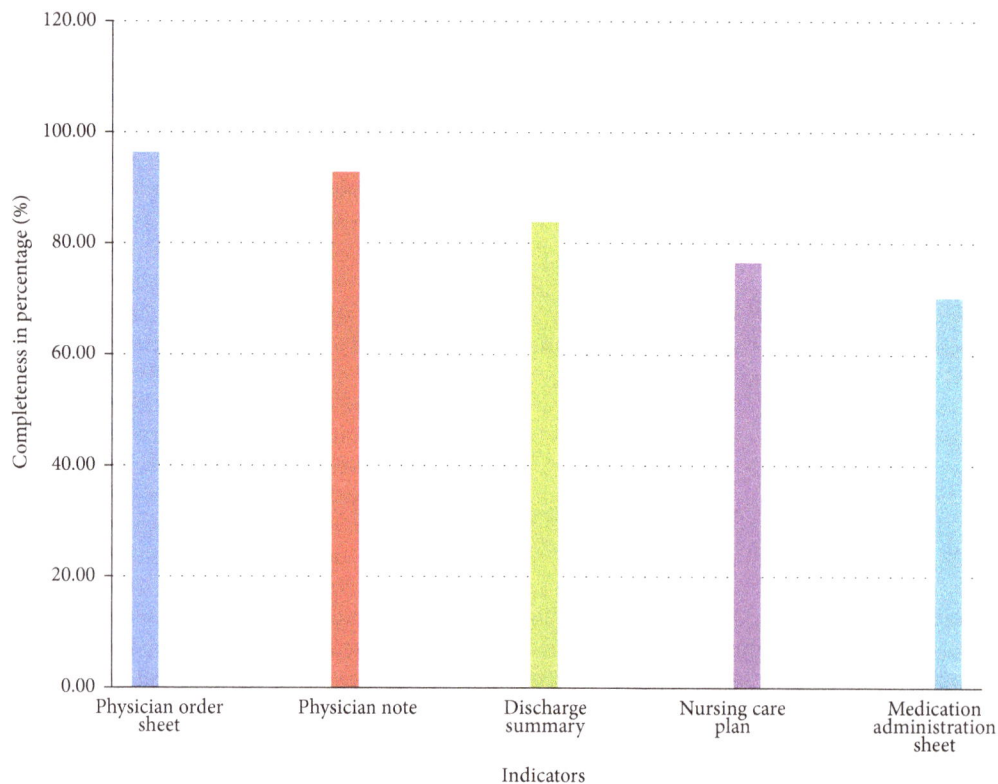

FIGURE 1: Status of completeness of medical record completeness in Menelik II Referral Hospital, Addis Ababa, Ethiopia, May 2016.

TABLE 1: Pre- and postintervention changes in medical record completeness in Menelik II Referral Hospital, Addis Ababa, Ethiopia, May 2016.

Indicators	Preintervention, September 2015	Postintervention, May 2016
Inpatient physician note	96%	92.8%
Physician order sheet	96%	96.4%
Nursing care plan	70%	76.6%
Medication administration sheet	40%	70.3%
Discharge summary	64%	83.8%
Total	73%	84%

medical records and applying simple set of intervention can bring changes [6].

The study done in a Dalefage Primary Hospital, West Afar, Ethiopia, shows that an enhancement of completeness and reporting of inpatient medical record completeness improved significantly from the baseline 0% to 73.6% during postintervention evaluation. Similar to our study after introduction of simple intervention inpatient medical record completeness improves from the baseline 73% to 84% during postintervention evaluation. This implies that, by implementing a set of intervention, it can bring improvement in completeness of medical records [8].

5. Conclusion

The overall inpatient medical record completeness in Menelik II Referral Hospital was 84% and the higher rate of completeness was seen in inpatient physician order sheet 96.4%

completed whereas the least completed was inpatient medication administration sheet 70.3% completed. The finding of this project suggests that a simple set of intervention availing inpatient medical record format and training healthcare provider improves the inpatient medical record completeness. This project indicates that applying strategic problem solving to medical record completeness can be effective in improving quality of healthcare.

6. Recommendations

(1) It is better if the Health Management Information System Department takes special consideration on full implementation and proper management of inpatient medical records.

(2) Intensive and continuous training should be given for the healthcare provider by responsible body.

(3) The Quality Officer and Chief Executive Officer at the administrative positions of the study hospital are recommended to design and launch intervention programs to improve medical record completeness.

(4) Effective long-term follow-up is needed to assess the sustainability of intervention by inpatients department head.

(5) Quality improvement project of this approach should be encouraged to be applied in other departments of hospital to enhance quality of healthcare services by quality team.

Authors' Contributions

Kasu Tola conceived the study, undertook statistical analysis, and drafted the paper. Dr. Haftom Temesgen, Yemane Gebremariam, and Birhanu Jikamo made major contributions to the study design and statistical analysis. All authors contributed to the writing of the paper and approved its submitted version.

Acknowledgments

The authors appreciate the management of Menelik II Referral Hospital and Healthcare provider working in inpatient departments. Kasu Tola also extends his thanks to Dr. Haftom Temesgen, Mr. Yemane Gebremariam, Mr. Dawit Tatek, and Mr. Birhanu Jikamo for their inspiration and technical support in many ways.

References

[1] M. Helfand and M. Freeman, *Evidence-Based Synthesis Program Assessment and Management of Acute Pain in Adult Medical Inpatients: Portland VA Health Care System, Oregon Evidence-Based Center: A Systematic Review*, 2008.

[2] WHO, *Medical Records Manual: A Guide For Developing Countries Revised and Updated*, 2006.

[3] M. Zegers, M. C. De Bruijne, P. Spreeuwenberg, C. Wagner, P. P. Groenewegen, and G. Van Der Wal, "Quality of patient record keeping: an indicator of the quality of care?" *BMJ Quality and Safety*, vol. 20, no. 4, pp. 314–318, 2011.

[4] I. T. Adeleke, A. O. Adekanye, K. A. Onawola et al., "Data quality assessment in healthcare: a 365-day chart review of inpatients' health records at a Nigerian tertiary hospital," *Journal of the American Medical Informatics Association*, vol. 19, no. 6, pp. 1039–1042, 2012.

[5] AHRQ, "Making health care safer II: an updated critical analysis of the evidence for patient safety practices," AHRQ Evidence Report 211, 2013.

[6] R. Wong and E. H. Bradley, "Developing patient registration and medical records management system in Ethiopia," *International Journal for Quality in Health Care*, vol. 21, no. 4, pp. 253–258, 2009.

[7] K. Tadesse, E. Gebeye, and G. Tadesse, "Assessment of health management information system implementation in Ayder referral hospital, Mekelle, Ethiopia," *International Journal of Intelligent Information Systems*, vol. 3, no. 4, pp. 34–39, 2014.

[8] N. M. Dima, *Improving the completeness of medical records at inpatient department of Dalefage Primary Hospital, west Afar, Ethiopia [Masters of Hospital and Health Care Administration]*, School of Graduate Studies of Addis Ababa University, 2014.

[9] N. Tavakoli, M. Jahanbakhsh, M. Akbari, and M. Baktashian, "The study of inpatient medical records on hospital deductions: an interventional study," *Journal of Education and Health Promotion*, vol. 4, article 38, 2015.

[10] AHRQ, "Enabling patient-centered care through health information technology," U.S. Department of Health and Human Services Report, 2012.

[11] P. C. Tang, M. P. Larosa, and S. M. Gorden, "Use of computer-based records, completeness of documentation, and appropriateness of documented clinical decisions," *Journal of the American Medical Informatics Association*, vol. 6, no. 3, pp. 245–251, 1999.

[12] H. Wang, "Sample size calculation for comparing proportions," in *Wiley Encyclopedia of Clinical Trials*, pp. 1–11, John Wiley & Sons, 2007.

[13] MOH Federal Democratic Republic of Ethiopia, *Hospital Performance Monitoring and Improvement Manual*, 2011.

[14] K. Legault, J. Ostro, Z. Khalid, P. Wasi, and J. J. You, "Quality of discharge summaries prepared by first year internal medicine residents," *BMC Medical Education*, vol. 12, no. 1, article 77, 2012.

[15] M. Greiver, J. Barnsley, R. H. Glazier, B. J. Harvey, and R. Moineddin, "Measuring data reliability for preventive services in electronic medical records," *BMC Health Services Research*, vol. 12, no. 1, article 116, 2012.

18

Knowledge, Attitude, and Practice regarding HIV/AIDS among People with Disability in Hawassa City, Southern Ethiopia

Mekdes Mekonnen, Tsigereda Behailu, and Negash Wakgari ⓘ

School of Nursing and Midwifery, College of Medicine and Health Sciences, Hawassa University, Hawassa, Ethiopia

Correspondence should be addressed to Negash Wakgari; negashwakgari@yahoo.com

Academic Editor: Hsin-Yun Sun

Background. People with disabilities are vulnerable group to be infected with HIV/AIDS and are challenged to utilize HIV/AIDS services. Hence, this study assessed knowledge, attitude, and practice about HIV/AIDS among disabled people in Hawassa city. *Methods.* A community-based cross-sectional study was conducted among 250 disabled people. All disabled people residing in Hawassa city during the study period were included. Pretested and structured questionnaire was used for data collection. Logistic regression analyses were used to identify the associated factors. *Results.* A high percentage (197 (79.8%)) of disabled people were knowledgeable about HIV/AIDS. Similarly, 190 (76%) of the respondents had a favorable attitude towards HIV/AIDS. In addition, being married (AOR = 2.20; 95% CI: 1.14, 4.27) and being employed (AOR = 2.85; 95% CI: 1.19, 6.81) were positively associated with knowledge about HIV/AIDS. Moreover, being a male (AOR = 2.83; 95% CI: 1.61, 2.90) and being married (AOR = 2.13; 95% CI: 2.25, 3.26) were also positively associated with having a favorable attitude towards HIV/AIDS. *Conclusions.* Significant numbers of disabled people were knowledgeable and had a favorable attitude towards HIV/AIDS.

1. Background

Disability is a complex phenomenon, reflecting the interaction between features of a person's body and features of the society in which he or she lives [1]. People living with disabilities are vulnerable groups to be infected with HIV/AIDS because of sexual violence and social exclusion factors such as being deprived of information, education, and communication [2]. People with disability lack basic knowledge about HIV and how it could be transmitted [2–7]. Discrimination and inequality also impair every aspect of their decision-making power and lives [2–4, 6–10]. Furthermore, disability affects sexual and reproductive health functions of women, consequently increasing the risk of sexual violence, unwanted pregnancy, and unsafe abortion [1–3, 5].

Health institutions where comprehensive HIV/AIDS service is provided are physically inaccessible and certain channels of communication are not appropriate for disabled people [7, 8]. Similarly, special schools for those with sensorial impairments are excluded from prevention campaigns [9–13].

Moreover, infrastructure is another challenge of disabled people to utilize HIV/AIDS services even after getting access to the healthcare facilities because the rooms are not suitable for the free movement [8].

There are an estimated 15 million people with disabilities in Ethiopia, comprising physical and intellectual disability, deafness, and blindness [14]; however, this study only focused on people with physical disability, deafness, and blindness. Very little is known about knowledge, attitude, and practice of disabled people towards HIV/AIDS in the study area. Hence, this study is aimed to assess knowledge, attitude, and practice regarding HIV/AIDS among people with disability in Hawassa city, southern Ethiopia. In addition, it is also intended to assess factors associated with the knowledge and attitude towards HIV/AIDS among disabled people.

2. Materials and Methods

2.1. Study Setting and Population. A community based cross-sectional study was conducted to assess knowledge, attitude, and practice about HIV/AIDS among disabled people in

Hawassa city, southern Ethiopia, from May to July 2015. Hawassa is an administrative city of Southern Nation, Nationalities and People Regional State located 275 km to the south of Addis Ababa. This administration city comprises a total population of 133,097 [15]. Moreover, it contains two hospitals and nine health centres.

2.2. Sample Size and Sampling Procedure.

All people with physical disability, blindness, and deafness residing in Hawassa city during the study period were included in the study. To identify the study population, the preliminary survey was conducted by the principal investigators. Firstly, the principal investigators contact Southern Nation, Nationality and People Regional Health Bureau to identify all organizations participating in supporting disabled people in the city. Accordingly, Birhan Le Ethiopia disability association and Salu Meredadat and Blind people associations were identified as organizations providing different supports for disabled people in the city. Secondly, all people with physical disability, blindness, and deafness who are supported by these organizations were invited in the study and advised by staff of each organization and data collectors to avoid double count. Consequently, 193 people with physical disability, deafness, and blindness were invited to the study from this organization, while nine mentally disabled people were excluded from the study, since they were unable to provide the necessary data. Finally, respondents who were not incorporated under support organization were searched and included in the study, while they were begging around the mosque, church, and street during the study period. To do this, easily identifiable physical disabilities were used. Thus, 57 people with physical disability, blindness, and deafness were included in the study, while they were begging around the mosque, church, and street.

2.3. Data Collection Tools and Procedures.

Structured and pretested interviewer administered questionnaire was used for the data collection. Different literatures were reviewed to develop the tool and to include all the important variables that address the objectives of the study [2–8, 13, 14]. The instrument was pretested on 20 similar study participants who were living in the Shashemene town. Findings from the pretest were used to modify the instrument. Two B.S. nurses and one expert with sign language were recruited and facilitated the data collection process. Two-day training was given for the data collectors before the actual data collection. The questionnaire was designed to obtain information on sociodemographic characteristics, knowledge about sexually transmitted disease, HIV/AIDS, stigma towards people living with AIDS, risky sexual behavior and condom use, and attitude towards HIV/AIDS.

Knowledge about HIV/AIDS was measured by using six knowledge questions. Accordingly, the following knowledge questions were asked: Have you ever heard about HIV/AIDS? What was the source of information about HIV/AIDS? What is the difference between HIV and AIDS? Would you mention some modes of transmission for HIV? Can HIV be transmitted from mother to child? How HIV can be transmitted from mother to child? Does the use of latex condom by a person with sexually transmitted disease reduce a transmission of HIV? What is the importance of medical help for an individual having sexually transmitted disease? Have you ever heard about AIDS treatment? In order to produce a more objective assessment of knowledge about HIV/AIDS, a scoring method was devised and a knowledge score for each participant was obtained by adding up the score for correct response given to selected questions in the questionnaire. A score of mean value and above (3–6) to knowledge-related questions was considered as knowledgeable, while a score of less than mean value (0–2) was considered as not knowledgeable. In addition, the attitude of disabled people towards HIV/AIDS was assessed by using ten questions. A 5-point Likert scale (strongly agree, agree, neutral or uncertain, disagree, and strongly disagree) was used to measure their attitude; individuals responding with "strongly agree" for positive attitude questions were given scores of 5 and those who responded with "strongly disagree" were given scores of 1, while the above scores were reversed for negative attitude questions. Finally the total score ($5 \times 10 = 50$) was dichotomized into favorable and unfavorable attitude taking the mean score (25) as a cutoff point (mean score or more = favorable attitude; less than the mean score = unfavorable attitude).

2.4. Data Management and Analysis.

The collected questionnaire was checked manually for its completeness, coded and entered into Epi-Info version 3.5.1 statistical package, and then exported to SPSS version 20.0 for further analysis. Descriptive and summary statistics were presented by frequency tables. Both bivariate and multivariable logistic regression analyses were used to determine the association of each independent variable with the dependent variable. Significant variables in bivariate analysis ($P < 0.2$) were entered into a multivariable logistic regression model to adjust the effects of cofounders on the outcome variable. Odds ratios with their 95% confidence intervals were computed to identify the presence and strength of association, and statistical significance was declared if $P < 0.05$.

The quality of data was assured by proper designing and pretesting the questionnaires. Proper categorization, coding, and skipping patterns of questionnaires were used. Training was given for data collectors and supervisor before the actual data collection. Each piece of data was reviewed and checked for completeness, accuracy, clarity, and consistency by the principal investigator daily and the supervisor immediately after data were collected. The necessary feedback was offered to the data collectors in the next morning. Data cleanup and cross-checking were done before the analysis.

2.5. Ethical Considerations.

Ethical clearance was obtained from the Institutional Review Board of College of Medicine and Health Sciences, Hawassa University. Permission letter was granted from the Zonal Health Department to respective health institutions. Verbal consent was obtained from each study subject prior to the data collection process. Those who were not willing to participate in the study were not forced to be involved. Their privacy was maintained. To keep their confidentiality, personal identifiers were not used.

3. Results

3.1. Background Information of the Respondents. A total of 250 people with disability were included in the study. About half (127 (50.8%)) of the respondents were males. The major ethnic composition of the study population was Wolaita (63 (25.2%)). 106 (42.4%) of them were Orthodox religion followers. Nearly half (122 (48.8%)) were single. Regarding educational status, 100 (40%) of them completed secondary education. About two-thirds (157 (62.8%)) of them had physical disability and 29 (11.6%) had more than one sexual partner (Table 1).

3.2. Knowledge of Respondents about HIV/AIDS. A high percentage (197 (79.8%)) of disabled people in this study were knowledgeable about HIV/AIDS. Most of the respondents (243 (97.2%)) heard about HIV/AIDS. The sources of information were mass media (32 (12.8%)) and healthcare facility (26 (10.4%)) and in 181 (72.4%) of the respondents the sources of the information were more than one. More than half (140 (56%)) of the respondents did not know the difference between HIV and AIDS. 51 (24.4%) of them responded that HIV can be transmitted through mosquito bite; and 36 (14.4%) of them replied that HIV can be transmitted by eating in the same eating utensils HIV-positive people use. Similarly, 69 (52.8%) of them said that HIV can be transmitted through kissing HIV-positive person. Majority (204 (81.6%)) of respondents knew that HIV can be transmitted from mother to child and only 77 (30.8%) of them mentioned the mode of transmission as during pregnancy, delivery, and breast-feeding. A small proportion (21 (8.4%)) stated that there is no need for medical help for an individual having sexually transmitted disease and 32 (9.2%) of them replied that they could not reduce HIV transmission by using latex condom. 102 (40.8%) were not aware of AIDS treatment.

3.3. Attitude and Practice of Respondents about HIV/AIDS. In this study, 190 (76%) of the respondents had a favorable attitude towards HIV/AIDS. Most (219 (87.6%)) of people with disabilities perceived themselves as at risk of contracting HIV. Similarly, 168 (67.2%) of them felt that their disability could increase risk of contracting HIV and majority of the respondents (231 (92.4%)) thought that sexually active disabled people should go for HIV testing only before having sex. Moreover, 85 (24%) of the respondents believed that condom promotion encourages sex. About two-thirds (171 (68.4%)) of them disagreed with the idea of condom being safe to use (Table 2).

Regarding practice about HIV/AIDS, more than two-thirds (188 (75.2%)) of the respondents did not test for HIV in the last three months (Table 3).

3.4. Factors Associated with Knowledge about HIV/AIDS among Disabled People. In bivariate analysis, the factors found to be significantly associated with the knowledge about

HIV/AIDS were sex, marital status, occupation, and type of disability. However, in multiple logistic regression analysis, marital status and occupation of disabled people were significantly associated with knowledge about HIV/AIDS. Those who were married were about two times more likely to be knowledgeable about HIV/AIDS than their counterparts (AOR = 2.20; 95% CI: 1.14, 4.27). Similarly, those who were employed were about three times more likely to be knowledgeable about HIV/AIDS compared to those who were unemployed (AOR = 2.85; 95% CI: 1.19, 6.81) (Table 4).

3.5. Factors Associated with Attitude towards HIV/AIDS among Disabled People. In bivariate analysis, the factors found to be significantly associated with the attitude towards HIV/AIDS were age, sex, marital status, and type of disability. However, in multiple logistic regression analysis, sex and marital status of disabled people were significantly associated with the attitude towards HIV/AID among disabled people. Those who were male were about three times more likely to have a favorable attitude than females (AOR = 2.83; 95% CI: 1.61, 2.90). In addition, those who were married were about two times more likely to have a favorable attitude compared to unmarried counterparts (AOR = 2.13; 95% CI: 2.25, 3.26) (Table 5).

4. Discussion

The study assessed the knowledge, attitude, and practice regarding HIV/AIDS among people with disability in Hawassa city, southern Ethiopia. In this study, 79.8% of people with disability were knowledgeable about HIV/AIDS (95% CI: 75.3–83.6). The present finding is lower than the studies conducted among people without disabilities. For instance, the study done in Lao, Japan, reported that 97.7% and 92.0% of the respondents knew that HIV can be transmitted by sexual intercourse and through sharing needles, respectively [16]. Similarly, the study conducted in Mekelle, Ethiopia, also reported that 85.5% of the respondents had a good level of knowledge about HIV/AIDS [13]. The possible explanation for this difference might be the fact that people with physical and intellectual disabilities are less likely to be knowledgeable than people without disabilities. For example, people with hearing impairments are not reached by the usual HIV/AIDS awareness, as they are not a part of these communication networks [5, 7]. However, this finding is higher than the study conducted in Johannesburg, South Africa (49%) [3], and lower than the study done in Addis Ababa, Ethiopia (83.6%) [4]. This difference might be due to difference in the study population, because the study of Johannesburg was conducted among mentally ill patients, which could be associated with cognitive impairment [5]. The other possible explanation for this difference might be the difference in the age of the respondents. For instance, the study of Addis Ababa was conducted among young disabled people.

This study reported that 76% of the respondents had a favorable attitude towards HIV/AIDS (95% CI: 71.8–80.4). This finding is higher than the studies done in Addis

TABLE 1: Sociodemographic characteristics of the study respondents, Hawassa city, 2016.

Variables ($n = 250$)	Frequency	Percentage
Sex		
Male	127	50.8
Female	123	49.2
Age		
15–19	22	8.8
20–24	78	31.2
25–29	54	21.6
30–34	40	16.0
35–39	22	8.8
40 and above	34	13.6
Ethnicity		
Sidama	62	24.8
Wolaita	63	25.2
Gurage	36	14.4
Amhara	50	20.0
Oromo	18	7.2
Tigrie	8	3.2
Others*	13	5.2
Religion		
Orthodox	106	42.4
Protestant	97	38.8
Muslim	26	10.4
Catholic	9	3.6
Others**	12	4.8
Occupation		
Governmental	30	11.9
Nongovernmental	117	46.4
Student	84	33.3
Others***	17	6.7
Income per month with birr		
<500	23	9.1
500–1000	67	26.6
1001–1500	23	9.1
1501–2000	13	5.2
2001–3000	19	7.5
>3000	9	3.6
Has no income	96	38.1
Marital status		
Unmarried	122	48.8
Married	64	25.6
Divorced	35	14.0
Widowed	29	11.6
Educational status		
Read and write only	17	6.7
Primary education	57	22.6
Secondary education	100	39.7
College/university	65	25.8

TABLE 1: Continued.

Variables ($n = 250$)	Frequency	Percentage
Type of disability		
Physical disability	157	62.8
Blindness	45	18.0
Deafness	41	16.4
More than one disability	7	2.8
Cause of disability		
Vehicle accident	47	19.0
Disease	134	54.0
Congenital/inborn	67	27.0
Number of sexual partners		
Have one sexual partner	70	28.0
Have two and more sexual partners	29	11.6
Have no sexual partners	151	60.4

*Kambata, Hadiya, and Dawuro; **Pagan and Waqeffata; ***trader and private worker.

Ababa (21.6%) [4] and Leo, Japan (55.7%) [16]. The possible explanation for this difference might be the difference in the sociodemographic characteristics of the respondents and time of the study. For instance, in the study of Addis Ababa, only young disabled people participated with a less likelihood to perceive about HIV acquisition. In addition, the study of Leo, Japan, was conducted among male school students without disability in 2010.

In the present study, only 62 (24.8%) and 42 (16.8%) of the respondents were tested for HIV in the last three months of the study and ever used condom during sex, respectively. This finding is in line with studies conducted in Addis Ababa, Ethiopia [4], and Nigeria [5]; however, it is lower than the study conducted in Leo, Japan [16], and Mekelle city, Ethiopia [13]. The difference observed between these studies might be due to difference in the study population and variable measurement.

Furthermore, marital status was found to be significantly associated with knowledge about HIV/AIDS among disabled people. Those who were married were about two times more likely to be knowledgeable about HIV/AIDS than unmarried counterparts. This might be due to the information gained during HIV testing and counseling before marriage and the level of the attention taken for the health of the family. Moreover, those who were employed were about three times more likely to be knowledgeable about HIV/AIDS compared to unemployed counterparts. The possible explanation could be the fact that those who are employed are often literate and economically independent compared to unemployed counterparts, which would improve accessibility to information. Also, higher disability rates are associated with higher rates of illiteracy and unemployment and lower occupational mobility [9, 10, 14].

In this study, being a male was also significantly associated with having a favorable attitude towards HIV/AIDS. This might be due to the fact that males with disabilities attend school more frequently than females with disabilities and most of girls with disabilities are illiterate [17, 18].

TABLE 2: Attitude of respondents towards HIV/AIDS, Hawassa city, 2016 ($n = 250$).

Variables	Strongly agree	Agree	Neutral or uncertain	Disagree	Strongly disagree
Do you feel that people treat you differently because of your disability?	45 (18%)	140 (56%)	24 (9.6%)	38 (15.2%)	3 (1.2%)
A person with disability is vulnerable to HIV infection	89 (35.6%)	130 (52%)	10 (4%)	18 (7.2%)	3 (1.2%)
A person with disability who is sexually active should go for HIV testing only before having sex	78 (31.2%)	153 (61.2%)	14 (5.6%)	4 (1.6%)	1 (.4%)
A person with disability who is sexually active should go for HIV testing at any time	52 (20.8%)	171 (68.4%)	19 (7.6%)	7 (2.8%)	1 (.4%)
A person with disability should protect themselves against HIV/AIDS	95 (38%)	139 (55.6%)	11 (4.4%)	5 (2%)	0
A person with disability needs to have knowledge about HIV/AIDS to make an informed decision before having sexual intercourse	114 (45.8%)	129 (51.8%)	2 (0.8%)	5 (2%)	0
My disability increases the risk of contracting HIV	51 (20.4%)	117 (46.8%)	16 (6.4%)	63 (25.2%)	3 (1.2%)
I receive pressure from my parents not to have sexual relationship	9 (3.6%)	82 (33.1%)	40 (16.1%)	97 (39.2%)	22 (8%)
Condoms encourage sex	17 (6.8%)	68 (27.2%)	28 (11.2%)	93 (37.2%)	44 (17.6%)
Condom is not safe to use for disabled people	6 (2.4%)	46 (18.4%)	27 (10.8%)	105 (42%)	66 (26.4%)

TABLE 3: Practice of respondents about HIV/AIDS, Hawassa city, 2016 ($n = 250$).

Practice of disabled people about HIV/AIDS		Frequency	Percentage
Did you visit the healthcare facility for the past six months to enquire about HIV/AIDS matter?	Yes	76	30.4
	No	174	69.6
Have you tested for HIV in the last three months?	Yes	62	24.8
	No	188	75.2
Have you had sex in the last six months?	Yes	98	39.2
	No	152	60.8
Have you ever used condom during sex?	Yes	42	16.8
	No	208	83.2
How often have you been using condom?	Usually	26	10.4
	Occasionally	16	6.4

In addition, those who were married were more likely to have a favorable attitude towards HIV/AIDS compared to unmarried counterparts. This might be due to the fact that male individuals are more economically independent and educated compared with females, which might influence their level of knowledge and attitude towards HIV/AIDS [9, 10].

This study has some limitations. Firstly, even if disabled people who were not included under support organization were tried to be identified by staff working at supporting organization, there might be missed respondents, particularly those who were not begging at mosque, church, and street. Secondly, the current study did not include mentally disabled individuals or people with intellectual disability. Lastly, since information about HIV/AIDS practice was obtained from respondents through an interview, response and social desirability bias are also potential limitations of this study. In addition, this study did not assess factors determining practice regarding HIV/AIDS.

5. Conclusions

This study found that the disabled participants in this study were reasonably knowledgeable with regards to HIV and AIDS and that their attitudes were also largely positive in nature. However, more than two-thirds of the respondents did not visit the healthcare facility for HIV/AIDS matter in the last three months. A higher level of knowledge was associated with being employed and being married. Further male participants and those who were married were more likely to have positive attitudes. In the light of these findings, it is recommended that ensuring access of HIV/AIDS counseling and testing services for disabled people is crucial to improve HIV/AIDS practices.

TABLE 4: Bivariate and multivariate analyses of factors associated with knowledge about HIV/AIDS among disabled people in Hawassa city, southern Ethiopia ($n = 250$).

Variables	Knowledgeable	Not knowledgeable	COR (95% CI)	AOR (95% CI)	P value
Age					
15–19	20	2	0.38 (0.72, 2.05)	**	
20–24	68	10	0.56 (0.19, 1.64)		
25–29	36	18	1.92 (0.70, 5.27)		
30–34	31	9	1.12 (0.36, 3.41)		
35–39	15	7	1.80 (0.53, 6.11)		
40 and above	27	7	1		
Sex					
Male	104	23	1.45 (0.79, 2.69)	**	
Female	93	30	1		
Marital status					
Married	92	36	2.41 (1.27, 4.58)	2.20 (1.14, 4.27)	0.013
Not married*	105	17	1		
Type of disability					
Deafness	35	4	1		
Other types of disability	162	49	2.65 (0.89, 7.81)	**	
Employment					
Employed	179	41	2.91 (1.11, 5.77)	2.85 (1.19, 6.81)	0.024
Unemployed	18	12	1		

*Single, divorced, and widowed. **Not significant in backward stepwise logistic regression. 1: reference.

TABLE 5: Bivariate and multivariate analyses of factors associated with attitude towards HIV/AIDS among disabled people in Hawassa city, southern Ethiopia ($n = 250$).

Variables	Favorable attitude	Unfavorable attitude	COR (95% CI)	AOR (95% CI)	P value
Age					
15–19	17	5	0.62 (0.18, 2.10)	**	
20–24	55	23	0.87 (0.36, 2.08)		
25–29	43	11	0.53 (0.20, 1.42)		
30–34	34	6	0.36 (0.12, 1.13)		
35–39	18	4	0.46 (0.12, 1.70)		
40 and above	23	11	1		
Sex					
Male	102	21	2.15 (1.17, 3.93)	2.83 (1.61, 2.90)	0.001
Female	88	39	1		
Marital status					
Married	50	14	1.17 (1.89, 2.56)	2.13 (2.25, 3.26)	0.024
Not married*	140	46	1		
Type of disability					
Deafness	30	9	1*		
Other types of disability	160	51	1.37 (0.76, 2.47)	**	

1: reference. *Not married. **Not significant in backward stepwise logistic regression.

Authors' Contributions

Mekdes Mekonnen and Tsigereda Behailu participated in the design of the study and data collection, analyzed the data, and drafted the paper. Negash Wakgari participated in the analysis and drafted and revised subsequent drafts of the paper. All authors read and approved the final manuscript.

References

[1] N. E. Groce, "HIV/AIDS and people with disability," *The Lancet*, vol. 361, no. 9367, pp. 1401-1402, 2003.

[2] J. Hanass-Hancock, "Disability and HIV/AIDS - a systematic review of literature on Africa," *Journal of the International AIDS Society*, vol. 12, no. 1, p. 34, 2009.

[3] G. Jonsson, M. Y. H. Moosa, and F. Y. Jeenah, "Knowledge, attitudes and personal beliefs about HIV and AIDS among mentally ill patients in Soweto, Johannesburg," *Southern African Journal of HIV Medicine*, no. 41, pp. 14–20, 2011.

[4] T. A. Kassa, T. Luck, A. Bekele, and S. G. Riedel-Heller, "Sexual and reproductive health of young people with disability in Ethiopia: A study on knowledge, attitude and practice: A cross-sectional study," *Globalization and Health*, vol. 12, no. 1, article no. 5, 2016.

[5] T. J. Aderemi, B. J. Pillay, and T. M. Esterhuizen, "Differences in HIV knowledge and sexual practices of learners with intellectual disabilities and non-disabled learners in Nigeria," *Journal of the International AIDS Society*, vol. 16, Article ID 17331, 2013.

[6] E. E. Tarkang, S. Gbogbo, and P. Lutala, "HIV/AIDS-Related Knowledge among Persons with Physical Disability inCameroon: A Qualitative Study," *Journal of AIDS and HIV Infections*, vol. 1, no. 2, 2015.

[7] C. Lefèvre-Chaponnière, "Knowledge, attitudes and practices regarding HIV/AIDS amongst disabled youth in Maputo (Mozambique)," *Santé Publique*, vol. 22, no. 5, pp. 517–528, 2010.

[8] K. Kelly and P. Ntlabati, "Early adolescent sex in South Africa: HIV intervention challenges," *Social Dynamics*, vol. 28, no. 1, pp. 42–63, 2002.

[9] N. E. Groce, "Adolescents and Youth with Disability: Issues and Challenges," *Asia Pacific Disability Rehabilitation Journal*, vol. 5, no. 2, pp. 12–32, 2004.

[10] N. E. Groce, "HIV/AIDS and disability: Preliminary findings from the World Bank/Yale University global survey," in *Proceedings of the Symposium HIV and disability - a global challenge*, pp. 189–200, IKO Verlag, 2004.

[11] S. K. Tororei, B. Chirchir, J. Matere, and Y. W. Machira, "Addressing the balance of burden of AIDS in people with disabilities in Kenya -a review of literature on HIV/AIDS and people with disabilities," 2008.

[12] T. Brown, B. Franklin, J. MacNiel, and S. Mills, *Effective Prevention Strategies in Low HIV Prevalence Settings*, UNAIDS Best Practice Key Materials, 2001.

[13] A. Tadese and B. Menasbo, "Knowledge, attitude and practice regarding HIV/AIDS among secondary school students in Mekelle City, Ethiopia," *African Journal of AIDS and HIV Research*, vol. 1, no. 1, pp. 001–007, 2013.

[14] World Health Organization, "World Report on Disability," Geneva, Switzerland, 2011, http://www.who.int/disabilities/world_report/2011/report.pdf.

[15] World Population Review, "Population of Cities in Ethiopia," 2017, http://worldpopulationreview.com/countries/.

[16] B. Thanavanh, M. Harun-Or-Rashid, H. Kasuya, and J. Sakamoto, "Knowledge, attitudes and practices regarding HIV/AIDS among male high school students in Lao People's Democratic Republic," *Journal of the International AIDS Society*, vol. 16, Article ID 17387, 2013.

[17] United Nations, "Fact Sheet: Youth with Disabilities. United Nations International year of youth," 2010, http://social.un.org/youthyear/links.html.

[18] A. K. Yousafzai, K. Edwards, C. D'Allesandro, and L. Lindström, "HIV/AIDS information and services: the situation experienced by adolescents with disabilities in Rwanda and Uganda.," *Disability and Rehabilitation*, vol. 27, no. 22, pp. 1357–1363, 2005.

19

Predictors of Neonatal Deaths in Ashanti Region of Ghana

Gertrude Nancy Annan ⓘ[1] and Yvonne Asiedu[2]

[1]*Nursing and Midwifery Training College, Kumasi, Ghana*
[2]*SDA Midwifery Training College, Asamang, Ghana*

Correspondence should be addressed to Gertrude Nancy Annan; afuaannan@outlook.com

Academic Editor: Ronald J. Prineas

Background. Neonatal mortality continues to be a public health problem, especially in sub-Saharan Africa. This study was conducted to assess the maternal, neonatal, and health system related factors that influence neonatal deaths in the Ashanti Region, Ghana. *Methods.* 222 mothers and their babies who were within the first 28 days of life on admission at Mother and Baby unit (MBU) at the Komfo Anokye Teaching Hospital (KATH) in Kumasi, Ashanti Region of Ghana, were recruited through systematic random sampling. Data was collected by face to face interviewing using open and closed ended questions. A logistic regression analysis was conducted to determine the influence of proximal and facility related factors on the odds of neonatal death. *Results.* Out of the 222 mothers, there were 115 (51.8%) whose babies did not survive. Majority, 53.9%, of babies died within 1–4 days, 31.3% within 5–14 days, and 14.8% within 15–28 days. The cause of death included asphyxia, low birth weight, congenital anomalies, infections, and respiratory distress syndrome. Neonatal deaths were influenced by proximal factors (parity, duration of pregnancy, and disease of the mother such as HIV/AIDS), neonatal factors (birth weight, gestational period, sex of baby, and Apgar score), and health related factors (health staff attitude, supervision of delivery, and hours spent at labour ward). *Conclusion.* This study shows a high level of neonatal deaths in the Ashanti Region of Ghana. This finding suggests the need for health education programmes to improve on awareness of the dangers that can militate against neonatal survival as well as strengthening the health system to support mothers and their babies through pregnancy and delivery and postpartum to help improve child survival.

1. Introduction

Child survival remains an urgent concern globally [1]. Despite the enormous progress made in improving child survival, this has not reflected in the decline in neonatal mortality [1, 2]. Since 1990, under-five mortality rate has been reduced nearly by half from 90 to 46 deaths per 1,000 live births in 2013 and the global under-five mortality rate is currently falling faster than at any other time over the past two decades [1]. The decline in neonatal deaths has however been slower than the decline in the postneonatal (1–59 months) mortality rate, leading to neonatal deaths currently representing a larger share of the total under-five deaths than in 1990. In 2013, about 44% of all under-five deaths occurred in the first 28 days of life, increasing from 37% in 1990 [1]. This proportion rose to 45% in 2015 [3]. Although every region in the world is experiencing an increase in the proportion of neonatal deaths, the burden is highest in West and Central Africa, where the risk of a baby dying within the first 28 days of life is almost 10 times higher than the risk facing a baby born in a high-income country [1].

In Ghana, neonatal mortality rate in the most recent period (2009–2014) stood at 29 deaths per 1,000 live births [4]. This rate is 2.2 times the postneonatal rate (13 deaths per 1,000 live births) during the same period. This shows a slower pace in reduction than infant and child mortality and has resulted in an increase in the contribution of neonatal deaths to infant deaths from 53% in 1998 to 71% in 2014. Sixty-eight percent of all deaths among children under age 5 in Ghana take place before a child's first birthday, with 48% occurring during the first month of life. This means that one in every 24 children in Ghana dies before reaching age 1, while one in every 17 does not survive to her or his fifth birthday [4].

The WHO's standard definition of neonatal death is the death of any live born infant within 28 days of his/her birth [5]. Almost 66% of neonatal deaths occur in the first week of life. Of those who die within the first week, approximately 66% die in the first 24 hours of life [6]. The initial 24 hours of a child's life are the most dangerous with over one million newborns around the world dying each year on their first and only day of life [7]. Without urgent action, the progress in under-five mortality could stall without urgent action to tackle the high rate of newborns dying, which now account for more than 4 in 10 child under-five deaths [7]. The causes of neonatal deaths are numerous and are related to pregnancy, delivery, and infections. Each of these factors accounts for about one-third of newborn deaths. Birth intervals of less than 36 months significantly increase the risk of low birth weight, premature babies, and neonatal death. Asphyxia and congenital anomalies, infections, hemorrhage, and respiratory distress syndrome also contribute to a high proportion of neonatal deaths [8, 9].

Neonatal and maternal deaths place a significant burden on health systems as well as on women and families. Making motherhood safer is critical to saving newborns. Research shows that a significant number of neonatal deaths could be prevented if all women received good quality antenatal care as well as good quality care during delivery and the postpartum period. Characteristics of the health system including attitudes of staff, availability of care, and place of delivery contribute to maternal and delivery outcomes [10]. Even though maternity services are largely said to be "free" at government facilities, associated hidden costs contribute to low utilization of maternity services. According to UNFPA reports [11], many factors complicate women's access to skilled care in the sub-Saharan African region. The report further explained that often women give birth at home because of the prohibitive cost of medical care or cultural beliefs that promote home-based delivery. Some simply lack confidence in the health system. Difficult geographic terrain and limited transportation may present obstacles to reaching a skilled attendant [12, 13].

Whiles the national neonatal mortality rate also has seen a decrease from 2003 to 2014 [4], the same cannot be said in terms of the regional statistics. The Ashanti Region recorded an increase in neonatal death over the same period (increased by 1.8 per 1000 live births) and the regional rate in 2014 was higher than the national average (42 versus 29 per 1000 live births). There is, however, paucity of evidence on the maternal and child level predictors of neonatal mortality in the Ashanti region. This study was conducted to assess the maternal, neonatal, and health system related factors that influence neonatal deaths in the Ashanti Region, Ghana.

2. Methods

2.1. Study Design and Setting.
The research was a quantitative descriptive survey conducted at the Mother and Baby unit (MBU) at the Komfo Anokye Teaching Hospital (KATH) in Kumasi, Ashanti Region of Ghana. The city of Kumasi is the capital of the Ashanti Region and the centre of the Kumasi Metropolitan District in Ghana. KATH is the second-largest

hospital in the country and the only tertiary health institution in the Ashanti Region. It is the main referral hospital for the Ashanti, Brong Ahafo, and Northern, Upper East and Upper West, and Western regions as well as for neighboring countries. The hospital was built in 1954 as the Kumasi Central Hospital. It was later named Komfo Anokye Hospital after Okomfo Anokye, a legendary fetish priest of the Ashanti. It was converted into a teaching hospital in 1975 to train nurses, doctors, medical technologist, and paramedics. It is affiliated to the School of Medical Sciences of the Kwame Nkrumah University of Science and Technology (KNUST).

The MBU is under the Child Health directorate, one of the 11 directorates of the hospital. It has a bed capacity of seventy-one (71) cots and six (6) incubators and admits babies from day of delivery to about 3 months. The unit runs a twenty-four (24) hour emergency service throughout the week. Cases are referred from regional hospitals, district hospitals, general practitioners, and maternity homes and from other regions. At the MBU, there are three subunits, the high dependency, premature/low dependency, and septic. The most common cases admitted at MBU are preterm/low birth weight and asphyxia. However neonatal infections, birth traumas, congenital abnormalities, jaundice, Vitamin K deficiency, and heart failure cases are also admitted, HIV/AIDS being the least case admitted.

2.2. Sampling Techniques and Sample Size.
The study population was mothers and their babies who were within the first 28 days of life on admission at MBU, KATH, Kumasi.

Sample size was estimated using Cochran's sample size formula [14]. The prevalence of neonatal mortality in the general population was assumed to be 14%.

As per the formula,

$$N = \frac{Z^2 Pq}{d^2}, \tag{1}$$

where

N is sample size

Z is the reliability coefficient for 95% confidence level set at 1.96

P is proportion of babies who die

$q = 1 - P = 86.0\%$ or 0.86

d is degree of freedom

$$N = \frac{1.96^2 \times (0.14) \times (0.86)}{0.05^2} = 185. \tag{2}$$

Considering nonresponse of 20%, we arrived at total of 222.

A systematic random sampling technique was used to recruit study participants, by defining a random starting point and a fixed sampling interval. Based on the number of expected attendance at the facility and the period of data collection, the average respondents needed per day were estimated. Mothers with their babies within 28 days of life and who consented to be part of the study were randomly selected.

During the visit hours, the first participant was identified and interviewed as the starting point followed by the Kth respondent. In cases when babies did not meet the inclusion criteria, the next and following participants were contacted. This was repeated until the required sample size was attained.

2.3. Data Collection Tools. A face to face interview using open and closed ended questions was adopted. Three (3) field assistants were recruited and trained in the data collection techniques and skills. Participants were recruited daily and the questionnaire was administered. All respondents were made to answer the same questions which were constructed in English. However for respondents who could not read and write, questions were asked in the dialect and their responses were written. Difficult technical terms were avoided in the preparation of the questionnaire. The field assistants were trained to ensure standardization of the questions across sites.

The study instrument (questionnaires) was pretested in Suntreso Government Hospital which has similar characteristics as the study site. This was done to check the clarity, consistency, and acceptability of people other than those interviewed for the study. This was further to train the interviewers and also ensure that the questionnaire met the stated objective. After pretesting, problems such as ambiguity associated with the questionnaire were rectified.

2.4. Assessment of Neonatal Mortality. Neonatal mortality was defined as death of a newborn within 28 days of his/her birth. A checklist was developed for all neonates admitted to the MBU during the period of the study and all of the neonates among that group who died before they were discharged from the hospital. The checklist included various characteristics of the neonates, such as the type of delivery (vaginal or Caesarian section), birth weight, single or multiple births, diagnoses of any diseases, and the duration of survival. These checklists were completed based on the available medical records.

2.5. Data Handling and Analysis. Regular verification and validation of data were done with all inconsistencies being checked and resolved with the researcher, research assistants, and the data entry clerk. All data were entered into and analysed with SPPSS Version 22 Software [15]. Result of the analysis were generated using descriptive and some analytical statistics. Bivariate associations were tested using Pearson chi-square or Fischer's exact test. Univariable and multivariable logistic regression analyses were also conducted to determine the influence of proximal and facility related factors on the odds of neonatal mortality. Proximal risk factors are risk factors that precipitate a condition. They represent an immediate vulnerability for a particular condition or event and they represented the maternal and neonatal factors in this study. The proximal factors considered in this study were maternal factors (age, parity, number of children, birth interval, duration of pregnancy, and disease of mother) and neonatal factors (birth weight, gestational period, sex, birth anomaly, Apgar score, respiratory distress, and crying immediately after birth). The health related factors were ANC visits, attitude of health staff, waiting time, delivery supervision, and labour conditions.

3. Ethical Considerations

Ethical clearance for this study was obtained from Department of Community Health-KNUST, the Ethics Committee of KNUST, and Komfo Anokye Teaching Hospital. In addition, written and informed consent was obtained from the individuals who agreed to be part of the study. Privacy and confidentiality were ensured during data collection and assured afterwards.

4. Results

4.1. Background Characteristics of the Respondents. The mean (standard deviation, SD) age of respondents was 22 years (0.710) and majority 50.9% of respondents interviewed were between the ages of 21 and 30 years, Table 1. Majority of the mothers had basic education (60.8%), were Christians (73.4%), and were married (62.6%). Fifty-nine mothers (26.6%) had monthly income less than GH¢100.00. Traders formed 29.3% of respondents.

Babies of 107 mothers, representing 48.2%, survived, while babies of 115 mothers (51.8%) died. Among mothers whose babies did not survive, the majority, 54.8%, were in the age group of 21–30 years. There was a statistically significant association ($p = 0.046$) between age of a mother and child survival. Among mothers whose babies did not survive, the majority, 56.5%, were married while 41.7% were single and there was a statistically significant association ($p = 0.034$) between marital status and child survival. Marital status ($p = 0.034$) and occupation ($p = 0.035$) of respondents also had a significant association with child survival (Table 1).

4.2. Neonatal Deaths. Majority (53.9%) of babies died within 1–4 days and 31.3% within 5–14 days while 14.8% died within 15–28 days. Most (37.4%) of the babies died from asphyxia. About 32.7% also died from low birth weight and 10.3% died due to prematurity, 9.3% congenital anomalies, 5.6% infections, and 3.7% respiratory distress syndrome (Figure 1).

4.3. Proximal Factors and Neonatal Death

4.3.1. Maternal Factors. As described in Table 2, though the age of mother had a significant association with child survival, this was not observed in the logistic regression analysis. In terms of parity, 47.8% and 47% of babies who did not survive were of primigravida and multigravida mothers, respectively, $p = 0.042$.

Among mothers with duration of pregnancy of 35–40 weeks, 67.3% had babies who survived compared to 34.8% whose children died, $p = 0.026$. Regression analysis indicated that mothers with duration of 35–40 weeks of pregnancy had 3.15 higher odds of their babies surviving (OR = 3.15, CI = 2.21, 6.79) as compared to those within duration of 24–30 weeks of pregnancy. The odds of child survival increased to 3.62 in the adjusted model. Babies whose mothers were not hypertensive also had higher odds of survival as compared to those whose mothers were hypertensive (adjusted odds ration [AOR] = 1.41, CI = 1.20, 1.68).

TABLE 1: Background characteristics of the mothers of children who died and those who survived.

Variable	Baby survived $n = 107$ N (%)	Baby did not survive $n = 115$ N (%)	Total $n = 222$ N (%)	p value
Age				
Mean (SD)	22 (0.710)			
15–20 yrs	15 (14.0)	21 (18.3)	36 (16.2)	
21–30 yrs	50 (46.7)	63 (54.8)	113 (50.9)	
31–40 yrs	42 (39.3)	28 (24.3)	70 (31.5)	0.046
Above 40 yrs	0 (0.0)	3 (2.6)	3 (1.4)	
Education				
None	5 (4.7)	7 (6.1)	12 (5.4)	
Basic	71 (66.4)	64 (55.7)	135 (60.8)	
Secondary	19 (17.8)	29 (25.2)	48 (21.6)	0.419
Tertiary	12 (11.2)	15 (13.0)	27 (12.2)	
Religion				
Christian	83 (77.6)	80 (69.6)	163 (73.4)	
Islam/Muslim	22 (20.6)	32 (27.8)	54 (24.3)	0.582
Traditionalist/others	2 (1.8)	3 (2.6)	5 (2.3)	
Marital status				
Single	32 (29.9)	48 (41.7)	80 (36.0)	
Separated	0 (0.0)	2 (1.7)	2 (0.9)	0.034
Divorced	1 (0.9)	0 (0.0)	1 (0. 05)	
Married	74 (69.2)	65 (56.5)	139 (62.6)	
Income of mother				
Unknown	59 (55.1)	54 (47.0)	113 (50.9)	
Less than GH¢100	28 (26.2)	31 (27.0)	59 (26.6)	
GH¢100–GH¢300	14 (13.1)	19 (16.5)	33 (14.9)	(0.509)
GH¢300–GH¢500	6 (5.6)	11 (9.6)	17 (7.7)	
Occupation				
Self-employed	18 (16.8)	23 (20.0)	41 (18.5)	
Housewife/student	19 (17.8)	31 (27.0)	50 (22.6)	
Civil servant	12 (11.2)	13 (11.3)	25 (11.3)	
Farmer	1 (0.9)	7 (6.1)	8 (0.6)	0.035
Trader	37 (34.6)	28 (24.3)	65 (29.3)	
Artisans	20 (18.6)	12 (10.5)	32 (14.5)	

SD: standard deviation.

Study results indicated that there was a statistically significant association ($p = 0.024$) between mothers with HIV/AIDS and child survival. Mothers who did not have HIV/AIDS had 1.53 higher odds of survival (AOR = 1.53, CI = 1.28, 1.71) than those who had HIV/AIDS (Table 2).

4.3.2. Neonatal Factors. Average birth weight according to the study was 2.5 kg while minimum and maximum birth weights were 0.8 kg and 4.6 kg, respectively, Table 3. Child survival increased with appreciable increase in baby's weight but declined when baby's weight was more than 3 kg. The analysis indicated that babies whose weights were 3 kg had 2.75 higher odds of survival (OR = 2.75, CI = 1.56, 3.87) as

compared to babies whose weight were less than 1 kg. The odds however reduced to 2.29 in the adjusted model.

Out of the 115 babies who did not survive, 68.7% were preterm, while out of the 107 who survived 81.3% were term, Table 3. The odds of survival were 5.28 times higher among babies whose gestational period was term (AOR = 5.28, CI = 3.01, 10.05) as compared to babies whose gestational period was preterm. Female babies had 1.73 higher odds of survival (OR = 1.73, CI = 1.48, 2.63) compared to their male counterparts but this was not significant in the adjusted models.

Baby's Apgar score proved to be relevant in child survival. Most (40.5%) of the babies had an Apgar score of 4/10–6/10, and about 32.4% had 7/10–10/10, while 27.0% had 1/10–3/10.

TABLE 2: Relationship between maternal factors and baby survival.

Variable	Baby survived n = 107 (%)	Baby did not survive n = 115 (%)	Total n = 222 (%)	p value	OR (95% CI)	AOR (95% CI)
Age of mother at childbirth (years)						
15–20 years	15 (14.0)	21 (18.3)	36 (16.2)	0.046	1.00	1.00
21–30 years	50 (46.7)	63 (54.8)	113 (50.9)		1.13 (0.31, 1.61)	1.21 (0.43, 1.77)
31–40 years	42 (39.3)	31 (24.3)	73 (31.5)		1.41 (0.37, 4.11)	1.82 (0.58, 5.13)
Parity						
Primigravida	38 (35.5)	55 (47.8)	93 (41.9)	0.042	1.00	1.00
Multigravida (2–5)	59 (55.1)	54 (47.0)	113(50.9)		1.55 (0.66, 1.73)	1.06 (0.29, 1.70)
Grand multigravida (6+)	10 (9.3)	6 (5.2)	16 (7.2)		1.23 (0.47, 1.12)	1.03 (0.41, 1.15)
Number of children						
1-2	63 (58.9)	69 (60.0)	132 (59.5)	0.352	1.00	1.00
3-4	35 (32.7)	31 (27.0)	66 (29.7)		1.42 (0.52, 1.66)	1.15 (0.34, 2.01)
5-6	6 (5.6)	8 (7.0)	14 (6.3)		1.51 (0.38, 1.96)	1.11 (0.22, 1.90)
Above 6	3 (2.8)	7 (6.1)	10 (4.5)		1.11 (0.31, 1.21)	1.01 (0.13, 1.11)
Birth interval in relation to newborn						
Less than 1 year	3 (2.8)	9 (7.8)	12 (5.4)	0.038	1.00	1.00
1–2 years	17 (15.9)	34 (29.6)	51 (23.0)		1.38 (0.43, 1.61)	1.52 (0.93, 1.95)
3–4 years	33 (30.8)	31 (27.0)	64 (28.8)		1.71 (0.87, 2.49)	1.80 (0.99, 3.23)
5–6 years	54 (50.5)	41 (35.7)	95 (42.8)		1.55 (0.63, 1.79)	1.73 (0.89, 2.65)
Duration of pregnancy (in relation to newborn baby)						
24–30 weeks	15 (14.0)	34 (29.6)	49 (22.1)	0.026	1.00	1.00
31–34 weeks	18 (16.8)	31 (27.0)	49 (22.1)		1.86 (0.95, 1.89)	1.97 (0.98, 2.09)
35–40 weeks	72 (67.3)	40 (34.8)	112 (50.5)		**3.15 (2.21, 6.79)**	**3.62 (2.29, 7.11)**
Disease in the mother (hypertension)						
Yes	13 (12.1)	10 (8.7)	23 (10.4)	0.047	**1.51 (1.23, 1.99)**	**1.41 (1.20, 1.68)**
No	94 (87.9)	105 (91.3)	199 (89.6)		1.00	1.00
Disease in the mother (HIV/AIDS)						
Yes	3 (2.8)	7 (6.1)	10 (4.5)	0.024	**1.86 (1.33, 1.99)**	**1.53 (1.28, 1.71)**
No	104 (97.2)	108 (93.9)	212 (95.5)		1.00	1.00
Disease in the mother (diabetes)						
Yes	5 (4.7)	7 (6.1)	12 (5.4)	0.327	1.21 (0.71, 1.74)	1.07 (0.44, 1.52)
No	102 (95.3)	108 (93.9)	210 (94.6)		1.00	1.00

OR: odds ratio for baby survival; AOR: adjusted odds ratio; p values based on Pearson chi-square or Fischer's exact test.

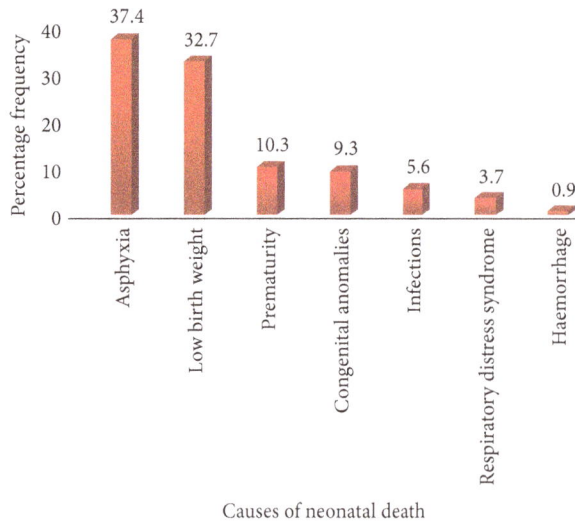

FIGURE 1: Percentage frequency distribution of causes of death.

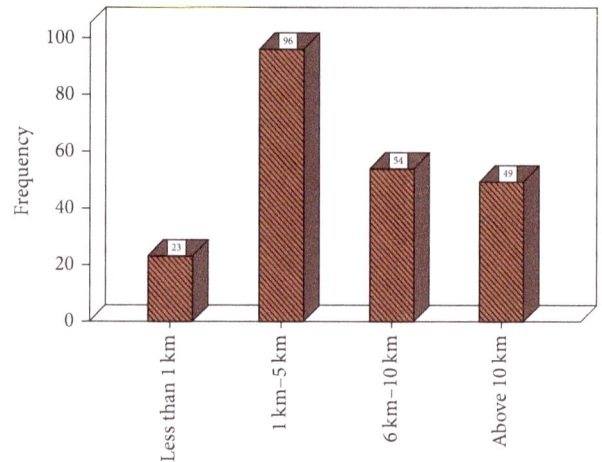

FIGURE 2: Nearest health centre from residence.

Out of 60 babies whose Apgar score was 1/10–3/10, 88.3% did not survive as compared to 77% out of 72 babies whose Apgar score was 7/10–10/10, $p = 0.038$. Regression analysis showed that babies whose Apgar score was 7/10–10/10 had 4.61 higher odds of survival (AOR = 4.61, CI = 3.02, 8.89) as compared to babies whose Apgar score was 1/10–3/10.

Eighty-six percent (86%) of babies were resuscitated. Although there was a significant association ($p = 0.047$) between neonatal resuscitation and child survival, regression analysis did not yield any marginal variations in the likelihood of child survival and neonatal resuscitation. Results of the study indicated that majority (66.7%) of babies did not have respiratory distress. Out of the 74 babies who had respiratory distress 71.6% did not survive, Table 3.

4.4. Socioeconomic Factors. Most (43.2%) of the mothers interviewed indicated that the nearest health centre from their residence was between 1 km and 5 km away. There was no significant association ($p = 0.522$) between distance of residence and child survival. Regression analysis did not reveal any variant likelihood of occurrence between child survival and distance of respondents' residence. As shown in Figure 2, 24.3% walk less than 1 km to the health centre nearest to respondent, 43.2% walk between 1 km and 5 km, 10.4% from 6 km to 10 km, and 2.1% above 10 km. Among the 222 interviewed, two hundred and nine representing 94.14% have registered for the National Health insurance. However, mothers' registration with the NHIS did not have any significant association ($p = 0.215$) with child survival. Majority, 74.8%, of the respondents do not know the amount paid during their visit to the health facility. This could be due to the NHIS. 12.6% paid an amount less than GH¢5.00 and 8.1% paid GH¢5.00 to GH¢10.00 while 4.5% paid more than GH¢10.00.

4.5. Health System Related Factors. Majority (50.9%) of mothers interviewed attended ANC 5–8 times, Table 4. However, some 4.5% did not attend ANC at all. Majority (51.8%)

of mothers interviewed delivered at KATH, 36.9% at another health facility (private and public), and 7.7% at a maternity home. The study revealed that there was a significant ($p = 0.038$) association between place of delivery and child survival.

Among health staff who attended to mothers during ANC visits, majority (74.8%) were midwives while 19.8% were doctors. There was a significant association ($p = 0.028$) between health staff attending to mothers at ANC visits and child survival. Neonates whose mothers were attended to by doctors were more likely to survive, as compared to those whose mothers were attend to by nurses. Generally, respondents judged staff attitude as good (54.1%), very good (37.4%), and excellent (2.3%). There was a significant association ($p = 0.028$) between service providers attitude and child survival. Very good staff attitude was associated with high odds of child survival as compared to average or poor staff attitude (AOR = 1.38, CI = 1.11, 2.93), Table 4.

41.9% of the mothers interviewed indicated that they spent 1 hour before health staff attended to them at the facility. Waiting time of mothers was significantly associated with baby survival in the crude model but was attenuated in the adjusted model. Majority (75.2%) of mothers were delivered by midwifes, while doctors delivered 19.8%. Babies who were delivered by doctors were 2.98 times more likely to survive as compared to those delivered by traditional birth attendants, TBA (AOR = 2.98, CI = 2.14, 4.57). Average hours spent at labour ward by mothers was 6 hours. There was a significant association ($p = 0.048$) between hours spent at labour ward and child survival.

5. Discussion

Out of the 222 respondents, babies of 107 mothers representing 48.2% survived, while babies of 115 mothers (51.8%) died. The proportion of neonatal deaths recorded in this study could however be higher than the general population, recognizing the fact that the facility where the study was conducted is a referral hospital and only worse cases might have been referred there. Nevertheless, Ghana is known

TABLE 3: Relationship between neonatal factors and baby survival.

Variable	Baby survived $n = 107$ N (%)	Baby did not survive $n = 115$ N (%)	Total $n = 222$ N (%)	p value	OR (95% CI)	AOR (95% CI)
Baby's birth weight						
Less than 1 kg	11 (10.3)	40 (34.8)	51 (23.0)		1.00	1.00
2 kg	31 (29.0)	34 (29.6)	65 (29.3)	0.022	2.17 (1.32, 3.33)	1.97 (1.12, 3.01)
3 kg	52 (48.6)	31 (27.0)	83 (37.4)		2.75 (1.56, 3.87)	2.29 (1.15, 3.23)
Above 3 kg	13 (12.1)	10 (8.7)	23 (10.4)		1.64 (0.78 1.91)	1.24 (0.53 1.62)
Gestational period						
Preterm	15 (14.0)	79 (68.7)	94 (42.3)		1.00	1.00
Term	87 (81.3)	34 (29.6)	121 (54.5)	0.038	4.48 (2.52, 9.21)	5.28 (3.01, 10.05)
Postterm	5 (4.7)	2 (1.7)	7 (3.2)		1.78 (0.56, 4.24)	2.44 (0.87, 6.09)
Sex of the baby						
Male	51 (47.7)	61 (53.0)	112 (50.5)	0.018	1.00	1.00
Female	56 (52.3)	54 (47.0)	110 (49.5)		1.73 (1.48, 2.63)	2.18 (1.88, 4.17)
Baby cried immediately after birth						
Yes	99 (92.5)	35 (30.4)	134 (60.4)	0.042	1.00	1.00
No	8 (7.5)	80 (69.6)	88 (39.6)		1.73 (1.34, 2.54)	1.41 (0.98, 2.14)
Birth anomaly						
Yes	6 (5.6)	19 (16.5)	25 (11.3)	0.047	1.00	1.00
No	101 (94.4)	96 (83.5)	197 (88.7)		1.55 (1.22, 3.01)	1.31 (0.78, 2.55)
Baby's Apgar score						
1/10–3/10	7 (6.5)	53 (46.1)	60 (27.0)		1.00	1.00
4/10–6/10	45 (42.1)	45 (39.1)	90 (40.5)	0.038	2.57 (1.64, 3.99)	3.64 (2.85, 5.01)
7/10–10/10	57 (51.4)	17 (14.8)	72 (32.4)		3.18 (2.35, 7.61)	4.61 (3.02, 8.89)
Neonatal resuscitation						
Yes	95 (88.8)	96 (83.5)	191 (86.0)	0.047	1.00	1.00
No	12 (11.2)	19 (16.5)	31 (14.0)		1.26 (0.13, 1.62)	1.41 (0.73, 1.82)
Respiratory distress						
Yes	21 (19.6)	53 (46.1)	74 (86.0)	0.034	1.00	1.00
No	86 (80.4)	62 (53.9)	148 (66.7)		1.36 (0.48, 1.41)	0.98 (0.12, 1.12)

OR: odds ratio for baby survival; AOR: adjusted odds ratio; p values based on Pearson chi-square or Fischer's exact test.

TABLE 4: Relationship between health systems related factors and baby survival.

Variable	Baby survived n = 107 (%)	Baby did not survive n = 115 (%)	Total n = 222 (%)	p value	OR (95% CI)	AOR (95% CI)
ANC visits						
None	2 (1.9)	8 (7.0)	10 (4.5)	0.614	1.00	1.00
1–4 times	15 (14.0)	54 (47.0)	69 (31.1)		**1.37 (1.01, 1.66)**	1.24 (0.81, 1.12)
5–8 times	68 (63.6)	45 (39.1)	113 (50.9)		1.45 (0.75, 3.77)	1.33 (0.63, 2.52)
Above 8 times	22 (20.6)	8 (7.0)	30 (13.5)		1.84 (0.48, 2.99)	1.41 (0.12, 2.99)
Place of delivery						
Home	4 (3.7)	2 (1.7)	6 (2.7)	0.038	1.00	1.00
KATH	71 (66.4)	44 (38.3)	115 (51.8)		**1.51 (1.21, 2.56)**	1.26 (0.86, 1.99)
Health facility (public/private)	25 (23.4)	57 (49.6)	82 (36.9)		1.27 (0.79, 2.14)	0.98 (0.32, 1.07)
Maternity home	7 (6.5)	12 (10.4)	19 (7.9)		1.39 (0.83, 2.38)	1.18 (0.57, 1.62)
Health staff attended to respondent when they visited ANC						
Nurse	2 (1.9)	2 (1.7)	4 (1.8)	0.038	1.00	1.00
Doctor	38 (35.5)	6 (5.2)	44 (19.8)		**1.51 (1.21, 2.56)**	**1.69 (1.36, 5.31)**
Midwife	65 (60.7)	101 (87.8)	166 (74.8)		1.27 (0.79, 2.14)	**1.92 (1.33, 3.08)**
Others	2 (1.9)	6 (5.2)	8 (3.6)		1.39 (0.83, 2.38)	1.92 (0.99, 3.18)
Service providers' attitude towards respondent						
Excellent	5 (4.7)	0 (0.0)	5 (2.3)	0.027	-	-
Very good	75 (70.1)	8 (7.0)	83 (37.4)		**1.27 (1.04, 1.87)**	**1.38 (1.11, 2.93)**
Good	26 (24.3)	94 (81.7)	120 (54.1)		**1.13 (1.08, 2.33)**	1.24 (0.85, 3.41)
Average/poor	1 (0.9)	13 (11.3)	14 (6.4)		**1.00**	1.00
Hours spent by health staff till attending to a respondent						
1 hr	52 (48.6)	41 (35.7)	93 (41.9)	0.021	1.00	1.00
2 hrs	18 (16.8)	24 (20.9)	42 (18.9)		**1.12 (1.01, 1.36)**	0.82 (0.73, 1.06)
3 hrs	19 (17.8)	22 (19.1)	41 (18.5)		**1.31 (1.21, 1.25)**	1.17 (1.00, 1.31)
Above 3 hrs	18 (16.8)	28 (24.3)	46 (20.7)		**1.44 (1.31, 1.61)**	1.21 (0.97, 1.55)
Delivery supervision						
TBA	4 (3.7)	4 (3.5)	8 (3.6)	0.031	1.00	1.00
Midwife	65 (60.7)	102 (88.7)	167 (75.2)		**1.87 (1.31, 2.69)**	**1.25 (1.09, 2.43)**
Doctor	38 (35.5)	9 (7.8)	47 (21.2)		**3.47 (2.53, 5.47)**	**2.98 (2.14, 4.57)**
Hours spent at the labour ward						
Less than 5 hrs	62 (57.9)	13 (11.3)	75 (33.8)	0.048	1.00	1.00
5 hrs–8 hrs	29 (27.1)	49 (42.6)	78 (35.1)		**1.38 (1.07, 1.41)**	1.12 (0.86, 1.31)
8 hrs–12 hrs	9 (8.4)	27 (23.5)	36 (16.2)		**1.41 (1.18, 1.67)**	1.21 (0.97, 1.38)
Above 12 hrs	7 (6.5)	26 (22.6)	33 (14.9)		**1.29 (1.14, 1.49)**	**1.13 (0.92, 1.38)**
Drugs or injection given in labour						
Yes	62 (57.9)	70 (60.9)	132 (59.5)	0.068	1.00	1.00
No	45 (42.1)	45 (39.1)	90 (40.5)		**1.54 (1.31, 1.75)**	**1.60 (1.19, 1.72)**

OR: odds ratio for baby survival; AOR: adjusted odds ratio; p values based on Pearson chi-square or Fischer's exact test; TBA: traditional birth attendant; KATH: Komfo Anokye Teaching Hospital; ANC: antenatal care.

to still record high rates of neonatal mortality [16]. In corroborating Lawn et al.'s findings, this study revealed that majority (53.9%) of babies died within 1–4 days and 31.3% within 5–14 days. The babies died from asphyxia, low birth weight, prematurity, congenital anomalies, infections, and respiratory distress syndrome. WHO Report [17] indicated that major causes of newborn deaths worldwide are preterm, pneumonia/infection, asphyxia, congenital abnormalities, tetanus, diarrhoea, and others. Low birth weight, which is related to maternal malnutrition, is a causal factor in 60–80% of all neonatal deaths.

5.1. Maternal Factors Influencing Neonatal Mortality. There was a statistically significant association between mothers' parity and child survival. 47.8% and 47.0% of babies who did not survive were of primigravida and multigravida mothers, respectively. Other studies have also shown that children born after a short interval are likely to have mothers in poor health, and such children tend to have low birth weight and increased chances of neonatal mortality [18]. This is consistent with findings from a systematic review and meta-analysis that found an increased risk of preterm and neonatal and infant mortality [19]. Multigravida increases competition for family resources and attention and also increases exposure to infectious childhood diseases.

Duration of pregnancy also influenced child survival. Mothers with pregnancy duration of 35–40 weeks were more likely to have babies who will survive. This finding means that babies born before term and after term stand a high risk of not surviving. This is congruent with findings from a recent study by Mengesha et al. [20], where preterm delivery was an independent predictor of neonatal mortality in Northern Ethiopia. This could be explained by the fact that preterm and postterm babies are unable to adjust to extrauterine life and therefore are prone to specific complications like breathing difficulties, intracranial bleeding, infections, hypothermia, and jaundice [21]. This study also found an influence of pregnancy complications on child survival. Mothers who were hypertensive were more likely to have children who did not survive. As stated by Lawn et al. [22], complications during the antenatal period like pregnancy induced hypertension, eclampsia, cardiac failure, diabetes, and renal diseases cause a median increased risk of 4.5 for neonatal death, with eclampsia posing the biggest risk.

5.2. Neonatal Factors. The study revealed statistically significant relationship between birth weight and child survival. The finding corroborates findings of a study of factors affecting the survival of "at risk" newborn at Korle Bu Teaching Hospital, in Accra, Ghana, which reported that 83.6% of 128 babies weighed less than 1 kg died while babies weighing beyond 2 kg were less likely to die [23]. Gestational age (GA) is known to contribute to neonatal mortality. This study found a significant association between gestational period and child survival. This concurs with the study by Khashu et al. [24], which elaborated that infants born before 37 weeks of gestation are at greater risk of mortality compared with term newborns and attributes this directly to specific complications like breathing difficulties, intracranial bleeds, infections, hypothermia, and jaundice.

Bromen and Jöckel [25] estimated in their study that mortality rates for boys in the early neonatal period are higher than those for girls, and that biological differences between the sexes tend to result in higher male mortality than female mortality. Similarly, this current study found that, out of the 107 babies who survived, majority, 52.3%, were females. Regression analysis slightly tilted in favour of survival of female babies.

Baby's Apgar score also proved to be relevant in child survival. There was a statistically significant association between a baby's Apgar score and child survival. This corroborates findings from the study by Li et al. [26], which found a relationship between five-minute Apgar scores and infant survival. In their study, the Apgar score showed its predictive value for infant death of both very preterm, preterm, and term infants in postneonatal period. They concluded that the Apgar score could still be a good and convenient predictor of infant death.

5.3. Health System Related Factors. Research shows that a significant number of neonatal deaths could be prevented if all women received good quality care during antenatal, delivery, and the postpartum period [27]. Majority of mothers interviewed delivered at the health facility and there was a significant association between place of delivery and child survival. These findings support the findings of Lawn et al. [22] which reported that skilled professional care during pregnancy and child birth and postnatal care are highly recommended as a critical measure to save the life of the mother and the baby. Skilled professional care during pregnancy, at birth and during the postnatal period, is as critical for both the mother and baby. Skilled attendance and institutional delivery rates are lowest in countries with the highest neonatal mortality rates [22]. Children delivered at home are likely to experience higher mortality than children delivered at the hospital or medical facilities because these facilities usually provide a sanitary environment and medical equipment to assist birth. However, home deliveries without a skilled attendant are chosen or occur for a variety of reasons, including long distances or difficult access to a birth facility, costs of services, and perceived lack of quality of care in a health facility [12, 28].

The general impression of respondents about staff attitude was good and there was a significant association between service providers' attitudes and child survival. Very good staff attitude increased the likelihood of child survival. A recent systematic review of literature documented a broad range of negative maternal health care providers' attitudes and behaviours affecting patient well-being, satisfaction with care, and care seeking [29]. Negative attitudes and behaviours of maternal health care providers lead to inadequate care seeking and reduce the quality of care, leading to rise in maternal and child mortality and morbidity. Majority (75.2%) of mothers were delivered by midwifes, while doctors delivered 19.8%. These figures for skilled supervised delivery are very good as they are way above the national average of 57% [30]. Babies who were delivered by doctors were more likely to survive compared to those delivered by nurses.

A unique strength of this study is that it provides important evidence on the predictors of neonatal mortality in Ghana. The choice of cross-sectional study design however could not permit us to make direct inferences on the relationship between the outcome variable and the covariates studied. Recruiting mothers from only one MBU could also present a selection bias and could affect the generizability of the findings. This study might also have suffered some recall bias in previous pregnancy experiences of participants. We however believed that this did not affect the study much, since our questionnaire had validation questions to most of the possible bias questions.

6. Conclusion

This study shows a high neonatal mortality rate in the Ashanti Region of Ghana, 51.8%, with majority dying within 5–14 days. The causes of death included low birth weight, prematurity, congenital anomalies, infections, and respiratory distress syndrome. Findings also reveal that neonatal deaths are influenced by neonatal, maternal, and health service related factors. This suggests the need for the health service providers and other stakeholders to organize intensive health education programmes to improve awareness of the dangers that can militate against neonatal survival. Inasmuch as the education, it should target the general population using local media, ANC and PNC clinic sessions, women in second cycle institutions, and tertiary institutions. The education should highlight some significant maternal factors such as appropriate birth interval for pregnancies and the need to manage properly all infectious and noninfectious diseases. There is also the need for strengthening the health system to support mothers and their babies through pregnancy and delivery and postpartum to help improve child survival.

Abbreviations

MBU: Mother and Baby unit
MDG: Millennium Development Goal
MOH: Ministry of Health
GDHS: Ghana Demographic Health Survey
GHS: Ghana Health Services
KATH: Komfo Anokye Teaching Service
NMR: Neonatal Mortality Rate.

Authors' Contributions

Gertrude Nancy Annan conceptualized and designed the study and collected the data. Both authors analysed and interpreted the data and wrote the draft manuscript. Both authors read and approved the final manuscript.

Acknowledgments

The authors appreciate very much the support and contributions by Dr. Alex Osei-Akoto Lecturer, Head of Child Health Department, KATH. Their suggestions and priceless editorial help motivated the authors to produce this useful work. They also thank Dr. Peter Adjei Baffour, a lecturer at the Department of Community Health, KNUST, and Mr. Emmanuel Owusu-Sekyere, a lecturer at University of Development Studies, Wa campus, for their suggestions and comments which made this work a great success. Their sincere thanks also go to the Nurse Manager and all the staff of MBU, KATH.

References

[1] T. Wardlaw, D. You, L. Hug, A. Amouzou, and H. Newby, "UNICEF Report: Enormous progress in child survival but greater focus on newborns urgently needed," *Reproductive Health*, vol. 11, no. 1, article 82, 2014, https://data.unicef.org/wp-content/uploads/2015/12/Enormous-progress-in-child-survival_220.pdf.

[2] UNICEF, "UNICEF Data: Monitoring the situation of children and women," 2014, https://data.unicef.org/.

[3] World Health Organization, *Neonatal Mortality*, World Health Organization, 2017, http://www.who.int/gho/child_health/mortality/neonatal/en/.

[4] Ghana Statistical Service, Ghana Health Service, and ICF International, *Ghana Demographic and Health Survey 2014*, Rockville, MD, USA, 2015, https://dhsprogram.com/pubs/pdf/FR307/FR307.pdf.

[5] World Health Organization, *Neonatal Mortality Rate (per 1 000 Live Births)*, World Health Organization, Geneva, Switzerland, 2005, http://www.who.int/healthinfo/morttables.

[6] C. Maccormack and T. S. Murphy, *State of the World'S Newborns: A Report from Saving Newborn Lives*, Washington, DC, USA, 2001, http://www.savethechildren.org.

[7] World Health Organization, *One Million Babies Die Within 24 Hours Of Birth*, World Health Organization, 2014, http://www.who.int/workforcealliance/media/news/2014/end_new_born_death/en/.

[8] R. E. Black, S. S. Morris, and J. Bryce, "Where and why are 10 million children dying every year?" *The Lancet*, vol. 361, no. 9376, pp. 2226–2234, 2003.

[9] H. R. Chowdhury, S. Thompson, M. Ali, N. Alam, M. Yunus, and P. K. Streatfield, "Causes of neonatal deaths in a rural subdistrict of bangladesh: implications for intervention," *Journal of Health, Population and Nutrition*, vol. 28, no. 4, pp. 375–382, 2010.

[10] M. E. Kruk, M. Paczkowski, G. Mbaruku, H. De Pinho, and S. Galea, "Women's preferences for place of delivery in rural Tanzania: A population-based discrete choice experiment," *American Journal of Public Health*, vol. 99, no. 9, pp. 1666–1672, 2009.

[11] UNFPA, "Providing emergency obstetric and newborn care," 2012, [cited 2017 Jun 8], https://www.unfpa.org/sites/default/files/resource-pdf/EN-SRHfactsheet-Urgent.pdf.

[12] K. N. Atuoye, J. Dixon, A. Rishworth, S. Z. Galaa, S. A. Boamah, and I. Luginaah, "Can she make it? transportation barriers to accessing maternal and child health care services in rural Ghana," *BMC Health Services Research*, vol. 15, article 333, 2015.

[13] G. B. Nuamah, P. Agyei-Baffour, K. M. Akohene, D. Boateng, D. Dobin, and K. Addai-Donkor, "Incentives to yield to obstetric referrals in deprived areas of Amansie West district in the Ashanti Region, Ghana," *International Journal for Equity in Health*, vol. 15, no. 1, article 117, 2016, http://equityhealthj.biomedcentral.com/articles/10.1186/s12939-016-0408-7.

[14] W. G. Cochran, *Sampling Techniques*, Probability and Mathematical Statistics Applied, John Wiley & Sons, New York, NY, USA, 3rd edition, 1977.

[15] IBM Corp Released, "IBM SPSS Statistics for Windows, Version 22.0," 2011.

[16] A. Ibrahim, "Ghana still recording high maternal, neonatal mortality," Myjoyonline, 2017, https://www.myjoyonline.com/lifestyle/2017/October-29th/ghana-still-recording-high-maternal-neonatal-mortality-health-minister.php.

[17] World Health Organization, *Newborn Death and Illness*, World Health Organization, 2011, [cited 2017 Jun 26], http://www.who.int/pmnch/media/press_materials/fs/fs_newborndealth_illness/en/.

[18] V. Sharma, J. Katz, L. C. Mullany et al., "Young maternal age and the risk of neonatal mortality in rural Nepal," *Archives of Pediatrics & Adolescent Medicine*, vol. 162, no. 9, pp. 828–835, 2008.

[19] N. Kozuki, A. C. Lee, M. F. Silveira et al., "The associations of birth intervals with small-for-gestational-age, preterm, and neonatal and infant mortality: a meta-analysis," *BMC Public Health*, vol. 13, supplement 3, 2013.

[20] H. G. Mengesha, W. T. Lerebo, A. Kidanemariam, G. Gebrezgiabher, and Y. Berhane, "Pre-term and post-term births: Predictors and implications on neonatal mortality in Northern Ethiopia," *BMC Nursing*, vol. 15, no. 1, article 48, 2016.

[21] D. J. Gallacher, K. Hart, and S. Kotecha, "Common respiratory conditions of the newborn," *Breathe*, vol. 12, no. 1, pp. 30–42, 2016.

[22] J. E. Lawn, S. Cousens, and J. Zupan, "4 Million neonatal deaths: when? Where? Why?" *The Lancet*, vol. 365, no. 9462, pp. 891–900, 2005.

[23] J. Welbeck, R. Biritwum, and G. Mensah, "Factors affecting the survival of the "at risk" newborn at Korle Bu Teaching Hospital, Accra, Ghana," *West African Journal of Medicine*, vol. 22, no. 1, 2003, https://www.ajol.info/index.php/wajm/article/viewFile/27981/21788.

[24] M. Khashu, M. Narayanan, S. Bhargava, and H. Osiovich, "Perinatal outcomes associated with preterm birth at 33 to 36 weeks' gestation: a population-based cohort study," *Pediatrics*, vol. 123, no. 1, pp. 109–113, 2009.

[25] K. Bromen and K. Jöckel, "Change in male proportion among newborn infants," *The Lancet*, vol. 349, no. 9054, pp. 804-805, 1997.

[26] F. Li, T. Wu, X. Lei et al., "The Apgar Score and Infant Mortality," *PLoS ONE*, vol. 8, no. 7, p. e69072, 2013.

[27] A. Tinker, K. Finn, and J. Epp, *Improving Women's Health Issues and Interventions*, Washington, DC, USA, 2000, [cited 2017 Jun 27], http://siteresources.worldbank.org/HEALTHNUTRITIONANDPOPULATION/Resources/281627-1095698140167/Tinker-ImprovingWomens-whole.pdf.

[28] Y. M. Adamu and H. M. Salihu, "Barriers to the use of antenatal and obstetric care services in rural Kano, Nigeria," *Journal of Obstetrics & Gynaecology*, vol. 22, no. 6, pp. 600–603, 2002, http://www.ncbi.nlm.nih.gov/pubmed/12554244.

[29] P. Mannava, K. Durrant, J. Fisher, M. Chersich, and S. Luchters, "Attitudes and behaviours of maternal health care providers in interactions with clients: a systematic review," *Global Health*, 2012, http://download.springer.com/static/pdf/749/art%253A10.1186%252Fs12992-015-0117-9.pdf?originUrl=http%3A%2F%2Fglobalizationandhealth.biomedcentral.com%2Farticle%2F10.1186%2Fs12992-015-0117-9&token2=exp=1496155013~acl=%2Fstatic%2Fpdf%2F749%2Fart%25253A10.1186%25252Fs-12992-015-0117-9.pdf*~hmac=d77e3e210f683c14d05998195476-264569d823c72521c3aea7446089bd576d30.

[30] Ghana Statistical Service and Ghana Health Service, "Ghana Demographic and Health Survey 2008. Ghana Statistical Service (GSS) Ghana Demographic and Health Survey," 2009.

20

Determinants of Skilled Birth Attendance in the Northern Parts of Ghana

Kwamena Sekyi Dickson[1] and Hubert Amu[2]

[1]*Department of Population and Health, College of Humanities and Legal Studies, University of Cape Coast, Cape Coast, Ghana*
[2]*Department of Population and Behavioural Sciences, School of Public Health, University of Health and Allied Sciences, Hohoe, Ghana*

Correspondence should be addressed to Kwamena Sekyi Dickson; nadicx@gmail.com

Academic Editor: Jennifer L. Freeman

Background. An integral part of the Sustainable Development Goal three is to ensure universal access to sexual and reproductive healthcare services which include skilled delivery by the year 2030. We examined the determinants of skilled delivery among women in the Northern part of Ghana. *Methods*. The paper made use of data from the Demographic and Health Survey. Women from the Northern part of Ghana were included in the analysis. Bivariate descriptive analyses coupled with binary logistic regression estimation technique were used to analyse the data. *Results*. Region of residence, age, household wealth, education, distance to a health facility, religion, parity, partner's education, and getting money for treatment were identified as the determinants of skilled delivery. While the probability of having a skilled delivery was higher in the Upper East Region, it was lower in the Northern and Upper West Regions compared to the Brong Ahafo Region. *Conclusion*. Our findings call for more attention from the Ghana Health Service and the Ministry of Health in addressing the skilled delivery gaps among women particularly in the Northern and Upper West Regions in ensuring attainment of the Sustainable Development Goal target related to reproductive health care accessibility for all by the year 2030.

1. Introduction

Access to skilled care during delivery is crucial to reducing maternal mortality [1]. This is based on the premise that, worldwide, about 830 women die every day due to complications resulting from pregnancy and childbirth [2]. Almost all of these deaths occur in low-resource settings and are preventable [2]. Out of the 830 deaths recorded, for instance, 550 occurred in sub-Saharan Africa and 180 in southern Asia, compared to five in developed countries [2]. The implication is that the risk of a woman dying due to obstetric causes during her lifetime in a developing country is about 33 times higher than for a woman living in a developed country [2]. Many studies have, for instance, indicated that more than three-fourths of maternal deaths recorded in developing countries are associated with direct obstetric causes such as haemorrhage, sepsis, abortion, hypertensive diseases of pregnancy, and ruptured uterus, and that over 77% of such deaths occur during childbirth or soon after delivery (within 24 hours) [2–4].

A major reason for the high maternal deaths in developing countries is the low utilization of skilled delivery services provided by skilled birth attendants (SBAs) for the majority of the women [5]. A skilled birth attendant is defined as "an accredited health professional – such as a midwife, doctor or nurse – who has been educated and trained to proficiency in the skills needed to manage normal (uncomplicated) pregnancies, childbirth, and the immediate postnatal period, and in the identification, management and referral of complications in women and newborns" [6].

The issue of maternal utilization of skilled delivery services is based on a conceptual framework for health-seeking behavior by Andersen and Newman [7]. The tenets of the model are predisposing, need, and enabling factors which influence the utilization of healthcare services. Predisposing factors include religion, sex, education, social networks, age, previous experience with illness, attitudes, and values [8]. Enabling factors are described as being external to the individual, but important in influencing his/her decisions concerning the use of healthcare services. They include income, availability of health facilities and personnel, waiting time at health facilities, quality and extent of social relationships, and health [9]. The need factors according to Andersen and Newman [7] refer to perceptions of the seriousness of a disease or health condition and include people's view of their own general health and functional state as well as the availability of help for care and support [7]. Existing predisposing factors according to the model combined with enabling and need factors to influence a person's utilization of healthcare facilities and services [8, 9].

Studies have shown that maternal and newborn mortalities are usually low when higher proportions of deliveries are attended by SBAs [10–12]. SBAs play significant roles in decreasing maternal mortality, as they offer timely obstetric care for life-threatening complications [13]. The low levels of utilization of skilled delivery services which lead to high rates of maternal mortality have been attributed to various factors including access to health facilities, health worker attitude towards women during delivery, cultural issues, maternal age, and parity [14, 15]. Primiparous women are, for instance, more likely to access skilled delivery while multiparous women also opt for unskilled support during delivery due to the perception of being experienced [15]. Transportation factors influencing the low utilization of skilled birth attendance also include poor road network, lack of a vehicle, and the high cost of transport [16].

In 2015, the Sustainable Development Goals (SDGs) were constituted to replace the Millennium Development Goals to which Ghana was a signatory [17, 18]. The Millennium Development Goals were eight goals which sought to propel the socioeconomic development of developing countries from 2000 to 2015 [19]. At the end of 2015, however, most of the developing countries, including Ghana, were unable to meet their MDG targets including those related to maternal health (MDG 5) [17–19]. Seventeen new SDGs were, therefore, developed to replace the MDGs. The SDG Goal three seeks to ensure healthy lives and promote well-being for all of all ages by the year 2030 [18, 20]. An integral part of this goal is to ensure universal access to sexual and reproductive healthcare services which include skilled delivery services [20]. To achieve this target, an understanding of the skilled delivery service utilization among women of all sociodemographic and economic backgrounds is imperative.

Ghana is usually categorized into a north-south divide based on the level of development and also for comparison [21–23]. The Greater Accra, Central, Volta, Western, Ashanti, and Eastern regions constitute the southern part while the Brong Ahafo, Northern, Upper East, and Upper West regions form the Northern part. Several studies have in the past found utilization of health care services including skilled delivery as being higher in the southern part of the country than in the Northern part [24–27]. In this regard, Abor et al. [28] for instance argued that geographical location is an important factor which influences the utilization of maternal health services. Also, Addai [29] in a study on the determinants of use of maternal-child health services in rural Ghana posited that living in the Central and Western regions (both located in the southern part of the country) increased the probability of consulting a physician for antenatal care services compared to living in the Northern part of the country. Addai [29] also noted that, compared to the Northern parts of Ghana, women residing in rural areas of western and central regions were two times more likely to see a physician for prenatal care compared with women in the Northern part. This is largely attributable to the adequacy and ease of access to health personnel and facilities among women living in rural areas of the southern parts of the country compared to those in the Northern part of the country [29–32]. Our study contributes to the body of knowledge available on skilled delivery by examining the determinants of skilled delivery in the Northern part of Ghana and making useful recommendations for policy and practice.

2. Materials and Methods

The study made use of data from the individual recode file of the Ghana Demographic and Health Survey (GDHS) 2014. Ghana Demographic and Health Survey is a nationwide survey which covers all the ten regions in Ghana and is designed and conducted every five years. The GDHS focuses on child and maternal health and is designed to provide adequate data to monitor the population and health situation in Ghana. GDHS gathers information on antenatal care, delivery care and postnatal care, fertility contraceptive use, child health, family planning, and much more.

The survey was carried out by the Ghana Statistical Service and the Ghana Health Service with technical support from ICF International through the MEASURE DHS program. In the 2014 version 9,396 women between the ages 15 and 49 from 12,831 households covering 427 clusters throughout Ghana were interviewed. It had a response rate of 97% [33]. For the purpose of this study, only women from the Northern part of Ghana who gave birth within five years prior to the survey were considered; sample of 1786 women was used. Permission to use the data set was given to us by MEASURE DHS following the assessment of a concept note. The dataset is available to the public (https://dhsprogram.com/).

Ten explanatory variables were used. These comprised maternal age, education, distance to health facility, ethnicity, parity (birth order), partner's education, getting money for treatment, religion, marital status, and household wealth. Maternal age was categorized into 15–19, 20–24, 25–29, 20–34, 35–39, 40–44, and 45–49. Education was classified into four categories: no education, primary education, secondary education, and higher education. Marital status was recoded as single (never married, widowed, and divorced), married, and cohabitating (living together). Distance to a health facility was coded as a big problem and not a big problem. Household wealth was created from wealth status in DHS dataset, which is an accumulation using factor analysis of various household belongings including agricultural land, car, refrigerator, materials used in constructing housing, bicycle, television, type of household cooking fuel, and radio [33]. Household wealth status was categorized as poorest, poorer, middle, richer, and richest. Parity (birth order) was categorized as zero birth, one birth, two births, three births, and four births or more. Partner's education was classified into four categories: no education, primary education, secondary education, and higher education. Getting money for treatment was captured as big problem and not a big problem.

3. Analysis

Since our interest was to examine the probability of utilizing skilled delivery services, the outcome variable employed for this study was assisted skilled delivery. This was derived from the question "who assisted with the delivery?" Responses of those who received assistance from a doctor, nurse/midwife, and community health officer/nurse were captioned as assisted skilled delivery. The outcome variable was coded as 1 = "Yes" and 0 = "No" since it was a dichotomous variable. A logit model was employed to show how the explanatory variables correlated with the outcome variable. Specifically, the binary logistic regression was employed since it allows the predictions of a mixture of continuous and categorical variables. Binary logistic regression is based on the assumption that the dependent variable should be a dichotomous variable and the data should not contain outliers. The formulae behind the binary logistic regression are given as follows.

Let Y be a dichotomous variable which is defined as

$$Y = \frac{1 \text{ for users of skilled birth attendants}}{0 \text{ for non-users of skilled birth attendants}},$$

$$p = \Pr\left(Y = 1 \mid X_1, \ldots, X_k\right),$$

$$p = \frac{1}{1 + \exp\left[-\left(\beta_0 + \beta_1 X_1 + \beta_2 X_2 + \cdots + \beta_k X_k\right)\right]}, \quad (1)$$

$$\widehat{p} = \frac{1}{1 + \exp\left[-\left(\widehat{\beta}_0 + \widehat{\beta}_1 X_1 + \widehat{\beta}_2 X_2 + \cdots + \widehat{\beta}_k X_k\right)\right]}.$$

Note. With no predictors, $\widehat{p} = \sum_{i=1}^{n} Y_i/n = \overline{Y}$.

The model was employed to show how the explanatory variables correlated with the outcome variable. Two models were used for the binary logistic regression. Model 1 was a bivariate analysis of each explanatory variable with the outcome variable, to check the effects of the individual explanatory variables on the outcome variable. Model 2 was a multivariate analysis of all the explanatory variables with the outcome variables.

Survey weights, which are typical of nationally representative studies, were factored into both inferential and descriptive analyses conducted. The weights helped to offset the challenges of under- and oversampling usually associated with national surveys. All analyses were conducted with STATA, version 13. The level of significance used in the study was at 95% or <0.05.

4. Results

Table 1 presents the utilization of skilled birth attendants based on sociodemographic characteristics. Nine of the explanatory variables showed significant associations with

the dependent variable: age, household wealth, education, region, distance to a health facility, religion, parity, partner's education, and getting money for treatment. It was observed that women aged 25–29 years had the highest proportion of skilled delivery (25%). Utilization of skilled delivery at birth declined with increasing household wealth.

Women with no formal education had the highest proportion of skilled delivery (59.8%) while those with the highest form of education had the least (1.8%). Regarding region, women from the Northern Region had the highest proportion of skilled deliveries (43.6%) compared to women from the Upper West Region, who had the least (10%). The Brong Ahafo and Upper East Regions also had proportions of 30.4% and 16%, respectively. Women who did not consider distance to a health facility as a big problem had a higher proportion of skilled deliveries (63.1%) compared to those who consider it a big problem (36.9%). Christian women (49.5%), women with four or more births (50.3%), those whose partners had no education (53%), those who considered getting money for treatment as a big problem (50.8%), and married women (78.3%) had the highest proportion of skilled deliveries in terms of religion, parity, partner's education, getting money for treatment, and marital status, respectively.

Table 2 presents results of the logistic regression analyses conducted for skilled delivery and the explanatory variables. For region, model 1 shows that the odds of accessing skilled delivery were higher for women in the Upper East Region (OR = 1.74, 95% CI = 1.08–2.21), while it was lower for those in the Northern (OR = 0.20, 95% CI = 0.15–0.26) and Upper West regions (OR = 0.56, 95% CI = 0.41–0.77) compared with women in the Brong Ahafo Region. We, however, observed that when the other variables were added, the odds of accessing skilled delivery increased for all three regions. This time, however, women in the Upper West Region were more likely to access skilled delivery (AOR = 1.35, 95% CI = 0.91–2.01) compared with women in the Brong Ahafo Region.

Regarding household wealth, we realized in the bivariate analysis that women in the richer wealth quintile were 34.79 times more likely to utilize skilled delivery services than those in the poorest wealth quintile. This probability, however, declined when the other variables were added in model 2 (AOR = 7.70, 95% CI = 2.62–22.66). Women with primary and secondary education were more likely to utilize skilled delivery services than those with no formal education. In both models, however, women with primary and secondary education were more likely to utilize skilled delivery services than those with no education.

In both models, we observed that women in all the other age cohorts (ranging from 20 to 49), were less likely to utilize skilled delivery services compared to those aged 15–19 years. A similar finding was made regarding parity, where, in both models, women with two births, three births, and four or more births were all less likely than those with one birth to utilize skilled delivery services. While the relationship between parity and the dependent variable was found to be significant at $P < 0.01$ and $P < 0.001$ in the first model, it became insignificant upon addition of the other explanatory variables in the second model.

TABLE 1: Background characteristics.

Variable	Correlates	$n = 1786$	Percentage	P value
Age	15–19	40	2.2	<0.001
	20–24	294	16.5	
	25–29	446	25.0	
	30–34	393	22.0	
	35–39	343	19.2	
	40–44	188	10.5	
	45–49	82	4.6	
Household wealth	Poorest	1043	58.4	<0.001
	Poorer	341	19.1	
	Middle	204	11.4	
	Richer	138	7.7	
	Richest	60	3.4	
Education	No education	1067	59.8	<0.001
	Primary	288	16.1	
	Secondary	399	22.3	
	Higher	32	1.8	
Region	Brong Ahafo	543	30.4	<0.001
	Northern	778	43.6	
	Upper East	286	16.0	
	Upper West	180	10.0	
Distance to health facility	Big problem	659	36.9	<0.001
	Not a big problem	1127	63.1	
Religion	Christianity	883	49.5	<0.001
	Islam	680	38.1	
	Traditional/spiritual	143	8.0	
	No region	80	4.4	
Parity	One birth	255	14.3	<0.001
	Two births	318	17.8	
	Three births	314	17.6	
	Four births or more	899	50.3	
Partner's education	No education	947	53.0	<0.001
	Primary	206	11.5	
	Secondary	523	29.3	
	Higher	110	6.2	
Getting money for treatment	Big problem	906	50.8	<0.001
	Not a big problem	880	49.2	
Marital status	Single	95	5.4	0.63
	Married	1399	78.3	
	Cohabiting	292	16.3	

In model 1, we observed that the probability of women utilizing skilled birth delivery increased with the level of education of their partners: primary (OR = 2.97, 95% CI = 2.15–4.12), secondary (OR = 4.62, 95% CI = 3.55–6.01), and higher (OR = 11.50, 95% CI = 5.95–22.21). Even though a similar pattern was realized in model 2, we observed that both the level of significance and probability declined due to addition of the other explanatory variables: primary (AOR = 1.52, 95% CI = 1.04–2.22), secondary (AOR = 1.62, 95% CI = 0.39–1.09), and higher (AOR = 1.65, 95% CI = 0.41–1.21). Women who lived in rural residences were less likely to utilize skilled delivery services as observed in both models 1 (OR = 0.19, 95% CI = 0.14–0.25) and 2 (AOR = 0.46, 95% CI = 0.31–0.67) (Table 2).

5. Discussion

We found that the probability of having a skilled delivery was higher in the Upper East Region than in the Brong Ahafo Region. The reverse, however, occurred where women in the Northern and Upper West Regions were less likely to access skilled assistance. This reflects the variations which exist

TABLE 2: Binary logistic regression on skilled delivery among women in the Northern part of Ghana.

Explanatory variable	Model 1 OR	95% confidence interval	Model 2 AOR	95% confidence interval
Region				
Brong Ahafo	Ref	Ref	Ref	Ref
Northern	0.20***	0.15–0.26	0.48***	0.33–0.69
Upper East	1.30*	1.08–2.21	3.02***	1.96–4.66
Upper West	0.56***	0.41–0.77	1.35	0.91–2.01
Household wealth				
Poorest	Ref	Ref	Ref	Ref
Poorer	2.11***	1.61–2.77	1.38	0.99–1.92
Middle	5.71***	3.74–8.72	2.11**	1.25–3.60
Richer	34.79***	12.8–94.56	7.70***	2.62–22.66
Richest	1	1	1	1
Education				
No education	Ref	Ref	Ref	Ref
Primary	3.71***	2.75–5.01	1.75**	1.22–2.50
Secondary	6.27***	4.59–8.57	1.79**	1.20–2.66
Higher	1	1	1	1
Age				
15–19	Ref	Ref	Ref	Ref
20–24	0.54	0.23–1.28	0.67	0.25–1.82
25–29	0.45	0.20–1.05	0.59	0.21–1.61
30–34	0.42*	0.18–0.97	0.59	0.21–1.68
35–39	0.38*	0.16–0.89	0.58	0.20–1.69
40–44	0.38*	0.15–0.91	0.68	0.23–2.04
45–49	0.20**	0.08–0.51	0.46	0.15–1.48
Parity				
One birth	Ref	Ref	Ref	Ref
Two births	0.59**	0.40–0.87	0.65	0.40–1.07
Three births	0.52**	0.35–0.76	0.65	0.39–1.09
Four births or more	0.31***	0.22–0.44	0.70	0.41–1.21
Partners education				
No education	Ref	Ref	Ref	Ref
Primary	2.97***	2.15–4.12	1.52*	1.04–2.22
Secondary	4.62***	3.55–6.01	1.62**	0.39–1.09
Higher	11.50***	5.95–22.21	1.65	0.41–1.21
Distance to health facility				
Not a big problem	Ref	Ref	Ref	Ref
Big problem	3.20***	2.61–3.93	1.41*	1.06–1.86
Money needed for treatment				
Not a big problem	Ref	Ref	Ref	Ref
Big problem	2.72***	2.21–3.34	1.19	0.90–1.58
Religion				
Christianity	Ref	Ref	Ref	Ref
Islam	0.99	0.79–1.23	1.02	0.77–1.37
Traditional/spiritual	0.12***	0.07–0.18	0.26***	0.16–0.44
No religion	0.18***	0.11–0.30	0.37**	0.20–0.66
Residence				
Urban	Ref	Ref	Ref	Ref
Rural	0.19***	0.14–0.25	0.46***	0.31–0.67

Computed from 2014 GDHS; Ref: reference; $^*P < 0.05$ $^{**}P < 0.01$ $^{***}P < 0.001$; model 1 is a bivariate analysis of the individual explanatory variables and the outcome variable; model 2 is a multivariate analysis of all the explanatory variables and the outcome variable.

among the four regions in the Northern part of Ghana, even though various studies have lumped all four of them together and ascribed the same characteristics for them in relation to sexual and reproductive health which include utilization of skilled delivery services [24, 25]. The findings where the Northern and Upper West Regions had lower probabilities of utilizing skilled attendance compared to the Brong Ahafo Region may be due to risk perception among women in those regions as the two are known to be poorer regions compared to the latter and lack the basic health facilities [25]. Thus, because women in the two regions are aware of the nonavailability of health facilities in their areas, they do everything they can to access the services in the towns where they are located in time to avoid avoidable deaths which arise from delays in seeking health care [34].

The fact that partner's education predicted delivery even better than the women's own education level points to the significant mediating roles men play in women's health decision-making. This finding is in agreement with studies on influences of partners' characteristics on women's health previous decision-making [35–37]. The implication of this finding is that utilization of skilled delivery services may continue to be low in the Northern parts of the country if male partner involvement is not promoted in the country. This is because societal ascriptions of gender roles for men and women strongly influence access to skilled delivery care for pregnant women [38]. These ascriptions normally make male partners the heads of their respective households. As heads of households, the males mainly decide the means of healthcare accessibility including where the women should seek care [39]. Male partner involvement refers to "the various ways in which men relate to reproductive health problems and programmes, reproductive rights, and reproductive behavior" [40]. Male partner involvement in maternal health care also refers to the direct assistance provided by men to improve their partners' and children's health through the perinatal, antenatal, labor, and delivery period [41].

We also observed that household wealth predicted utilization of skilled delivery. This gives an indication of conceivable significant differences among the respective groupings of the variables. The fact that women who lived in rural residences were less likely to utilize skilled delivery services than urban women is probably due to the fact that the plethora of health facilities are disproportionately located in urban centers. This makes it easier for urban women to utilize such services compared to women who live in rural areas and are largely deprived of such facilities and their accompanied skilled delivery services/skilled birth attendants. This points to various studies which have shown very wide disparities between rural and urban areas with rural areas being the disadvantaged [2, 42].

The fact that most of the background characteristics were found to have predicted utilization of skilled delivery among the women surveyed points to the relevance of Andersen and Newman's [7] proposition that predisposing factors such as age, religion, education, social networks, previous experience with illness, attitudes, and values are significant in informing people's decisions to utilize health care services and facilities.

Despite the important findings made in our study, the limitations inherent in the data and methods used are worth mentioning. Due to the fact that we relied on data which was collected cross-sectionally, we were unable to account for unobserved heterogeneity. Also, the relationships we established between the explanatory and dependent variables may vary over time.

6. Conclusion

Our findings which point to the low probability of skilled delivery services utilization among women in the Northern and Upper West Regions call for more attention from the Ghana Health Service, Ministry of Health, and Nongovernmental Organisations (NGOs) involved in maternal and reproductive health issues in addressing the gaps related to the utilization of skilled delivery services among women in those regions. Specifically, efforts should be made to improve the level of education of women on the need for skilled delivery, convince male partners to encourage their spouses to utilize skilled delivery services, and cite more health posts and skilled birth attendants (particularly midwives) in rural areas found in these regions. Ghana's Community-Based Health Planning and Services (CHPS) program which was established in the year 2000 to improve access and quality of healthcare including skilled delivery services throughout the country should also be strengthened in the affected regions. These efforts when implemented would contribute immensely to ensuring the attainment of the Sustainable Development Goal target which requires the country to reduce the maternal mortality ratio to less than 70 maternal deaths per 100,000 live births by the year 2030.

Authors' Contributions

Kwamena Sekyi Dickson and Hubert Amu conceived the study. Hubert Amu reviewed the relevant literature. Kwamena Sekyi Dickson designed and performed the analysis and methods section. Hubert Amu drafted the manuscript. Both authors proof-read the final manuscript and approved it.

Acknowledgments

The authors acknowledge MEASURE DHS for granting access to using the DHS data for their analysis.

References

[1] R. K. Esena and M. M. Sappor, "Factors Associated with the utilization of skilled delivery services in the Ga East Municipality of Ghana Part 2: barriers to skilled delivery," *International Journal of Scientific and Technology Research*, vol. 2, no. 8, pp. 195–207, 2013.

[2] World Health Organisation, *Global health observatory data: maternal mortality*, 2015, http://www.who.int/gho/maternal_health/mortality/maternal_mortality_text/en/.

[3] Family Care International, "Testing approaches for increasing skilled care during childbirth: the skilled care initiative," Family Care International, New York, NY, USA, 2007.

[4] United Nations Population Fund (UNFPA), *Trends in maternal health in Ethiopia: challenges in achieving the MDG for maternal mortality*, United Nations Population Fund, Addis Ababa, Ethiopia, 2012.

[5] B. Choulagai, S. Onta, N. Subedi et al., "Barriers to using skilled birth attendants' services in mid- and far-western Nepal: a cross-sectional study," *BMC International Health and Human Rights*, vol. 13, article 49, 2013.

[6] World Health Organization, *Skilled birth attendants, factsheet*, World Health Organization, Geneva, Switzerland, 2008.

[7] R. Andersen and J. F. Newman, "Societal and individual determinants of medical care utilization in the United States," *Milbank Memorial Fund Quarterly. Health & Society*, vol. 51, no. 1, pp. 95–124, 1973.

[8] R. M. Andersen, "Revisiting the behavioral model and access to medical care: does it matter?" *Journal of Health and Social Behavior*, vol. 36, no. 1, pp. 1–10, 1995.

[9] R. Andersen and J. F. Newman, "Societal and individual determinants of medical care utilization in the United States," *The Milbank Quarterly*, vol. 83, no. 4, pp. 1–28, 2005.

[10] A. S. Teferra, F. M. Alemu, and S. M. Woldeyohannes, "Institutional delivery service utilization and associated factors among mothers who gave birth in the last 12 months in Sekela District, North West of Ethiopia: a community—based cross sectional study," *BMC Pregnancy and Childbirth*, vol. 12, article 74, 2012.

[11] M. Abera, A. Gebremariam, and T. Belachew, "Predictors of safe delivery service utilization in Arsi Zone, South-East Ethiopia," *Ethiopian Journal of Health Sciences*, vol. 21, no. 1, pp. 95–106, 2011.

[12] E. Lule, G. N. V. Ramana, N. Ooman, J. Epp, D. Huntington, and J. E. Rosen, *Achieving the millennium development goal of improving maternal health: determinants, interventions, and challenges*, World Bank, Washington, DC, USA, 2005.

[13] S. Onta, B. Choulagai, B. Shrestha, N. Subedi, G. P. Bhandari, and A. Krettek, "Perceptions of users and providers on barriers to utilizing skilled birth care in mid- and far-western Nepal: a qualitative study," *Global Health Action*, vol. 7, article 24580, 2014.

[14] H. V. Doctor, "Intergenerational differences in antenatal care and supervised deliveries in Nigeria," *Health & Place*, vol. 17, no. 2, pp. 480–489, 2011.

[15] M. Amoakoh-Coleman, E. K. Ansah, I. A. Agyepong, D. E. Grobbee, G. A. Kayode, and K. Klipstein-Grobusch, "Predictors of skilled attendance at delivery among antenatal clinic attendants in Ghana: a cross-sectional study of population data," *BMJ Open*, vol. 5, no. 5, Article ID e007810, 2015.

[16] P. M. Lerberg, J. Sundby, A. Jammeh, and A. Fretheim, "Barriers to skilled birth attendance: a survey among mothers in rural Gambia.," *African Journal of Reproductive Health*, vol. 18, no. 1, pp. 35–43, 2014.

[17] Council for International Development (CID), *Sustainable Development Goals: Changing the world in 17 steps – interactive*, 2015, http://www.cid.org.nz/news/sustainable-development-goals-changing-the-world-in-17-steps-interactive/.

[18] H. Amu and S. H. Nyarko, "Preparedness of health care professionals in preventing maternal mortality at a public health facility in Ghana: a qualitative study," *BMC Health Services Research*, vol. 16, article 252, 2016.

[19] United Nations, *The Millennium development goals report*, United Nations, New York, NY, USA, 2015, http://www.un.org/millenniumgoals/2015_MDG_Report/pdf/MDG%202015%20rev%20(July%201).pdf.

[20] The Guardian, "Sustainable development goals: changing the world in 17 steps – interactive," 2015, http://www.theguardian.com/global-development/ng-interactive/2015/jan/19/sustainable-development-goals-changing-world-17-steps-interactive.

[21] S. K. Mort, "Unveiling the Secrets of the North-South Development Gap of Ghana," 2009, http://www.ghanaweb.com/GhanaHomePage/features/Unveiling-the-Secrets-of-the-North-South-Development-Gap-of-Ghana-161705.

[22] D. Fusheini, G. Marnoch, and A. M Gray, "The implementation of the National Health Insurance Programme in Ghanaan institutional approach," in *Proceedings of the The implementation of the National Health Insurance Programme in Ghanaan institutional approach*, pp. 3–5, 2012.

[23] R. K. Alhassan, E. Nketiah-Amponsah, and D. K. Arhinful, "A review of the national health insurance scheme in Ghana: What are the sustainability threats and prospects?" *PLoS ONE*, vol. 11, no. 11, Article ID e0165151, 2016.

[24] B. O. P. Asamoah, A. Agardh, and E. K. Cromley, "Spatial analysis of skilled birth attendant utilization in Ghana," *Global Journal of Health Science*, vol. 6, no. 4, pp. 117–127, 2014.

[25] S. K. Annim, S. Mariwah, and J. Sebu, "Spatial inequality and household poverty in Ghana," *Economic Systems*, vol. 36, no. 4, pp. 487–505, 2012.

[26] D. K. Ofosu, *Assessing the spatial distribution of health facilities in the Eastern Region of Ghana*, Kwame Nkrumah University of Science and Technology, Kumasi, Ghana, 2012.

[27] J. Heyen-Perschon, *Report on current situation in the health sector of Ghana and possible roles for appropriate transport technology and transport related communication interventions*, Institute for Transportation and Development Policy, New York, NY, USA, 2005.

[28] P. A. Abor, G. Abekah-Nkrumah, K. Sakyi, C. K. D. Adjasi, and J. Abor, "The socio-economic determinants of maternal health care utilization in Ghana," *International Journal of Social Economics*, vol. 38, no. 7, pp. 628–648, 2011.

[29] I. Addai, "Determinants of use of maternal-child health services in rural Ghana," *Journal of Biosocial Science*, vol. 32, no. 1, pp. 1–15, 2000.

[30] I. Addai, "Demographic and sociocultural factors influencing use of maternal health services in Ghana.," *African Journal of Reproductive Health*, vol. 2, no. 1, pp. 73–80, 1998.

[31] D. Buor, "Determinants of utilisation of health services by women in rural and urban areas in Ghana," *GeoJournal*, vol. 61, no. 1, pp. 89–102, 2004.

[32] G. B. Fosu, "Childhood morbidity and health services utilization: Cross-national comparisons of user-related factors from DHS data," *Social Science & Medicine*, vol. 38, no. 9, pp. 1209–1220, 1994.

[33] "Ghana Statistical Service (GSS), Ghana Health Service (GHS), ICF International, Ghana demographic and health survey 2014, Maryland, United States, 2015".

[34] S. Thaddeus and D. Maine, "Too far to walk: Maternal mortality in context," *Social Science & Medicine*, vol. 38, no. 8, pp. 1091–1110, 1994.

[35] K. S. Dickson, E. K. M. Darteh, and A. Kumi-Kyereme, "Providers of antenatal care services in Ghana: Evidence from Ghana demographic and health surveys 1988-2014," *BMC Health Services Research*, vol. 17, no. 203, pp. 1–9, 2017.

[36] A. Kumi-Kyereme and J. Amo-Adjei, "Effects of spatial location and household wealth on health insurance subscription among women in Ghana," *BMC Health Services Research*, vol. 13, no. 221, 2013.

[37] L. A. Rempel and J. K. Rempel, "Partner influence on health behavior decision-making: Increasing breastfeeding duration," *Journal of Social and Personal Relationships*, vol. 21, no. 1, pp. 92–111, 2004.

[38] T. Ensor and S. Cooper, "Overcoming barriers to health service access: Influencing the demand side," *Health Policy and Planning*, vol. 19, no. 2, pp. 69–79, 2004.

[39] H. Amu and K. S. Dickson, "Health insurance subscription among women in reproductive age in Ghana: do socio-demographics matter?" *Health Economics Review (HER)*, vol. 6, article 24, 2016.

[40] A. Kumar, "Role of males in reproductive and sexual health decisions," *The Bihar Times*, 2007, http://www.bihartimes.com/articles/anant/roleofmales.htm.

[41] F. Ampt, M. M. Mon, K. K. Than et al., "Correlates of male involvement in maternal and newborn health: a cross-sectional study of men in a peri-urban region of Myanmar," *BMC Pregnancy and Childbirth*, vol. 15, p. 122, 2015.

[42] M. Alemayehu and W. Mekonnen, "The prevalence of skilled birth attendant utilization and its correlates in North West Ethiopia," *BioMed Research International*, vol. 2015, Article ID 436938, 8 pages, 2015.

21

Comparison of General Practice and Pharmaceutical Dispensing Data for Pharmacoepidemiological Research: Assessing the Risk of Urinary-Tract Infections with Sodium Glucose Cotransporter 2 Inhibitors for Diabetes

Svetla Gadzhanova (ID) **and Elizabeth Roughead**

Quality Use of Medicines and Pharmacy Research Centre, University of South Australia, Australia

Correspondence should be addressed to Svetla Gadzhanova; svetla.gadzhanova@unisa.edu.au

Academic Editor: Jennifer L. Freeman

Background. This study compared results of a study undertaken using Australia's general practice electronic health record database, MedicineInsight, to assess risk of urinary-tract infections with sodium glucose cotransporter 2 inhibitors (SGLT2) for diabetes, by undertaking the same study in a 10% random sample of data from the national Pharmaceutical Benefits Scheme data. *Methods.* Cohort studies were undertaken using deidentified data from the two national datasets. In each dataset, initiators of SGLT2 inhibitors were compared to initiators of dipeptidyl peptidase 4 (DPP-4) inhibitors in the period Jan 2012 to Sep 2015. The risk of urinary-tract infections (UTI) was assessed in six-month follow-up after initiation of SGLT2 and DPP-4. *Results.* There were 1,977 people in the SGLT2 and 1,964 people in the DPP-4 cohort (MedicineInsight data) and 3,120 in the SGLT2 and 12,359 in the DPP-4 cohort (10% PBS data). In both datasets, the risk of UTI after initiation of SGLT2 was not significantly increased in comparison to DPP-4 cohort (MedicineInsight: 3.6% versus 4.9%; aHR=0.90, 95% CI 0.66-1.24; PBS: 3.0% versus 3.9%; aHR=0.90, 95% CI 0.72-1.13, 10%). *Conclusions.* Comparison of MedicineInsight data to PBS national pharmacy data demonstrated highly comparable results for the specific study question. MedicineInsight is a reliable source of data that can be used for pharmacoepidemiological studies.

1. Introduction

In 2011, the Australian Government Department of Health funded NPS MedicineWise "to establish and manage a longitudinal general practice data platform to improve the post-marketing surveillance of medicine use in Australia and support quality improvement activities in general practices" [1].

NPS MedicineWise began to introduce a database (MedicineInsight) from 2013 onwards, with the aim of establishing a database comprising electronic health records for postmarketing surveillance of medicines and devices. Longitudinal deidentified patient data are regularly extracted from the medical record software of 500 general practices across Australia. Over 3000 general practitioners (which is 10% of all GPs in Australia [2]) participate in the program,

with data representing more than 4.8 million patients [3, 4] which is 20% of the total population in Australia in 2015 [5]. MedicineInsight data provides information on prescribed medicines, pathology results and clinical observation, and diagnosis/reason for the GP visit. For all prescribed medicine, the prescribing date, type, dose, strength, quantity, and number of repeats are recorded as well as reason for prescribing. This has the potential to be a significant advance of existing Australian datasets for pharmacoepidemiological studies and health service research as the data include clinical information.

The existing datasets in Australia were administrative health claims data, namely, the Medicare Benefits Schedule data, which is a national claims dataset for medical practitioner attendances (with no reason for encounter) and diagnostic and pathology services provided (with no clinical data), and the Pharmaceutical Benefits Scheme (PBS) data, which includes records of all subsidised medicines under the national scheme for treatment of most health conditions of all Australian residents. PBS data are collected from community pharmacies, private hospitals, and most public hospitals. Patient information includes gender, age, beneficiary status (general or concessional), and geographic location. Prescription information include date of supply, drug code, therapeutic class, generic name, form, quantity dispensed, and number of prescription repeats. Since the middle of 2012, PBS data represents full capture of dispensing records for both general and concessional beneficiaries. One advantage of the PBS dataset over the MedicineInsight dataset is the frequency of records for prescription medicines. In Australia, the majority of medicines for chronic conditions are supplied in quantities of one month's supply with pharmacists allowed to refill the prescription another five times, providing six month's supply in total with a record in the dataset approximately every month. By comparison MedicineInsight data has the record of the original prescription; thus, unless changes to medicines are made, one record appears approximately every six months. Another difference between the two datasets is that the Pharmaceutical Benefits Scheme data include all 24 million persons in Australia, while MedicineInsight data involve a sample of patients based on GP practices volunteering to participate.

Given that MedicineInsight data contains health records, it has the potential to be used for health outcome studies and other advanced pharmacoepidemiological research in Australia. The data for the database is sourced from voluntary participation of general practices. While the number of practices participating is large, resulting in a large number of patients, whether the data gives consistent results with other Australian datasets is unknown. For this reason, we chose to triangulate the results from a study using the MedicineInsight database with the results using the same study design but using the national PBS dataset. We chose to use the national PBS dataset for comparison as it represents complete capture of medicines information for all Australians (24 million persons), as all Australians are provided with medicines via the national Pharmaceutical Benefits Scheme. It would be advantageous to determine the comparative performance of the MedicineInsight and PBS datasets because they are complementary with regard to their data collection on medicine utilisation, yet their source data are substantially different. Thus, consistent findings from both datasets gives more support to observational research findings. In this research, we aimed to compare the results of a study undertaken using Australia's general practice electronic health record database, MedicineInsight, to assess risk of urinary-tract infections with sodium glucose cotransporter 2 inhibitors for diabetes [6] by undertaking the same study in a 10% random sample of data from the national Pharmaceutical Benefits Scheme data. This example was chosen, as one of the main purposes of establishing the MedicineInsight data collection was to improve the postmarketing surveillance of medicines in Australia. The SGLT 2 inhibitors were subject to a risk management plan to monitor safety, including the incidence of urinary infections, when they were approved for

marketing in Australia by the Australian Therapeutic Goods Administration.

2. Materials and Methods

2.1. Study Populations. Retrospective longitudinal studies were conducted utilising the two national datasets. In both datasets all patients with a SGLT2 inhibitor initiation between 1 Jan 2013 and 1 Sep 2015 were identified. A new user design was used which included all patients with prior history in the 12 months prior to the first prescription of an SGLT2 or DPP-4. Initiation was defined as no record of any SGLT2 or DPP-4 medicine in the previous 12 months. For MedicineInsight data prior history was defined as having at least one visit to the GP in the 12 months prior to medicine initiation, while for the PBS data it was defined as having at least one dispensing for any medicine. All people who initiated dipeptidyl peptidase 4 (DPP-4) inhibitor in the same period were included as a comparison cohort. The date of initiation of either SGLT2 or DPP-4 inhibitors was considered as index date. People who were initiated on both products within 18 months were excluded to avoid overlap of pre- and post-periods.

2.2. Medicines Included in the Analysis. There are three SGLT2 inhibitors available in Australia. The Anatomical Therapeutic Chemical (ATC) code [2] was used to identify them. Dapagliflozin is available as 10 mg only (ATC code: A10BX09); Empagliflozin is available as 10 mg and 25 mg (ATC code A10BX12); and Canagliflozin is available as 100 mg or 300 mg (ATC code A10BX11).

Saxagliptin, sitagliptin, linagliptin vildagliptin, alogliptin, and linagliptin (either as a single agent product or a combination product) are the dipeptidyl peptidase 4 inhibitors available in Australia. They were selected by ATC code A10BH and A10BD07- A10BD11.

2.3. Statistical Analysis. We utilised both MedicineInsight and the 10% PBS dataset to investigate the strength of the SGLT2 inhibitor at initiation and the use of other diabetes medicines in the year prior to index SGLT2 as well as the use of potentially interacting medicines. Angiotensin Converting Enzyme (ACE) inhibitors, Angiotensin II receptor blockers (ARB), nonsteroidal anti-inflammatory drugs (NSAIDs), and loop diuretics may potentially interact with the SGLT2 inhibitors and their use was analysed [6]. Concurrent use of interacting medicines was defined as a record of a prescription in the three months prior to or the six-month period after initiation of the SGLT2 or DPP 4 inhibitors. This period of time was chosen as PBS prescriptions are for one-month supply and allow for up to five repeats; thus a six-month period is the minimum period required to see a record in the prescribing dataset.

The risk of urinary-tract infections (UTIs) was the main outcome measure of interest. It was assessed for the 6 months after SGLT2 and DPP-4 initiation. For MedicineInsight data we investigated prescribing of UTI specific medicines (trimethoprim, nitrofurantoin, norfloxacin) as well as reasons for the visit to the GP and recorded diagnosis/condition

TABLE 1: Cohorts' demographics.

	MedicineInsight data			10% PBS data		
	SGLT2 (N=1977)	DPP-4 (N=1964)	p-value	SGLT2 (N=3120)	DPP-4 (N=12359)	p-value
Mean age	59.8 (SD=11.4)	60.6 (SD=12.5)	0.027 [a]	60.2 (SD=11.0)	62.9 (SD=13.4)	<0.0001 [a]
Gender						
Females	887 (45%)	800 (41%)	0.009 [b]	1333 (43%)	5333 (43%)	0.667 [b]
Males	1090 (55%)	1164 (59%)		1787 (57%)	7026 (57%)	
Comorbidity (prior 12 months)						
No comorbidity	148 (8%)	300 (15%)		279 (9%)	719 (6%)	
One or two	564 (28%)	659 (34%)	<0.0001 [b]	1016 (33%)	4285 (35%)	<0.0001 [b]
Three or more	1265 (64%)	1005 (51%)		1825 (58%)	7355 (59%)	
Prior UTIs (prior 6 months)	67 (3.4%)	82 (4.2%)	0.196 [b]	78 (2.5%)	441 (3.5%)	0.003 [b]

[a] Student's t-test; [b] Chi-square test.

Note: Prior UTIs were identified only by medicines specific for UTIs (trimethoprim, nitrofurantoin, norfloxacin) in the 10% PBS data, while in the MedicineInsight data we accounted for UTI medicines (74% of all cases) and diagnosis/reasons for encounters (26% of all cases).

using definite terms to identify urinary-tract infections. For PBS data we investigated only dispensing of UTI specific medicines (trimethoprim, nitrofurantoin, norfloxacin) as no diagnostic or encounter information was available. Furthermore, we performed sensitivity analysis and assessed the risk of UTIs in subjects who were only prescribed the three medicines specific for UTI in MedicineInsight data (i.e., excluding UTIs identified from clinical information).

Demographic characteristics of the cohorts from the two datasets were compared, including mean age, gender, number of comorbidities, and percent of prior infections. Comorbidities were determined based on prescription history using the Rx-Risk-V Comorbidity index [7]. Proportions were compared by chi-square tests and means were compared by Student's t-test.

Median time from initiation of SGLT2 or DPP-4 to first UTI in the follow-up period was determined using Kaplan Meier method. People were censored for death and end of study in the MedicineInsight data and only for end of study in the 10% PBS data as date of death is unavailable in the PBS dataset. Cox proportional hazards models were used to determine hazard ratios. The models were adjusted for gender, age, comorbidity, and prior UTI infections. All data analyses were performed using SAS software (version V9.4, SAS Institute Inc. Cary, North Caroline, USA).

The study was approved by the NPS MedicineInsight Data Governance Committee and the Australian Government Department of Human Services External Requests Evaluation Committee.

3. Results

There were 1,977 people initiated on SGLT2 inhibitors in the MedicineInsight data and 3,120 in the PBS data. There were 1,964 patients initiated on DPP-4 in MedicineInsight data and 12,359 in the PBS data. Demographics of the cohorts are presented in Table 1. In both datasets, the SGLT2 cohort

was younger and had more comorbidities than the DPP-4 cohort. The rates of prior UTI were slightly higher in MedicineInsight data but that could be due to the availability of diagnostic/encounter information in addition to prescribing information which accounted for one-quarter of the identified prior UTIs.

In both datasets, dapagliflozin accounted for the majority of SGLT2 initiation (Table 2). However, canagliflozin was initiated in higher proportion of people in PBS data (9% versus 3% in MedicineInsight, chi-square p<0.0001). The SGLT2 inhibitors strength use was similar in the two datasets. Vast proportion of SGLT2 initiators had prior diabetes therapy (90% in MedicineInsight and 80% in PBS), and similar proportions were coprescribed potentially interacting medicines (Table 2).

Post-UTIs were identified only by medicines specific for UTIs (trimethoprim, nitrofurantoin, norfloxacin) in the 10% PBS data, while in the MedicineInsight data we accounted for UTI medicines (74% of all cases) and diagnosis/reasons for encounters (26% of all cases). The frequency of urinary-tract infections after SGLT2 initiation was low: majority of people who had a UTI had just one occurrence in the 6 months after SGLT2 initiation happening in the first 12 weeks (Table 3).

In both datasets, the risk of UTIs was not increased in the SGLT2 initiators compared to DPP-4 initiators (Table 4):

(i) for MedicineInsight data: 3.6% versus 4.9%, adjusted hazard ratio (aHR)=0.90, 95% CI 0.66-1.24;

(ii) for 10% PBS data: 3.0% versus 3.9%, aHR=0.90, 95% CI 0.72-1.13.

Sensitivity analysis for MedicineInsight data assessing the risk of UTIs based only on the medicines specific for UTIs resulted in aHR=1.02, 95% CI 0.77-1.65.

4. Discussion

This study is the first to our knowledge to compare MedicineInsight results against another national dataset. In

TABLE 2: Other indicators.

	MedicineInsight	10% PBS
	SGLT2 cohort (N=1977)	SGLT2 cohort (N=3120)
Type of the index medicine	Dapagliflozin – 93% Canagliflozin – 3% Empagliflozin – 4%	Dapagliflozin – 87% Canagliflozin – 9% Empagliflozin – 4%
Strength at initiation	Dapagliflozin initiators – all on 10mg (one strength) Canagliflozin initiators – 78% on 300mg (higher strength) Empagliflozin initiators – 74% on 10mg (lower strength)	Dapagliflozin initiators – all on 10mg (one strength) Canagliflozin initiators – 77% on 300mg (higher strength) Empagliflozin initiators – 72% on 10mg (lower strength)
Prior diabetes therapy (prior 12 months)	90% had documented diabetes medicine 86% had metformin and/or sulfonylurea	80% had dispensing for diabetes medicine 69% had metformin and/or sulfonylurea
Interacting medicines (3 months prior and 6 months post index)	ACE/ARB – 61% NSAIDs – 14% Frusemide – 6%	ACE/ARB – 61% NSAIDs – 14% Frusemide – 7%

TABLE 3: Frequency of UTIs in the 6 months after SGLT2 or DPP-4 initiation.

	MedicineInsight data		10% PBS data	
	SGLT2 (N=1977)	DPP-4 (N=1964)	SGLT2 (N=3120)	DPP-4 (N=12359)
Proportion with at least one UTI	3.6% (N=71) Of those: 89% had just one infection; 64% had the 1st infection in the 12 weeks post index SGLT2	4.9% (N=97) Of those: 91% had just one infection; 58% had the 1st infection in the 12 weeks post index DPP-4	3.0% (N=94) Of those: 83% had just one infection; 64% had the 1st infection in the 12 weeks post index SGLT2	3.9% (N=479) Of those: 80% had just one infection; 59% had the 1st infection in the 12 weeks post index DPP-4

Note: Post-UTIs were identified only by medicines specific for UTIs (trimethoprim, nitrofurantoin, norfloxacin) in the 10% PBS data, while in the MedicineInsight data we accounted for UTI medicines (74% of all cases) and diagnosis/reasons for encounters (26% of all cases).

Terms used to identify UTIs in diagnoses and reason for encounters in MedicineInsight data: urinary tract infection, cystitis, genitourinary tract infection, pyelonephritis, urethritis, kidney infection, prostatitis.

this study we compared results from MedicineInsight data on SGLT2 inhibitors for type 2 diabetes and risk of infections [6] with results from the 10% PBS data. We investigated the use of prior diabetes therapies and interacting medicines, as well as safety concerns related to risk of urinary-tract infections. We found very similar results across both datasets, with a very high proportion of SGLT2 initiators having prior diabetes therapy, which is consistent with subsidy requirements, almost identical proportions receiving the potentially interacting medicines, and very similar but not significant hazard ratios for the risk of UTI post SGLT2 initiation. MedicineInsight data is superior to PBS data as it provides not only information on prescribed medicines but also clinical information about reasons for encounters and diagnosis (e.g., diagnoses for UTI), as well as pathology/laboratory results (e.g., HbA1c test results) and observation data (e.g., weight). This may account for some differences in the rates of prior and post-UTIs (slightly higher in MedicineInsight than in the PBS data) as diagnosis/reasons for encounters contributed to identification of extra patients with a UTI. However, the hazard ratios for the risk of UTI after SGLT2 initiation were very similar and nonsignificant in both datasets. Sensitivity analysis for MedicineInsight data assessing the risk of UTIs based only on the three medicines specific for UTIs resulted in a similar and nonsignificant hazard ratio.

Our results are consistent with existing evidence on UTI risk associated with use of SGLT2 inhibitors. With regard to dapagliflozin, the rate of UTI was not significantly increased in 12 randomized placebo-controlled trials (4.3% versus 3.7%, p=0.48) [8]. Meta-analyses of the use of SGLT2 inhibitors in comparison with insulin for diabetes found no increased risk of urinary-tract infections [9]. An indirect comparison between SGLT2 inhibitors (added to insulin) and DPP-4 inhibitors (added to insulin) from fourteen randomized controlled trials showed no differences in the risk of UTIs between SGLT2/insulin and DPP-4/insulin (RR=1.38, 95% CI 0.87-2.19, p=0.149) [10].

TABLE 4: Risk of UTIs.

	MedicineInsight data		10% PBS data	
	Unadjusted Hazard ratio (HR), 95% CI	Adjusted Hazard ratio (aHR), 95% CI	Unadjusted Hazard ratio (HR), 95% CI	Adjusted Hazard ratio (aHR), 95% CI
SGLT2 vs DPP-4 cohort	0.88 (0.65-1.19)	0.90 (0.66-1.24)	0.75 (0.60-0.94)	0.90 (0.72-1.13)

Note: In the 10% PBS data the adjusted hazard ratio (aHR) is adjusted for prior infection, age, gender, and comorbidity; in the MedicineInsight data the adjusted hazard ratio (aHR) is adjusted for prior infection, age, gender, weight, HbA1c, location, smoking status, and comorbidity.

A strength of this study is the direct comparison of two large national datasets on a number of indicators: one representing 500 general practices, 3000 GPs, and 4.8 million patients; the other capturing prescription data of 10% (2.5 million persons) of all Australians. Limitation of both datasets is the lack of information if the prescribed medicines were actually consumed. MedicineInsight provides no linkage information for patients visiting multiple GP practices which might lead to loss of patients to follow-up. This may indicate potential underestimation of the outcome events. While MedicineInsight data provide clinical and diagnosing information allowing identification of all patients with a UTI, the PBS data do not include diagnostic or encounter information which can result in underestimation of the outcome events in the PBS population. Another limitation is that the analysis based on PBS data was not censoring for death as these data were unavailable in the PBS dataset.

Even though the risk of genital infections has been assessed in MedicineInsight data, it was not possible to be assessed in the PBS data as fungal creams and tablets are not generally subsidised on the PBS and there is no diagnostic or encounter information in the data. This confirms again that MedicineInsight data is a more complete source of medical information.

5. Conclusion

Comparison of MedicineInsight data to PBS national pharmaceutical data demonstrated highly comparable results for the specific study question. MedicineInsight is a rich dataset providing clinical and diagnostic information as well as observation and pathology data in addition to pharmaceutical claims which makes it a valuable data source for pharmacoepidemiological research.

Abbreviations

ACE: Angiotensin Converting Enzyme
ARB: Angiotensin II receptor blockers
ATC: Anatomical Therapeutic Chemical
DPP-4: Dipeptidyl peptidase 4
GP: General practitioners
NSAID: Nonsteroidal anti-inflammatory drugs
PBS: Pharmaceutical Benefits Scheme
SGLT2: Sodium glucose cotransporter 2
UTI: Urinary-tract infections.

Disclosure

The authors declare that NPS had no involvement in the study design, in the analysis and data interpretation, in the manuscript writing, and in the decision to submit for publication.

Acknowledgments

The study was part of the employment of the authors by the University of South Australia. The data for the study was provided by NPS MedicineWise.

References

[1] NPS MedicineWise, "Using MedicineInsight data," 2017. https://www.nps.org.au/medicine-insight/using-medicineinsight-data.

[2] "Drug utilisation sub-committee (DUSC)," Medicines for the treatment of diabetes, 2017, http://www.pbs.gov.au/info/industry/listing/participants/public-release-docs/2017-02/medicines-diabetes-feb-2017.

[3] "MedicineInsight: Representativeness and overview of MedicineInsight data," NPS MedicineWise, Sydney, 2016.

[4] NPS MedicineWise, "What is MedicineInsight?" 2015. http://www.nps.org.au/health-professionals/medicineinsight.

[5] "Australian Bureau of Statistics," Australian Demographic Statistics, 2015, http://www.abs.gov.au/ausstats/abs@.nsf/mf/3101.0.

[6] S. Gadzhanova, N. Pratt, and E. Roughead, "Use of SGLT2 inhibitors for diabetes and risk of infection: Analysis using general practice records from the NPS MedicineWise MedicineInsight program," *Diabetes Research and Clinical Practice*, vol. 130, pp. 180–185, 2017.

[7] A. Vitry, S. A. Wong, E. E. Roughead, E. Ramsay, and J. Barratt, "Validity of medication-based co-morbidity indices in the Australian elderly population," *Australian and New Zealand Journal of Public Health*, vol. 33, no. 2, pp. 126–130, 2009.

[8] K. M. Johnsson, A. Ptaszynska, B. Schmitz, J. Sugg, S. J. Parikh, and J. F. List, "Urinary tract infections in patients with diabetes treated with dapagliflozin," *Journal of Diabetes and its Complications*, vol. 27, no. 5, pp. 473–478, 2013.

[9] Y. Yang, S. Chen, H. Pan et al., "Safety and efficiency of SGLT2 inhibitor combining with insulin in subjects with diabetes," *Medicine*, vol. 96, no. 21, p. e6944, 2017.

[10] S. H. Min, J.-H. Yoon, S. Hahn, and Y. M. Cho, "Comparison between SGLT2 inhibitors and DPP4 inhibitors added to insulin therapy in type 2 diabetes: a systematic review with indirect comparison meta-analysis," *Diabetes/Metabolism Research and Reviews*, vol. 33, no. 1, 2017.

22

Level of Knowledge and Associated Factors of Postnatal Mothers' towards Essential Newborn Care Practices at Governmental Health Centers in Add is Ababa, Ethiopia

Demis Berhanⓘ **and Hanna Gulema**ⓘ

Addis Continental Institute of Public Health, P.O. Box 26751/1000, Addis Ababa, Ethiopia

Correspondence should be addressed to Demis Berhan; demisber63@gmail.com

Academic Editor: Jagdish Khubchandani

Background. Globally 4 million newborns die every year before they reach the age of one month and approximately 3.4 million newborns die within the first week of life. Of these deaths, 66% occur during the 1st 24 hours. Late death, i.e., after 24 hours, still occurs 34% and may be prevented if mothers have knowledge about newborn care including dangers sign of newborn. *Objective.* The aim of the study was to assess level of knowledge and associated factors of postnatal mothers towards essential newborn care practices at governmental health centers in Addis Ababa. *Methodology.* Institutional-based cross-sectional study with internal comparison was conducted using multistage sampling method in AA health centers from December 5 to January 30, 2016. *Result.* A total of 512 mothers who came for postnatal visit were interviewed using structured pretest questionnaires. Knowledge was assessed using closed and open ended questions. Poor knowledge has strong association with women's occupation (**AOR** = 2.10, 95% CI : (1.38,3.20)). Parity of the women was found as one of significant predictors for poor knowledge of essential newborn care. Women who were primiparas are **1.99** times more likely to have poor knowledge of ENC compared to women who were multiparas **AOR** = 1.99,95% CI: (1.25,3.20). The other significant predictors for poor knowledge of ENC were ANC visit. Women who had less than four antenatal visits were 0.63 times less likely to have poor knowledge than those who visit four times and above. **AOR** = 0.63, 95% CI:(0.40,0.99). *Conclusion.* Maternal education programs should be given emphasis for the components of ENC for mothers' knowledge gaps. Special emphasis needs to be placed when educating vulnerable groups including those who failed to fully attend antenatal clinic visits.

1. Introduction

Essential newborn care (ENC) is a comprehensive strategy designed to improve the health of newborns through interventions before conception, during pregnancy, at and soon after birth, and in the postnatal period. This brief describes the components of ENC, criteria for prioritizing them, and strategies used in operationalizing them. Implementation of ENC will have a positive impact on neonatal and infant mortality. New born care comprises basic preventive newborn care such as temperature maintenance, eye and cord care, early and exclusive breastfeeding on demand day and night, immunization, and early detection of problems or danger signs [1].

Despite an established evidence base of simple, affordable and low-cost interventions to avert neonatal deaths, global progress in reducing neonatal mortality has stagnated in recent years. Clean cord care is one of the essential newborn care practices recommended by the World Health Organization to reduce morbidity and mortality amongst the World's newborns. Despite this, cord infections are still prevalent in developing countries because of the high rates of unhygienic cord care practices [2].

The burden of neonatal death is still high in developing countries where most of the causes could be prevented [3]. Globally 4 million newborns die every year before they reach the age of one month. Out of them 1.5 million newborns die in four countries of South Asia. Approximately 3.4 million newborns die within the first week of life. Of these deaths, 66% occur during the 1st 24 hours. Late death, i.e., after 24 hours, occurs in the rest 34% and this may be prevented if mothers have good knowledge about newborn care including danger signs of newborn [4]. Up-to-date information on the causes of child deaths is crucial to guide global efforts to improve child survival [5].

The main focus of studies of childhood mortality has been the infant and under-five mortality rates. Neonatal mortality (deaths <28 days of age) has received limited attention. The World Health Organization recommends that improving newborn care practices at birth is crucial in order to reduce morbidity and mortality [6]. The three major causes of neonatal deaths (infections, complications of preterm birth, and intrapartum-related neonatal deaths) account for almost 90% of all neonatal deaths. The highest impact interventions to address these causes of neonatal death are summarized with estimates of potential for lives saved. A major gap is care during the early postnatal period for mothers and babies. There are promising models that have been tested mainly in research studies in Asia that are now being adapted and evaluated at scale including through a network of African implementation research trials [6].

Worldwide mortality in children younger than 5 years has dropped from 11.9 million deaths in 1990 to 7.7 million deaths in 2010, consisting of 4 million neonatal deaths, 2.3 million postneonatal deaths, and 2.3 million childhood deaths (deaths in children aged 1-4 years). 33.0% of deaths in children younger than 5 years occur in south Asia and 49.6% occur in sub-Saharan Africa, with less than 1% of deaths occurring in high-income countries. Across 21 regions of the world, rates of neonatal, post neonatal, and childhood mortality are declining. The global decline from 1990 to 2010 is 2.1% per year for neonatal mortality, 2.3% for post neonatal mortality, and 2.2% for childhood mortality. In 13 regions of the world, including all regions in sub-Saharan Africa, there is evidence of accelerating declines from 2000 to 2010 compared with 1990 to 2000. Within sub-Saharan Africa, rates of decline have increased by more than 1% in Angola, Botswana, Cameroon, Congo, Democratic Republic of the Congo, Kenya, Lesotho, Liberia, Rwanda, Senegal, Sierra Leone, Swaziland, and Gambia [7].

Two priority opportunities to address newborn deaths through existing maternal health programs are highlighted. First, antenatal steroids have high impact, feasible, and yet underused in low resource settings. Second, with increasing investment to scale up skilled attendance and emergency obstetric care, it is important to include skills and equipment for simple immediate newborn care and neonatal resuscitation [8].

For sub-Saharan Africa, on average, there has been no statistically significant change in neonatal mortality over the past decade. In sharp contrast, five African countries have reduced neonatal deaths by over 25%, more than double their neighbors. Important lessons emerge from this supplement, especially around seizing opportunities to promote community-based newborn care and to integrate newborn care interventions into frontline health worker delivery platforms, and especially into facility-based maternity care,

which is already being scaled up. At the same time, there are dozens of countries, mostly middle-income countries in Eastern Europe and Latin America, which have halved neonatal deaths in the last decade. As advanced previously in *The Lancet* Neonatal Survival Series, the analysis in paper 1 of this supplement demonstrates that while rapid progress in neonatal survival in these countries was linked with economic progress, significant improvements occurred in the absence of economic progress. Sri Lanka, for example, halved neonatal deaths due to prematurity despite a destabilizing internal conflict and weak economic growth, through extending their strong primary care system with effective referral level newborn care [9].

Promotion of essential newborn care practices is one strategy for improving newborn health outcomes. In settings where a majority of births take place at home without a skilled attendant and care seeking rates are low, preventive interventions included in essential newborn care should also be promoted at the community level [10]. For example, promotion of preventive behaviors through home visits by community health workers has been shown to improve key newborn care practices such as early initiation of breast-feeding, skin-to-skin contact, delayed bathing to prevent hypothermia, and clean care of the umbilical cord [11].

In Ethiopia about 120,000 newborns die every year in the first weeks of life which accounts for 42% of all deaths of under-five mortality. The study conducted in Addis Ababa health centers also indicated that level of essential newborn care practices were low even though the majority of respondents practice early initiation of breast feeding and safe cord care [12]. In Ethiopian demographic health survey (EDHS) 2011 neonatal mortality was at 37 deaths per 1,000 live births which was 49 deaths per 1,000 live births in 2000. Neonatal deaths accounts for 63% of all infant deaths and 42% of all under-five deaths which makes the reduction of neonatal mortality a critical intervention. The Ethiopian minidemographic health survey (EMDHS) 2014 reported coverage of 18% for PNC within the recommended 6-week period among these women who received a postnatal checkup; 8% were examined within 4 hours of delivery, 3% within 4-23 hours, 2% within 1-2 days, and 5% within 3-41 days of delivery; this is the time when the mother and baby are most vulnerable to morbidity and mortality associated with child birth. Infants who receive postnatal care within the first six weeks after birth are only 18% [13].

As indicated in the sustainable development goals (SDG), Ethiopia will intensify reproductive, maternal, newborn, child, adolescent, and health (RMNCAH) interventions to end preventable maternal and child deaths by 2030. The targets set in the health sector transformation plan (HSTP) are in line with the global aspirations. The impact-level targets of (HSTP) by 2020 are to reduce maternal mortality rate (MMR) to 199/100,000 LB; reduce under five-year infant and neonatal mortality rates 30, 20, and 10 per 1,000 live births, respectively; reduce stunting, wasting, and under-weight in under-5 year to 26%, 4.9%, and 13%, respectively [14]. Study in four regions (Amhara, Oromia, Tigray and Southern Nations, and Nationalities and People Region) of Ethiopia revealed that mothers' unprompted knowledge of newborn danger signs was rather low, with only 29.3% of respondents able to name 3 or more danger signs out of a list of 11. Among women who delivered alive baby in the period 1 to 7 months prior to data collection found that exclusive breastfeeding was 87.6%, wrapping the baby before delivery of the placenta 82.3%, and dry cord care 65.2%. In Ethiopia reproductive, maternal, newborn, child, and adolescent health (RMNCAH) and nutrition will continue to be top priority for the next 5 years [15].

Study done in Eastern Tigray showed essential newborn care knowledge and practice of mothers revealed that 80.4% had good knowledge and 92.9% had good practice. Most mothers had good knowledge on temperature maintenance, breast feeding initiation, and first bathing time [16].

In addition to their knowledge, almost all mothers practiced the main essential newborn care except a substance (oil and butter) application to the cord stump. The majority of mothers apply oil and butter on the cord stump which may lead to many neonatal infections. However, mothers should not apply any preparations on the cord. 98% of Mothers had ANC follow-up though 18.2% mothers still delivered at home [17].

There has been an increasing trend towards early hospital discharge of the mother baby pair following delivery [18]. Two-thirds of babies in developing countries are born at home and the others are discharged from health facilities soon after birth [19].

There is very limited information about newborn care practices in Ethiopia because many key indicators are not currently measured by routine surveys like the Demographic and Health Survey. Improving neonatal survival and motivating healthcare providers to give information for pregnant mothers, postnatal mothers, and child care givers regarding essential newborn care practice help to reduce preventive neonatal mortality.

The ability to identify knowledge gaps early in the neonatal period would help healthcare workers identify and implement timely and appropriate interventions that would lead to better neonatal outcomes. Therefore, this study will be expected to investigate the mothers level of knowledge and associated factors towards essential newborn care practice which the researchers, policy makers, healthcare workers, and community and care givers use as a base line for their future interventions and activities.

The following conceptual framework is proposed after extensive review of different literatures which are mentioned as main factors/determinant of mothers' knowledge and associated factors of Essential Newborn Care (ENBC), which includes sociodemographic factors, obstetrics factors, knowledge and associated factors, tradition, source of information, and maternal health services (see Figure 1)

2. Methodology

2.1. Study Setting. The study was conducted in Addis Ababa, capital city of Ethiopia, with an estimated area of 540 square kilometers, lies between 2326-3000 meters above sea level with lowest and highest annual temperature about 10°C and 32°C respectively and annual rain fall around 1200mm. Based on Addis Ababa city administration health bureau 2016/2017

Woreda base plan, Addis Ababa is estimated to have a total population of 3,433,999 consisting of 1,524,696(44.4%) males and 1,909,303(55.6%) females and reproductive age group of 1,189,537. Addis Ababa city administration health bureau is responsible for both curative and preventive health care services in the city. There are 10 subcity health departments which are directly accountable to their respective subcity administrations. In the city, there are 92 public health centers and all of them provide delivery service and newborn care.

2.1.1. Study Design & Study Period. Institution-based descriptive cross sectional study with internal comparison was conducted in ten A.A health centers from December 5 to January 30, 2017.

2.1.2. Source and Study Population. Source populations were all mothers in A.A who came for their postnatal visit within six weeks.

Study subject were all mothers who came for their postnatal visit within six weeks period during the data collection period consecutively and meet the inclusion criteria.

2.1.3. Sample Size Determination. To assess postnatal mothers level of knowledge towards essential newborn care. The required sample size was determined by using a single population proportion sample determination formula considering the following assumptions.

Based on the study conducted on four regions of Ethiopia, Proportion of mothers that were knowledgeable about newborn danger signs was 29.3% [15].

Level of significance = 95%
Margin of error = 5%
Non-respondent rate = 10%
The formula for calculating the sample size is

$$n = \frac{(Z\alpha/2)^2\, p\,(1-p)}{d^2} \qquad (1)$$

where α-level of confidence is
p = % of postnatal mothers who were knowledgeable
q = (1-p)
n- Sample size
Z- Standard normal distribution curve value for 95% CI which is 1.96 (where $\alpha = 0.05$)
d- Tolerable margin of error = 5% (0.05)
DEFF-design effect = 1.5
Hence, $n = (1.96)^2 \times 0.293 \times (1 - 0.293)/(0.05)^2 \times 1.5 = \mathbf{466}$

Additional 10% allowance (nonresponse rate)
Hence, the calculated sample size was 466. Adding a 10% nonresponse rate gave the required minimum sample size (n) = 512.
Thus, total sample size = **512**.

2.1.4. Sampling Procedure. In the study area there were ten sub-cities and in all sub-cities there were 92 health centers, from each sub city to get adequate sample size those health centers who have more than ten years' service are selected and then simple random sampling (lottery method) was used to identify the health centers from each subcities. Ten health

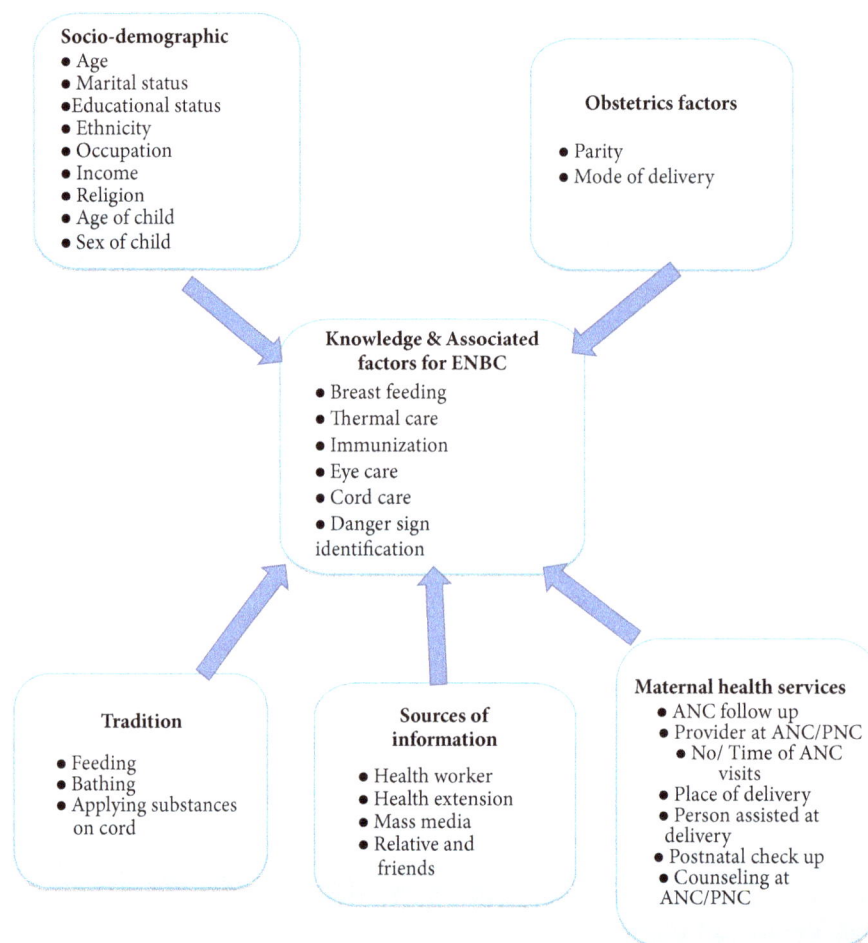

FIGURE 1: Conceptual frame work for factors that affects essential newborn care (adopted from Journal of perinatology 2002; 22:572–576).

centers, one from each subcities was selected using multi-stage sampling method. Study subject were all postnatal mothers who came for their postnatal visit within six weeks during the data collection period consecutively and meet the inclusion criteria.

The investigator identified those mothers who meet the eligibility criteria from the medical records and informed consent was obtained. Postnatal mothers of neonates born normal and alive and Post-natal mothers who give informed consent were included in the study. Postnatal mothers who refused to give informed consent and mentally ill were exclude form the study.

Data Collection Procedure. In each study area, one data collector from the staff nurse, who is able to communicate in Amharic was recruited. For effective and quality data collection, a two-day intensive training was given in Addis ketema health center for the selected nurses which covers study objectives, a thorough review of questionnaire, interview techniques, and directions as to how to administer the questionnaire.

Before starting the main data collection pretest by semi-structured interviews questionnaire were given for 5% (25) of Nifas-silk lafto (Woreda 09 Health center) postnatal mothers

coming to the health center within six weeks period. The questionnaire was first prepared in English and then translated in to Amharic. The questionnaire was translated back to English to observe consistency of the variables under question. The questionnaire consists of semistructured questionnaire addressing the neonate's and parents sociodemographic data, antenatal and birth history of the neonate, and mother's knowledge on the WHO essential newborn care practices.

2.2. Data Quality Control. The training was given for the data collectors and supervisors a week before they went to distribute and collect data from the participants. The questionnaire was pretested by maternal and child health (MCH) nurses on Woreda 09. Health center from Nifas Silk Lafto subcity 5% (25) of postnatal mothers who came within six weeks period, to ensure validity of the questionnaire before commencement of the study. Study tools were revised accordingly. As a result of the pretest, based on the findings, necessary corrections were given for some of the questions of the questionnaires. Moreover, during data collection supervisors checked in the field how the data collectors did their task. The principal investigator also closely supervised the field activity on daily basis. At the end of each data collection day, the principal investigator also checked the completeness of filled questionnaires and whether recorded information makes sense to ensure the quality of data collected. Besides this, the principal investigator carefully entered and thoroughly cleaned the data before the commencement of the analysis.

2.3. Data Processing and Analyzing. The quantitative collected data entered into EPI info version 7.2 and transported, cleaned and analyzed using SPSS version 20. Frequencies and percentages of different variables were computed for description as appropriate. Odds ratio with 95% confidence interval was computed to determine the degree of association between the dependent and independent variables; seven variables were examined independently using a bivariate analysis and then five variables those with a p-value of less than 0.20 were included into a logistic regression model to calculate the adjusted odds ratios and 95% confidence intervals while controlling for potential confounding factors. Level of significance was taken at p value < 0.05. A scoring system was used to analyze responses to closed ended questions on knowledge: 1 = coded as correct response (consistent with WHO essential newborn care guidelines).

0 = coded as incorrect response (inconsistent with WHO essential newborn care guidelines). Any mother who does not know the answer was considered to have an incorrect response.

Therefore, according to this study those scoring below the median are considered to have poor knowledge and above or equal to the median are considered to have good knowledge

The responses for the open ended questions summarized and descriptive statistics were carried out. During analysis for factors associated with maternal knowledge on newborn care, the median score was used as a cut off to distinguish between poor knowledge and good knowledge.

2.4. Ethical Considerations. The study was conducted after approval by Addis continental institute of public health (ACIPH) research ethical review committee and getting ethical paper from Addis Ababa health bureau ethical review committee. The researcher explained the purpose of the study to the mother before recruitment and informed consent was obtained. Any information pertinent to care of neonate was immediately communicated to the primary doctor. No invasive procedure was done as part of the study. No tissue specimen was collected as part of the study. Participation in this study was purely voluntary and there was no monetary gain. The postnatal mothers were expected to be free to withdraw from the study without any penalty. No compensation was offered for participation in the study. Once the primary caregiver discharged the mother and her neonate(s), no follow-up interviews were required. All the participants' response were kept confidential by using the information only for the purpose of the study and storing the study in a closed file. The rights of the respondents to refuse to answer for few or all of the questions were respected.

3. Results

3.1. Background Information of the Respondents. A total of 512 postnatal mothers were interviewed; among them 464

(90.6%) were married. Employed women accounted for 306(59.8%). The proportion of women who are illiterate is 42 (8.2%) as shown in Table 1. Orthodox Christians accounted for 304 (59.4%) of the respondents', while Muslims accounted for 126 (24.6%) and Protestants accounted for 82 (16%) (see Table 1).

3.2. Antenatal and Birth History. From the total 512 interviewed mothers, 504 (98.4%) had attended antenatal clinic. The mean gestation at first visit was 3-4 months with an average of 4 visits (SD=0.3). Of those interviewed, 355 (69.3%) of the mothers were primiparous. Vaginal deliveries accounted for 407 (79.5%) while Caesarean section accounted for 85 (16.6%). The proportion of male to female deliveries was almost equal with male neonates accounting for 259 (50.6%) and females 253 (49.4%).

3.3. Knowledge on Essential Newborn Care

3.3.1. Breast Feeding. Only 339 (66.2%) of mothers reported that their newborns were breastfed within the first hour after delivery. Additionally, 12 (2.3%) of mothers reported that they squeezed out the colostrum before breastfeeding the newborn; 89(17.4%) reported feeding their newborns food or liquid other than breast milk in the first two days. 350 (68.4%) of mothers knew about breastfeeding on demand, 436 (85.2%) reported exclusive breastfeeding for 6 months, and 500(97.7%) of mothers knew that colostrum should be given to their newborns. 139 (27.1%) of the mothers did not know that prelacteal feeds should not be given to neonates. Among those newborns that were given other foods, the most commonly food reported by mothers was cow's milk 332(64.8%), plain water 100 (19.5%), packed milk 61(11.9%), sugar water 17(3.3%), and others 2 (0.4%) (see Figure 2).

3.3.2. Immunization. 492 (96.1%) of mothers were aware of the need to vaccinate their newborns at birth while 461 (90%) knew that vaccines were given to prevent diseases. Only 199 (38.9%) knew that BCG vaccine was for prevention of tuberculosis and 246(48%) mothers reported that OPV was the vaccine given at birth to protect the child from polio (see Figure 3).

3.3.3. Cord Care. Among mothers interviewed, 339 (66.2%) correctly stated that the stump should be uncovered. Out of those interviewed, 384 (75%) of mothers believed that water should be used to clean the soiled umbilical stump, 340 (66.4%) of mothers believed that nothing should be applied to the cord, while 53 (10.4%) of mothers mentioned that butter should be applied to the stump, while 111 (21.7%) mother said they did not know, and 8 (1.6%) of mothers know that vaseline and oil was applied on the cord (see Figure 4).

3.3.4. Thermoregulation. 351 (68.6%) of mothers believed that warm cloth prevents heat loss from neonate, while 260 (50.8%) of mothers mentioned that mother-baby skin to skin contact prevents neonates from cold.

3.3.5. Eye Care. From the study participants, 410 (80.1%) of mothers are aware of signs of eye infection among which, 347

TABLE 1: Sociodemographic characteristics' of postnatal mothers in Addis Ababa health centers, Dec.1-Jan.30, 2017.

Variable	Frequency	Percentage
Age of the mother		
15-25	207	40.4
26-35	245	47.9
36-45	60	11.7
Marital status		
Married	464	90.6
Single/Divorce/widowed	48	9.4
Occupation of mother		
Employed	306	59.8
Unemployed	206	40.2
Education level		
Illiterate	42	8.2
1-10	250	48.8
Higher than 10	220	43
Religion		
Orthodox	304	59.4
Muslim	126	24.6
Protestant	82	16
Ethnicity of mother		
Amhara	189	36.9
Oromo	148	28.9
Gurage	101	19.7
Others	74	14.5
Families monthly income (in Birr)		
≤1000	80	15.6
1001-2000	114	22.3
>2000	318	62.1

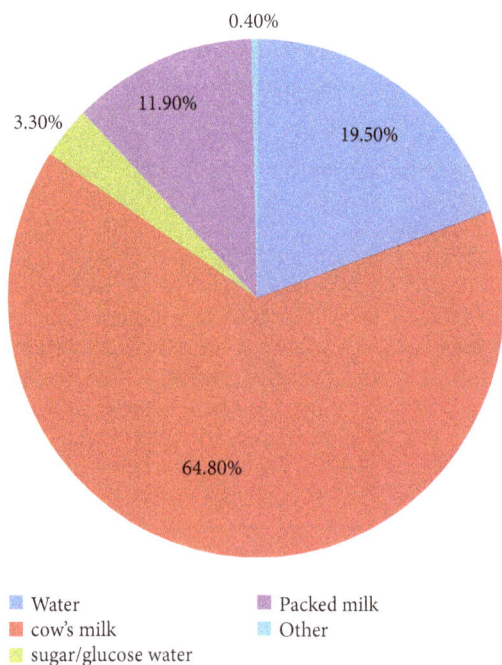

FIGURE 2: Knowledge of prelacteal feed given for neonate in Addis Ababa health centers, Dec. 1-Jan. 30, 2017.

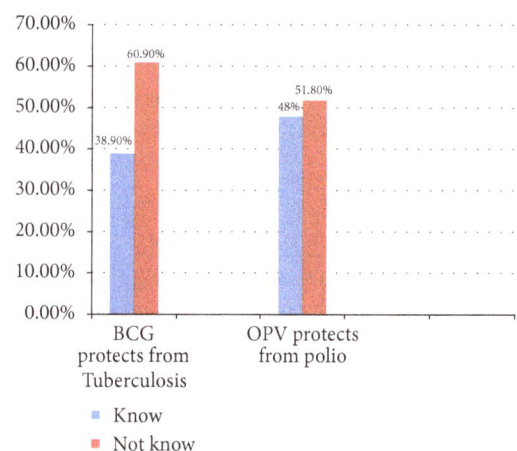

FIGURE 3: Proportion of postnatal mothers with knowledge on vaccines given at birth in Addis Ababa health centers, Dec. 1-Jan. 30, 2017.

(67.8%) of women reported that eye discharge is the main symptom while reddening of eye accounts for 305(59.2%), 179 (35%) mentioned swollen eye, and 3 (0.6%) for other symptoms (see Figure 5).

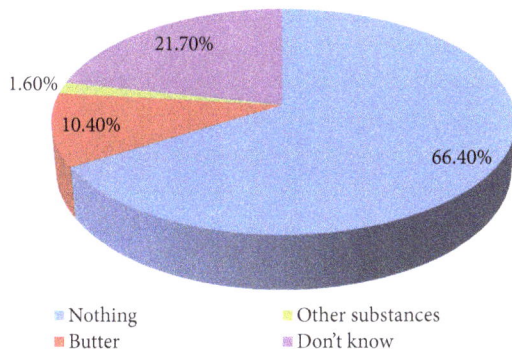

FIGURE 4: Substances applied on umbilical cord after cutting mentioned by postnatal mothers' in Addis Ababa health centers, Dec. 1-Jan.30, 2017.

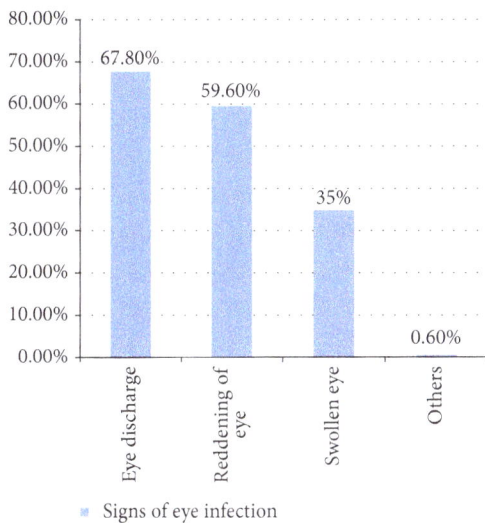

FIGURE 5: Knowledge of postnatal mothers' on sign of eye infection in Addis Ababa health centers, Dec.1-Jan. 30, 2017.

3.4. Knowledge on Danger Sign. Among 455 (88.9%) of mothers who have correct response towards danger sign, majority of them 382 (74.6%) recognized fever as a danger sign while few 77 (15%) of them recognized baby being too small/born being too early as a danger sign and 102(12.2%) did not have awareness on newborn danger signs. More than 74.6% of participants perceived that serious neonatal illness needs special attention to consult health personnel urgently.

3.5. Over All Knowledge Level of Mothers on ENC. Questions regarding knowledge of breast feeding, cord care, eye care, immunization, thermal care, and identification of danger sign measures for newborn care were scored and pulled together and the median score was computed to determine the overall knowledge of respondents.

The overall knowledge question composite showed that the median knowledge score was 25 with SD = 5.64 & mean 22.48. A woman who does not respond to all questions scored 0 and who responds to all questions scored 32, based on this

fact the minimum knowledge score, was 9 and maximum score was 32. Respondents who scored below the median are considered as having poor knowledge.

In this study among 512 post-natal mothers 60.2% of them had poor knowledge towards essential newborn care.

The multivariable logistic regression analysis showed that poor knowledge has strong association with women's occupation, parity, and number of ANC visits. Unemployed mothers had 2.10 times more chance of having poor knowledge than those who are employed (**AOR** =2.10, 95% CI: (1.38, 3.20).

Parity of the women was found as one of significant predictors for poor knowledge of ENC. Women who were primiparas were **1.99** times more likely to have poor knowledge of ENC compared to women who were multiparas **AOR** = 1.99,95% CI: (1.25,3.20).

The other significant predictors for poor knowledge of ENC was ANC visit. Women who had less than four antenatal visits were 0.63 times less likely to have poor knowledge than those who visited four times and above **AOR** = 0.63,95% CI: (0.40,0.99) (see Table 2).

4. Discussion

About 60.2% postnatal mothers had poor knowledge on essential new born care and those mothers who were unemployed, primiparous, and those mothers who had ANC visit greater than four had more likely poor knowledge. Similar study which was done in Fiche town shows that 53.6% of the respondents have poor knowledge towards essential newborn care; this shows that there is information gap.

The proportion of poor knowledge on essential new born care is lower than previous reports from Ethiopia, which was 85%. [12]. The suggested reason of this difference could be due to different sociodemographic characteristics of the study participants and the other possible explanation could be newborn health and maternal health are given due attention by the Government of Ethiopia, federal ministry of health (FMOH), NGO, and other stakeholder.

Education on newborn care practices was given in a lower rate when antenatal period is compared with postnatal period (70.5%, 83.6%), respectively. unless the information's were provided only regarding to pregnant mothers on birth preparedness. The importance of antenatal education shown by Darmstadt GL, Oot DA, Lawn JE, who demonstrated that antenatal education among expectant mothers resulted in sustained improvement in knowledge of newborn care in the postnatal period [7].

In this study majority of the newborn care education received among the study participants was related to exclusive breastfeeding and when to start immunization. Breastfeeding knowledge among mothers was encouraging with 85.2% of mothers are aware of exclusive breastfeeding and 68.4% are aware of breastfeed on demand and 72.9% of mothers are aware that Pre lacteal feeds should not be given to baby, Initiation of breastfeed immediately after birth accounts 66.2%.

Similar study in Cameroon on knowledge of postnatal mothers regarding initiation of breast feeding shows that 48% answered to initiate breast feed within one hour of

TABLE 2: Factors associated with poor maternal knowledge on newborn care in Addis Ababa health centers, Dec. 1-Jan. 30, 2017.

Variables	Knowledge of mothers		COR(95%CI)	AOR(95% CI)
	Good	Poor		
Age				
15-25	85 41.1%	122 58.9%	0.97(0.54,1.75)	0.73(0.37,1.42)
26-35	94 37.5%	151 62.5%	0.87(0.49,1.55)	0.73(0.39,1.37)
36-45	25 41.7%	35 58.3%	1	1
Education status				
Illiterate	9 21.4%	33 78.6%	0.35 (0.16,0.77)	0.77 (0.32,1.85)
1-10	99 39.6%	151 60.4%	0.85 (0.59,1.22)	1.21 (0.79,1.85)
Higher than 10	96 43.6%	124 56.4%	1	1
Marital status				
Married	188 40.5%	276 59.5%	1	1
Single/Divorce and widowed	16 33.3%	32 66.7%	1.36 (0.72,2.55)	1.40(0.72,2.71)
Occupation				
Employed	144 47.1	162 52.9%	1	1
Unemployed	60 29%	146 71%	2.16 (1.49,3.15)*	2.10 (1.38,3.20)*
Income				
≤1000	19 23.8	61 76.2%	0.42 (0.24,0.73)	0.60(0.32,1.10)
1001-2000	49 43%	65 57%	1.01 (0.65,1.55)	1.14(0.71,1.83)
>2001	136 42.8%	182 57.2%	1	1
Parity				
Primipara	158 44.5%	197 55.5%	1.93 (1.29,2.89)*	1.99 (1.25,3.20)*
Multipara	46 29.3	111 70.7%	1	1
No of antenatal visit				
< 4	36 31%	80 69%	0.59(0.38,0.92)*	0.63(0.40,0.99)*
≥ 4	168 43.2%	221 56.8%	1	1

*significant at p <0.05 1: reference category.

birth. This shows that there are information gaps on the initiation immediate breastfeeding [3]. Similar studies in Sri Lanka shows that all (100%) respondents have had knowledge and practice to feed colostrum and exclusive breast feeding and 70 (70%) knew about early initiation of breastfeeding [17], these findings were similar to those reported by Indira Narayanan, who also found that majority of Sri Lankan postnatal mothers were aware of early and exclusive breast-feeding. More than 90% of mothers knew about breastfeeding on demand, the advantages of colostrum and the duration of exclusive breastfeeding [1]. Study in Cameroon showed that 64% of the participants were not aware of the duration of exclusive breastfeeding; this is because there may be information gaps regarding exclusive breastfeeding and 44% of participants obtained knowledge regarding child care from health workers.

A study reported by Indira Narayanan indicated that colostrum is highly nutritious and protective to the newborn. More than half of mothers knew that colostrum should be given to their babies. Cultural beliefs play role to squeeze out colostrum; people believe that colostrum was not clean and not important and can cause a disease. These findings are more encouraging than an Indian setting where strong cultural beliefs hampered the use of colostrum. In this study in contrast to the above study due to cultural reasons, lack of awareness, and influence of neighbor, only 12 (2.3%) of

mothers did not give colostrum; this shows knowledge level on colostrum is very interesting [1].

WHO advocates for hygienic practices while handling the cord which is a potential source of infection. In this study, knowledge level was assessed by determining maternal factors on handling the cord. 75% of mothers are aware of the opinion that water should be used to clean a soiled cord. Only 66.4% of mothers agreed with the recommendation of using the cord clean and dry without applying any substances.

In the study done in Kenya only four mothers agreed with the recommendation of using the cord clean and dry without applying any substances. This variation in opinions among postnatal mothers is likely due to lack of knowledge on packages of essential newborn care especially on cord care [18]. Also study done in south india indicated that knowledge of mothers on on umblical cord care was inadequate, which was only 35%.

In this study, 96.1% of mothers were aware of the need to vaccinate their neonates. Only 38.9% of mothers were aware of disease prevented by vaccine given on left forearm at birth (BCG). Only 48% of mothers were aware of disease prevented by vaccine given orally at birth (OPV) to newborns.

Mothers in this study scored poorly when asked to match vaccine given with the disease it prevented. Findings suggest poor dissemination of immunization information to mothers by healthcare providers. Similar study done by Darmstadt

GL and Bhutta ZA showed regarding the mothers knowledge on immunization of their infant that 95% of the participants were aware of the need for immunization of their infant. Among participants 76% were not aware of the names of the individual vaccines given for the newborn babies. Only 8% of the mothers had adequate knowledge on the different immunization component even though the immunization coverage was good; these may be because of information gap on the name and advantage of each component of vaccine during immunization [2].

This study found that information on danger sign was not adequately disseminated to mothers 36.3% and 44.1% for both antenatal and postnatal, respectively. In a similar study conducted in Kenya, information on danger signs in the neonate was not adequately disseminated to mothers both antenatally and postnatally [17].

Recognition of danger signs in the newborn by mothers has been shown to be a cause of concern in several studies conducted in developing countries [5]. In this study, the danger signs that were identified by most mothers included fever, poor feeding/sucking and fast breathing. Similar study in Kenya, the danger signs that were identified by most mothers included fever, diarrhea and vomiting.

In this study, mothers who were unemployed more likely had poor knowledge more than those who are employed. Studies in India and Sri Lanka showed similarly that mothers' who have poor knowledge/awareness were associated with unemployed women than counterparts [17].

Primparous mothers more likely had poor knowledge than multiparous. Similar study done in Sri Lanka showed mother's knowledge was strongly associated with parity, occupational status and month of first ANC visits [17]. According to this study, women who had visited antenatal care less than four times were less likely to have poor knowledge than those who visited four time and above. Literatures that support this result were not found.

5. Conclusion

A national health program is incomplete without community participation and this holds good for reproductive and child health program as well. Awareness on postnatal and early neonatal care is a fundamental prerequisite to effective community participation. This study has revealed the presence of knowledge gap, in spite of the fact that reproductive and child health (RCH) program is given top priority by the government. Despite the fact that participant records show highest number of ANC attendance and institutional deliveries, the existing knowledge gap in key areas of neonatal care will greatly affect the success of child care services.

Better maternal education on essential newborn care was received in the antenatal period. In this study, provision of information on essential newborn care to antenatal mothers was lower when compared to postnatal with regards to essential newborn care.

Postnatal mothers are most likely to have poor knowledge on essential newborn care practices including those who failed to fully attend antenatal clinic visits and those who did not receive any source of newborn education during pregnancy. Antenatal clinics provide an opportunity to educate mothers on newborn care which results in sustained knowledge in the postnatal period. The main finding in this study was that 60.2% of mothers have poor knowledge towards essential newborn care. Sociodemographic and maternal factors that were significantly associated with mothers knowledge score were occupation, parity, and number of antenatal visits.

Authors' Contributions

Demis Berhan participated in the design of the study and data collection, analyzed the data, and drafted the paper. Hanna Gulema participated in revising subsequent drafts of the paper from the design to final draft of the paper. Both authors read and approved the final manuscript.

Acknowledgments

This is, in fact, a great moment to raise the corresponding author's deepest gratitude and appreciation to their dear advisor Hanna Gulema, for her unreserved support and constructive comments including timely Communication throughout the preparation of this thesis. Moreover, those experiences and Constructive ideas were marvelous. The author is also pleased to thank his beloved wife Helen Ayele, for her unreserved support, encouragement, and follow-up: "thank you very much, you are the reason for all my successes." The authors also greatly thank their classmates Mr. Alemayehu Wondimu and Kahsay G/kidan who play a great role in facilitating the health centers to provide them with genuine response during data collection and in helping during analysis on SPSS. Special appreciation goes to Addis Continental Institute of Public Health (ACIPH) Department of Public Health for teaching and guiding this research. Sincere thanks are also goes to all respondents, Addis Ababa Health Bureau Ethical Review Committee, administrations at all levels of Addis Ababa Health bureau, and the ten targeted health centers in each subcity.

References

[1] N. Indira, R. Mandy, and C. Dilberth, "The Components of Essential Newborn Care," *Basics Support Institutionalizing Child Surviv Proj BASICS II U S Agency Int Dev*, 2004.

[2] G. L. Darmstadt, Z. A. Bhutta, S. Cousens, T. Adam, N. Walker, and L. De Bernis, "Evidence-based, cost-effective interventions: how many newborn babies can we save?" *The Lancet*, vol. 365, no. 9463, pp. 977–988, 2005.

[3] F. Monebenimp, M. M. Enganemben, D. Chelo et al., "Mothers' Knowledge and Practice on Essential Newborn Care at Health Facilities in Garoua City, Cameroon," vol. 14, no. 12, 2013.

[4] S. P. Saraswati, "Knowledge and Practice of Postnatal Mothers on Newborn Care at Hospital Setting," *ARC Journal of Nursing and Healthcare*, vol. 2, no. 1, 2016.

[5] R. E. Black, S. Cousens, H. L. Johnson et al., "Global, regional, and national causes of child mortality in 2008: a systematic analysis," *The Lancet*, vol. 375, no. 9730, pp. 1969–1987, 2010.

[6] V. Kumar, A. Kumar, and G. L. Darmstadt, "Behavior Change for Newborn Survival in Resource-Poor Community Settings: Bridging the Gap Between Evidence and Impact," *Seminars in Perinatology*, vol. 34, no. 6, pp. 446–461, 2010.

[7] G. L. Darmstadt, D. A. Oot, and J. E. Lawn, "Newborn survival: Changing the trajectory over the next decade," *Health Policy and Planning*, vol. 27, no. 3, pp. iii1–iii5, 2012.

[8] J. E. Lawn, K. Kerber, C. Enweronu-Laryea, and O. M. Bateman, "Newborn survival in low resource settings - Are we delivering?" *BJOG: An International Journal of Obstetrics & Gynaecology*, vol. 116, no. 1, pp. 49–59, 2009.

[9] J. E. Lawn, M. V. Kinney, R. E. Black et al., "Newborn survival: a multi-country analysis of a decade of change," *Health Policy and Planning*, vol. 27, no. suppl_3, pp. iii6–iii28, 2012.

[10] M. Z. Oestergaard, M. Inoue, and S. Yoshida, "Neonatal mortality levels for 193 countries in 2009 with trends since 1990: a systematic analysis of progress, projections, and priorities," *PLoS Medicine*, vol. 8, no. 8, Article ID e1001080, 2011.

[11] P. I. Opara, T. Jaja, D. A. Dotimi, and B. A. Alex-Hart, "Newborn Cord Care Practices Amongst Mothers in Yenagoa Local Government Rea, Bayelsa State, Nigeria," *International Journal of Clinical Medicine*, vol. 03, no. 01, pp. 22–27, 2011.

[12] Alemayehu Mekonnen and Workinesh Daba, "Assessment of Magnitude and Determinants of Neonatal Care Practice among Mothers in Selected Health Centers of Addis Ababa, Administration, Ethiopia," 2015.

[13] Central Statistical Agency, *Ethiopia Mini Demographic and Health Survey 2014*, Central Statistical Agency, Addis Ababa, Ethiopia, 2014.

[14] FMOH, *The federal Democratic Republic of Ethiopia ministry of Health: Health sector transformation plan*, FMOH, 2015.

[15] J. A. Callaghan-Koru, A. Seifu, M. Tholandi et al., "Newborn care practices at home and in health facilities in 4 regions of Ethiopia," *BMC Pediatrics*, vol. 13, no. 1, 2013.

[16] H. G. Misgna, H. B. Gebru, and M. M. Birhanu, "Knowledge, practice and associated factors of essential newborn care at home among mothers in Gulomekada District, Eastern Tigray, Ethiopia, 2014," *BMC Pregnancy and Childbirth*, vol. 16, no. 1, 2016.

[17] P. Waiswa, M. Kemigisa, J. Kiguli, S. Naikoba, G. W. Pariyo, and S. Peterson, "Acceptability of evidence-based neonatal care practices in rural Uganda - Implications for programming," *BMC Pregnancy and Childbirth*, vol. 8, 2008.

[18] Lucia Amolo, "Knowledge and attitude of postnatal mothers on essential newborn care practices at kenyatta national hospital," H58/70087/11, 2013.

[19] WHO, *Maternal and newborn health, Safe motherhood, Report of a technical working group*, WHO, 1994.

23

Smoking, Alcohol Consumption, and Illegal Substance Abuse among Adolescents in Sri Lanka: Results from Sri Lankan Global School-Based Health Survey 2016

Sameera Senanayake (ID),[1] **Shanthi Gunawardena,**[2]
Mahesh Kumbukage (ID),[3] **Champika Wickramasnghe,**[3] **Nalika Gunawardena** (ID),[4]
Ayesha Lokubalasooriya,[1] **and Renuka Peiris**[5]

[1]*Family Health Bureau, Ministry of Health, Sri Lanka*
[2]*Non-Communicable Diseases Unit, Ministry of Health, Sri Lanka*
[3]*Ministry of Health, Sri Lanka*
[4]*World Health Organization, Sri Lanka*
[5]*Ministry of Education, Sri Lanka*

Correspondence should be addressed to Mahesh Kumbukage; mpkumbukage@gmail.com

Academic Editor: Carol J. Burns

Background. Adolescence is defined by the World Health Organization (WHO) as "the transition period from childhood to adulthood". Increases in autonomy during this period, willingness to experiment, and peer influence create an environment of taking high-risk decisions influencing adolescent health, such as substance abuse and smoking. The current study was conducted to estimate the prevalence of smoking, alcohol consumption, and illegal substance abuse and their determinants on in-school adolescents using data from the Global School-based Student Health Survey, Sri Lanka in 2016. *Methods.* A cross-sectional survey was conducted among 3,650 students using a self-administered questionnaire in government schools. Weighted prevalence was calculated, and logistic regression analysis was conducted to determine the correlates. *Results.* The prevalence of current alcohol, smoking, smokeless tobacco consumption, and substance abuse, 30 days before the survey, was 3.4% (95% CI 2.6 - 4.3), 3.6% (95% CI 2.5-5.0), 2.3% (95% CI 1.5-3.7), and 2.7% (95% CI - 1.7-4.2%). Male sex and involvement in physical fighting were independently associated with increased risk in all four substance categories assessed. Multivariate analysis using multiple logistic regression revealed that only the male sex and involvement in physical fighting were correlates for four substance categories assessed when confounding effects of other variables were accounted for. Being in the 16-17 age category, parents' tobacco use and seeing actors consuming alcohol on TV increased the risk of alcohol consumption, smoking, and smokeless tobacco. Having ever attempted suicide was positively associated with increased risk for alcohol consumption, smoking, and illegal substance abuse. *Conclusion.* Alcohol use, smoking, smokeless tobacco use, and illegal substance abuse by students remain a concern in Sri Lanka and implementing life skills-based interventions at schools is recommended.

1. Introduction

Adolescence is defined by the World Health Organization (WHO) as "the transition period from childhood to adulthood", ranging from ages 10 to 19 years. In Sri Lanka, adolescents consist of 16.1% of the total population, with 70% attending school [1].

Adolescence is one of the most rapid phases of human development where biological maturity precedes psychosocial maturity [2]. Both individual and the environmental characteristics influence changes taking place during adolescence. Increased autonomy during this period, willingness to experiment, and peer influence/pressure create an environment encouraging high-risk decisions which influence adolescents' health, such as substance abuse and smoking [3, 4].

During the past few decades, an increase in trends of smoking and substance abuse among adolescents has been reported worldwide [5, 6]. These behaviors are well-associated with various social, biological, economical, and psychological issues such as violence, crime, injuries, diseases, increased school dropout rates, and deaths in extreme cases [3]. However, every year, more than 12300 of Sri Lankan people are killed by tobacco-caused disease. Further, more than 6000 children (10-14 years old) and 1725000 adults (15+ years old) continue to use tobacco each day [7]. In Sri Lanka, the smoking prevalence among aged 13-15 years is believed to be around 2% [8]. Tobacco use includes use of both smoked (ganja, cigarette, bidi, cigars) and smokeless (chewing tobacco, betel with tobacco, babul, and madana modaka). Though the importing or selling is banned in Sri Lanka since 2016, smokeless tobacco products such as Babul, Beeda, Mawa, Pampara, and Gurkha are still available in the market. Understanding the usage pattern of illicit drug use among adolescents is useful in developing effective strategies to prevent initiation of these behaviors.

The Global School-Based Student Health Survey (GSHS) was initiated in 2001 by the WHO in collaboration with UNICEF, UNESCO, and UNAIDS with technical assistance from the US Centers for Disease Control and Prevention (CDC). Since 2003, this has been an important source of information to observe the prevalence of behavioral risk and protective factors among the adolescent school-attending population. In Sri Lanka, the GSHS was conducted both in 2008 and 2016. The GSHS in 2008 did not assess the usage patterns of alcohol, cigarettes, smokeless tobacco, or illegal substances. Realizing the importance of estimating the magnitude of these behaviors among school children, the survey in 2016 explored practices related to smoking, alcohol consumption, and illegal substance abuse. Furthermore, the Ministry of Health, Sri Lanka, is planning to carry out this survey periodically; thus the usage patterns of alcohol, cigarettes, smokeless tobacco, or addictive substances among adolescents could be found out.

In this milieu, the purpose of this paper is to estimate the prevalence and correlation of smoking, alcohol consumption, and illegal substance abuse among school-going adolescents ages 13-17 in Sri Lanka, using the data of the GSHS conducted in 2016.

2. Methods

This study involved analysis of data from the Sri Lankan GSHS conducted in 2016. Students of grades 8, 9, 10, 11, and 12 in government schools in Sri Lanka were recruited for the survey. Data collection was done during the period of October 1st to November 31st, 2016.

2.1. Sample Size and Sampling. A sample of 3,650 was selected, based on a desired precision of ±5 percent and an expected response rate of 80%. A two-stage cluster sample design was employed to produce a representative sample of students in grades 8 to 12 in the country. In the first stage, the

sampling frame consisted of all schools with grades 8-12 in Sri Lanka. Out of them, 40 schools were selected by probability proportional to school enrollment size. Systematic equal probability sampling with a random start was used to select classes from each selected school in the next step. All students in the selected classes were eligible to participate in the survey.

2.2. The Questionnaire. Data were collected via a self-administered, standard GSHS questionnaire adapted to the Sri Lankan culture and translated to Sinhala and Tamil. There were three separate sections in the questionnaire assessing the status of smoking, alcohol consumption, and illegal substance abuse. In the questions related to smoking, there were a total of 10 questions which inquired into aspects such as the commencement of smoking (e.g., ganja, cigarette, bidi, and cigars), current smoking status, and the use of smokeless tobacco (chewing tobacco, betel with tobacco, babul, madana modaka, Beeda, and Mawa). Alcohol consumption was assessed using seven questions, including aspects such as the initiation of drinking and current drinking status. In the three questions relating to substance abuse, the use of marijuana, amphetamines, cocaine, inhalants, babul, ganja, and madana modaka was assessed. Initiation of substances and current usage patterns were assessed using these questions. Current consumption was assessed by asking the students if they had consumed a substance 30 day prior to the survey. In addition to these questions, sociodemographic details and data related to students' mental health and parental engagement in students' life were collected. Adequate measures were taken to obtain quality data while ensuring minimal interference in school activities.

2.3. Data Analysis. Data were analyzed using SPSS version 21.0 software. A weight was associated with each questionnaire to reflect the likelihood of sampling each student and to reduce bias by compensating for differing patterns of nonresponse. The weight used for estimation is given by

W = W1 * W2 * f1 * f2 * f3;

W1 = the inverse of the probability of selecting the school;

W2 = the inverse of the probability of selecting the classroom within the school;

f1 = a school-level nonresponse adjustment factor calculated by school size (small, medium, large). The factor was calculated in terms of school enrollment instead of the number of schools;

f2 = a student-level nonresponse adjustment factor calculated by class;

f3 = a poststratification adjustment factor calculated by grade.

The prevalence of smoking, alcohol consumption, and illegal substance abuse in in-school adolescents in Sri Lanka is presented together with 95% confidence intervals. The correlates of smoking, alcohol consumption, and illegal substance abuse in in-school adolescents were determined by conducting bivariate analyses and a backward logistic regression analysis.

TABLE 1: Description of study participants of the 2016 Sri Lankan Global School-Based Survey (N=3262).

Characteristic	Total	
	n	(%)
Age		
12 years or younger	66	(2.1)
13-15 years	2197	(66.5)
16-17 years	977	(30.7)
18 and older	22	(0.7)
Sex		
Male	1437	(48.9)
Female	1805	(51.1)

2.4. Administrative Requirements and Ethical Clearance. Ethical clearance was obtained from the ethical review committee of Colombo Medical Faculty. Approval of the study protocol was obtained from the Ministry of Education and relevant zonal education directors and principals.

3. Results

Of the selected 3,650 sampled students, 3,262 questionnaires were usable after data editing, giving a response rate of 89%.

3.1. Description of the Study Sample. Most of the students who responded belonged to the 13-15-year age group (66.5%). The study group consisted of a slightly higher proportion of females (51.1%) than males (Table 1).

3.2. Prevalence of Current Alcohol Consumption, Smoking, Use of Smokeless Tobacco Products, and Illegal Substance Use. The prevalence of current alcohol consumption, 30 days prior to the survey, was 3.4% (95% CI 2.6 - 4.3). Compared to girls (1.1%, 95% CI 0.6 – 1.5), the prevalence among males (5.8%, 95% CI 4.6 – 7.1) was significantly higher (p<0.05). Prevalence in the older adolescents (16-17 years) (5.8%, 95% CI 4.2-7.9) was higher compared to the younger (13-15 years) (2.0%, 95% CI 1.4-2.9).

Current smoking prevalence among the study group was 3.6% (95% CI 2.5-5.0). Similar to alcohol consumption, significantly (p<0.05) more boys (6.4%, 95% CI 5.2-7.7) were engaged in smoking, compared to girls (0.7%, 95% CI 0.3-1.1). During the 30 days before the survey, 2.3% (95% CI 1.5-3.7) of the students consumed smokeless tobacco with more males consuming smokeless tobacco (4.5%, 95% CI 3.4-5.6) compared to females (0.4%, 95% CI 0.1 -0.7). Unlike alcohol consumption, the prevalence of current smoking consumption was similar among the younger and older adolescents.

The prevalence of illegal substance abuse among the school children was 2.7% (95% CI – 1.7-4.2%). The percentage among the male students (4.1%, 95% CI 3.1- 5.2) was significantly (p<0.05) higher compared to the females (1.1%, 95% CI 0.6-1.5). However, the consumption of substance between the age categories was almost equal (Table 2).

According to the survey, of those who had ever had a drink of alcohol other than a few sips, 42.5% had their first drink before the age of 14, with a significantly higher proportion of younger (64.7%) reporting the first drink before 14 years of age compared to the older (20.2%) adolescents (p<0.05). On inquiry as to the main reason for the first drink of alcohol, the desire to actually taste alcohol was the main reason for the first drink (41.9%).

Of those whoever had smoked, 54.8% had their first smoke before the age of 14 years, with no significant difference by age or sex.

3.3. Correlates of Alcohol Consumption, Smoking, Smokeless Tobacco, and Illegal Substance Abuse. Age and sex-matched analysis, using logistic regression, revealed that being physically attacked during past 12 months (OR 2.2, 95% CI 1.4-3.3), involvement in physical fighting within the past 12 months (OR 4.0, 95% CI 2.4-6.6), obtaining a serious injury within the past 12 months (OR 2.5, 95% CI 1.5-3.9), being bullied in school within the last 30 days (OR 2.3, 95% CI 1.5-3.6), attempted suicide within the last 12 months (OR 3.3, 95% CI 1.8-6.1), having seen actors consuming alcohol on TV (OR 3.4, 95% CI 2.2-5.4), engaging in leisure activities more than three hours (OR 3.4, 95% CI 2.2-5.4), and parental tobacco use (OR 2.2, 95% CI 1.4-3.4) were significantly associated with alcohol consumption. The same factors were associated with smoking and smokeless tobacco consumption. The factors significantly associated with substance abuse were being physically attacked within the past 12 months (OR 2.5, 95% CI 1.5- 4.0), involved in physical fighting within the last 12 months (OR 4.1, 95% CI 2.3- 7.2), obtaining a serious injury within the past 12 months (OR 5.7, 95% CI 3.1- 10.3), being bullied in school within the last 30 days (OR 3.6, 95% CI 2.1-6.1), attempted suicide within the last 12 months (OR 6.5, 95% CI 3.6- 11.6), and seen actors consuming alcohol on TV (OR 2.9, 95% CI 1.7- 4.9).

The age-matched analysis revealed that the male sex was significantly associated with current use of alcohol (OR 5.6, 95% CI 3.3-9.4), smoking (OR 9.6, 95% CI 5.2-17.6), smokeless tobacco (OR 11.2, 95% CI 5.1-24.6), and illegal substance abuse (OR 4.1, 95% CI 2.4-7.0). Similarly, sex-matched analysis revealed that, except for illegal substance abuse, being in the older age category (16-17 years) was significantly associated with the current use of alcohol (OR 3.1, 95% CI 2.0-4.7), smoking (OR 2.6, 95% CI 1.7-3.9), and smokeless tobacco (OR 2.7, 95% CI 1.6-4.3) (Table 3).

Multivariate analysis using multiple logistic regression revealed that only the male sex and involvement in physical fighting were correlates for four substance categories assessed when confounding effects of other variables were accounted for. Being in the 16-17 age category, parents' tobacco use and seeing actors consuming alcohol on TV increased the risk of alcohol consumption, smoking, and smokeless tobacco. Having ever attempted suicide was positively associated with increased risk for alcohol consumption, smoking, and illegal substance abuse (Table 4).

Male students had a 10.2 times higher risk of smoking (AOR 10.2; 95% CI 4.3-24.0), and 10.8 (AOR 10.8; 95% CI 3.8-30.8) times higher risk of using smokeless tobacco compared to females. Elder students have 2.5 times higher risk of smoking (AOR 2.5; 95% CI 1.5-4.2) and 2.4 times the risk of

TABLE 2: Prevalence of current use of alcohol consumption, smoking, smokeless tobacco, and illegal substances among the study participants (N = 3173).

	Current use of Alcohol		Current Smoking		Current use of smokeless tobacco		Current use of illegal Substances	
	n*	% (95% CI)	n*	% (95% CI)	n*	% (95% CI)	n*	% (95% CI)
Total	103	3.4 (2.6-4.3)**	107	3.6 (2.5-5.0)**	69	2.3 (1.5-3.7)**	79	2.7 (1.7-4.2)**
Age								
13-15 Years	49	2.0 (1.4-2.9)**	40	2.5 (1.6-3.9)**	30	1.5 (0.9-2.6)**	46	2.4 (1.4-3.9)**
16-17 Years	52	5.8 (4.2-7.9) **	55	5.5 (3.7-8.0)**	36	4.0 (2.4-6.4)**	30	3.3 (1.6 – 6.9)**
Sex								
Male	81	5.8 (4.6 – 7.1)* * *	92	6.4 (5.2-7.7)* * *	62	4.5 (3.4 -5.6)* * *	58	4.1 (3.1 – 5.2)* * *
Female	19	1.1 (0.6 – 1.5)* * *	12	0.7 (0.3-1.1)* * *	7	0.4 (0.1 – 0.7)* * *	19	1.1 (0.6 – 1.5)* * *

* denotes unweighted frequency; ** denotes weighted percentage; * * * denotes unweighted percentage.

TABLE 3: Factors associated with current use of alcohol consumption, smoking, smokeless tobacco, and illegal substances (age and sex matched Odds Ratios with 95% CI).

Characteristic		n	Current use of Alcohol	Current Smoking	Current use of Smokeless Tobacco	Current use of illegal Substances
Age**	16-17 Years	977	3.1 (2.0-4.7)	2.6 (1.7-3.9)	2.7 (1.6-4.3)	1.5 (0.9-2.4)
	13-15 Years	2196	1	1	1	1
Sex* * *	Male	1437	5.6 (3.3 – 9.4)	9.6 (5.2-17.6)	11.2 (5.1-24.6)	4.1 (2.4-7.0)
	Female	1805	1	1	1	1
Physically attacked [1]	Yes	1119	2.2 (1.4-3.3)	1.8(1.2-2.8)	2.2 (1.3-3.7)	2.5 (1.5-4.0)
	No	2120	1	1	1	1
Engage in physical fighting [1]	Yes	1420	4.0 (2.4-6.6)	4.4 (2.6-7.3)	2. 4 (1.4-4.2)	4.1 (2.3-7.2)
	No	1838	1	1	1	1
Serious Injury [1]	Yes	1044	2.5(1.5-3.9)	2.8 (1.8-4.4)	2. 1 (1.2-3.6)	5.7 (3.1-10.3)
	No	1981	1	1	1	1
Bullied in School [2]	Yes	1208	2.3 (1.5-3.6)	2. 6 (1.7-4.2)	1.8 (1.1-3.1)	3.6 (2.1-6.1)
	No	1988	1	1	1	1
Felt Lonely [1]	Yes	2021	1.5 (0.9-2.3) *	1.5 (0.9-2. 3) *	1.1 (0.6-1.6) *	1.2 (0.5-1.3) *
	No	1229	1	1	1	1
Considered Suicide [1]	Yes	298	2.1 (1.2-3.6)	2.0 (1.1-3.7)	1.3 (0.6-3.1) *	2.6 (0.6-3.1) *
	No	2923	1	1	1	1
Attempted Suicide [1]	Yes	214	3.3 (1.8-6.1)	4.2 (2.4-7.5)	2.7 (1.2-5.7)	6.5 (3.6-11.6)
	No	3006	1	1	1	1
Having close Friends	No	180	1.6 (0.7-3.7) *	1.3 (0.6-3.3) *	2. 1 (0.8-5.1) *	1.8 (0.7-4.3) *
	Yes	3065	1	1	1	1
Parent Tobacco Use	Yes	659	2.2 (1.4-3.4)	2.0 (2.7-6.4)	1.7 (1.1-3.0)	1.5 (0.9-2.5) *
	No	2589	1	1	1	1
Other activities >3 Hours	>3 Hours	1196	2.1 (1.3-3.2)	1.8(1.2-2.8)	1.8 (1.1-2.9)	1.4 (0.8-2.2) *
	<3 Hours	2044	1	1	1	1
Parents understood the problems	No	1217	1.6 (0.8-3.3) *	1.4 (0.7-2.6) *	1.1(0.5-2.4)*	1.0(0.5-1.7) *
	Yes	827	1	1	1	1
Played sports	No	824	1.3 (0.6-.3.0) *	1.0(0.5-2.3)*	3.3 (0.9-11.0) *	1.0 (0.4-2.6) *
	Yes	532	1	1	1	1
Seeing actors consuming alcohol on TV	Yes	849	3.4 (2.2-5.4)	2.4 (1.6-3.7)	2.9 (1.7-4.9)	2.9 (1.7-4.9)
	No	2389	1	1	1	1

*Not significant at p=0.05 level, **sex matched, and * * *age matched.
[1]During last 12 months. [2]During last 30 days.

TABLE 4: Factors associated with current use of alcohol consumption, smoking, smokeless tobacco, and illegal substances (Adjusted Odds Ratios with 95% CI).

Characteristic		Current use of Alcohol	Current Smoking	Current use of Smokeless Tobacco	Current use of illegal Substances
Sex	Male	3.7 (2.0-3.9)	10.2 (4.3-24.0)	10.8 (3.8 – 30.8)	3.4 (1.6 – 6.8)
	Female	1	1	1	1
Age	16-17 Years	2.4 (1.5-6.7)	2.5 (1.5-4.2)	1.7 (1.05-3. 1)	
	13-15 Years	1	1	1	
Physical Fighting [1]	Yes	3.6(2.0-6.5)	3.9 (2.0-7.4)	2.2 (1.1-4.5)	3.6 (1.6 -8.0)
	No	1	1	1	1
Attempted Suicide [1]	Yes	3.1 (1.5-6.2)	3.4 (1.6-7.0)		6.0 (3.0 – 12.0)
	No	1	1		1
Parents Smoking [1]	Yes	1.8 (1.1 – 2.9)	1.8 (1.1-3.0)	1.8 (1.09 – 3.5)	
	No	1	1	1	
Seen Actors Consuming Alcohol on TV	Yes	2.9 (1.7 – 4.9)	2.5 (1.5-4.1)	2.5 (1.3 – 4.5)	
	No	1	1	1	
Bullied in school [2]	Yes	1.6 (1. 09-2.7)			2.1 (1.0 3– 4.1)
	No	1			1
Being physically attacked [1]	Yes			1.8 (1.04-3.5)	
	No			1	
Other activities >3 Hours	>3 Hours			1.7 (1.07-3.0)	
	< 3 Hours			1	
Obtaining serious injuries [1]	Yes				2.5 (1.3 -5.1)
	No				

[1] During last 12 months. [2] During last 30 days.

alcohol consumption (AOR 2.4; 95% CI 1.5-6.7) compared to younger students (Table 4).

4. Discussion

4.1. Prevalence of Alcohol, Smoking, Smokeless Tobacco, and Illegal Substance Use. The survey inquired about alcohol use 30 days prior to the survey as an indicator for current use of alcohol. The current prevalence of alcohol consumption among the participants was 3.4% (95% CI: 2.6-4.3) and the prevalence was significantly higher among males (5.8%, 95% CI: 4.2-7.9) compared to females (1.1%, 95% CI: 0.6-1.5). In a similar survey conducted by UNICEF among Sri Lankan school-age adolescents in 2004, the current use of alcohol among adolescents was 5.7%, higher than the current study result [9]. In the National Youth Health Survey (NYHS) conducted by the Family Health Bureau, Sri Lanka, in 2014, the current alcohol prevalence among adolescents, both school going and nonschool going, was 10.2% (95%CI: 8.9-11.7) [10]. Further, alcohol prevalence was significantly higher among the nonschool-going adolescents (4.9%: 95% CI: 4.2-5.6) compared to schoolers (3.1%, 95% CI: 2.6-3.8). School is a place where students are nurtured, and tools are provided to make correct choices in life. Evidence indicates that less school bonding is associated with problem behaviors among adolescents [11].

Evidence indicates that the prevalence of alcohol use among school-going adolescents varies markedly among countries. In an analysis of 12 developing countries around the world, using the GSHS data revealed that the prevalence of alcohol consumption was ranging from 40-60% in Seychelles, St. Vincent, St. Lucia, Grenada, and Trinidad; 10-20% in Botswana, Thailand, Kenya, Philippines, and Uganda [12].

Current smoking among school children was 3.6% (95% CI: 2.5-5.0). This prevalence has been in a steady state since 2003, despite numerous steps taken by the relevant stakeholders. According to the Global Youth Tobacco Survey (GTYS) done in Sri Lanka in 2003, the prevalence of current cigarette use among adolescents was 2.5%, while it was 1.5% (95% CI: 0.8 – 2.7) in 2016 [13, 14]. Despite having laws to control the sale of tobacco products to youth, all the students enrolled in these surveys who used tobacco were under the age of 18, which indicates ineffective implementation of tobacco control laws in the country. Further, in the present survey, of those who had ever smoked, 54.8% had their first smoke before the age of 14. According to a multicounty study done in 61 countries, the median current tobacco smoking prevalence among students aged 13–15 years was 10.7%. The highest prevalence was reported in Timor-Leste (35.0%), followed by Bulgaria (27.4%) and Lithuania (26.4%). Of the South-East Asian countries, the highest was reported in Timor-Leste (35.0%) followed by Indonesia (19.4%) and Bhutan (16.6%) [8].

The prevalence of the current use of smokeless tobacco products has a declining trend among students. According to 2011 GYTS, the prevalence of current users of smokeless tobacco among students was 8.6% (95% CI 7.1 – 10.1), but both the present study (2.3%; 95% CI 3.4-5.6) and the GYTS (2.4%; 95% CI 1.2 – 4.7) which were conducted in 2016, show significantly lower rates [14, 15]. According to a study published comparing GYTS data available in South-East Asia region, the prevalence of current use of SLT among youth varied from 5.7% in Thailand to 23.2% in Bhutan; among boys, from 7.1% in Bangladesh to 27.2% in Bhutan; and among girls, from 3.7% in Bangladesh to 19.8% in Bhutan [16].

The addictive illegal drugs commonly used in Sri Lanka are babul (areca nut from India), madana modaka (Cannabis based product), cough syrup and cannabis (ganja), with cannabis being the most widely used illicit drug [17]. In Sri Lanka, 2.7% (95% CI: 1.7-4.2) of the students currently use addictive drugs, according to the current survey. According to a UNICEF study in 2004, the prevalence of illegal substances was 2.3%, which indicates that the above-prevalence has not changed much over the last decade.

4.2. Correlates of Alcohol, Smoking, Smokeless Tobacco, and Illegal Substance Use. Multivariate analysis shows male sex and involvement in physical fighting has positive association with current use of smoking, alcohol, smokeless tobacco and illegal substances. The risk of all the substances studied in the present study was significantly higher, and similar results have been reported elsewhere in the international literature [18–20]. Seeking higher levels of sensation during the developmental stage among males compared to greater inhibitory control among females is evident [20]. Thus, males are more likely to experiment with risky behaviors, and this could be one reason for the higher risk among males.

In the current study, alcohol, smoking, and smokeless tobacco use were positively associated with age. It is stated that teenagers who started smoking were more likely to become smokers as adults and less likely to quit smoking [21]. Therefore, it is very important to address these issues at young age. Early initiation of these substances can lead to many problems such as poor school performance, school drop-outs, health problems, and future risks for substance use disorders [22, 23].

During the GSHS, the students were asked how often they see actors consuming alcohol when they watch television, videos, or movies. The current study indicates these students had 2.9 times increased risk in engaging in alcohol consumption compared to the nonexposed. A US study reveals exposing adolescents on alcohol advertising was positively related to an increase in drinking. The research concluded that individuals who saw one more advertisement on average than other individuals had 1% more alcoholic drinks per month (AOR, 1.01; 95% CI, 1.01-1.02) [24]. This highlights the importance of strict advertising regulation on movies and videos, which now include alcohol and smoking advertising.

It is well documented that when children are exposed to smoking on a daily basis or are exposed to secondhand smoking, they are at greater risk of becoming cigarette users [25]. Parental smoking increases the risk of smoking by the student by 1.8 times in the current study. A similar result was observed in a study done in Hong Kong, where having a father who smoked increased the risk of the student smoking by 2.7 times (95% CI 2.2-10.2) [26]. These examples very clearly state that children tend to follow the actions of their parents and role models.

Attempted suicide is highly associated with illegal substance abuse (AOR 6.0, 95% CI 3.0-12.0), smoking (AOR 3.4, 95% CI 1.6-7.0) and alcohol intake (AOR 3.1, 95% CI 1.5-6.2) among school children. According to Kelly et al., alcohol and drug abuse is a risk factor for attempted suicide [27]. This is a very significant association, as it clearly indicates these substances have psychogenic properties and lead to adverse effects like suicide among their users. Therefore, finding these students and referring them for counselling are essential to avoid these mental health implications. As Sri Lanka is having one of the highest suicide rates in the world, it is important to note that addressing substance and alcohol abuse among adolescents will help to reduce it.

4.3. Conclusion and Recommendations. A comparison of the study findings with existing data shows that the proportion of alcohol and smokeless tobacco consumption among schooling adolescents though the prevalence of smoking and substance use has not changed. Males and those reported as having been involved in physical fights within the past 12 months were more likely to be current users of all illicit substances. Also, it is significant to note that alcohol, smoking, and substance abuse are associated with attempted suicide, parental substance abuse, and advertising.

School-based interventions to address these issues should be designed with the goal of increasing adolescents' awareness of the various social influences that support substance abuse and teaching them specific life skills for effectively resisting both peer and media pressures to smoke, drink, or use drugs. While direct advertising of alcohol is prohibited in Sri Lanka, indirect advertising by the media and at social gatherings is still in effect. Therefore, addressing these indirect alcohol promotions and full enforcement of Framework Convention of Tobacco Control (FCTC) recommendations banning advertisements of tobacco products is also important.

4.4. Limitations of the Study. The study had following limitations. Firstly, it was conducted only among school-going adolescents, limiting the ability to generalize the findings to the entire adolescent population. In Sri Lanka nearly 1/3 of the adolescent population were identified as nonschool goers according to FHB survey [10]. As discussed in the article, the prevalence of smoking and substance misuse is likely to be higher among nonschool-attending adolescents who are exposed to many adverse circumstances. Secondly, as a cross-sectional analysis was conducted, temporal direction between associations could not be established. As the data collection was done using a self-administered questionnaire, the answers depend on the participants' interpretations of the questions.

Acknowledgments

This study was funded by the World Health Organization.

References

[1] *Census of population and housing*, Department of Census and Statistics, Miistry of Finance and Planning, Colombo, Sri Lanka, 2015.

[2] World Health Organization, *Health for the world's adolescents a second chance in the second decade*, World Health Organization, 2018, http://apps.who.int/adolescent/second-decade/.

[3] D. P. Swanson, M. C. Edwards, and M. B. Spencer, Eds., *Adolescence: development during a global era*, Elsevier Academic Press, Amsterdam, The Netherlands, 2010.

[4] D. G. Moon, M. L. Hecht, K. M. Jackson, and R. E. Spellers, "Ethnic and gender differences and similarities in adolescent drug use and refusals of drug offers," *Substance Use & Misuse*, vol. 34, no. 8, pp. 1059–1083, 1999.

[5] United Nations Office for Drug Control and Crime Prevention, *World Drug Report 2004*, United Nations Office for Drug Control and Crime Prevention, Vienna, Austria, 2004.

[6] World Health Organisation, *Global Youth Tobacco Survey Guyana Report*, World Health Organisation, 2000.

[7] American Cancer Society, *The tobacco atlas - Sri Lanka*, American Cancer Society, Sri Lanka, 2018, https://tobaccoatlas.org/country/sri-lanka/.

[8] R. A. Arrazola, I. B. Ahluwalia, E. Pun, I. G. de quevedo, S. Babb, and B. S. Armour, "Current tobacco smoking and desire to quit smoking among students aged 13-15 years — Global youth tobacco survey, 61 countries, 2012-2015," *Morbidity and Mortality Weekly Report (MMWR)*, vol. 66, no. 20, pp. 533–537, 2017.

[9] UNICEF, *National Survey on Emerging Issues among Adolescents in Sri Lanka*, UNICEF, 2004, https://www.unicef.org/srilanka/Full_Report.pdf.

[10] Family Health Bureau, *National Youth Health Survey 2012/2013 Sri Lanka*, Family Health Bureau, 2015.

[11] B. G. Simons-Morton, A. D. Crump, D. L. Haynie, and K. E. Saylor, "Studentschool bonding and adolescent problem behavior," *Health Education Research*, vol. 14, no. 1, pp. 99–107, 1999.

[12] O. Balogun, A. Koyanagi, A. Stickley, S. Gilmour, and K. Shibuya, "Alcohol consumption and psychological distress in adolescents: A multi-country study," *Journal of Adolescent Health*, vol. 54, no. 2, pp. 228–234, 2014.

[13] P. W. Gunasekara, *Report on the results of the Global Youth Tobacco Survey (GYTS–Repeat)*, World Health Organization Regional Office for South East Asia, Sri Lanka, 2003.

[14] World Health Organization, *Global Youth Tobacco Survey (GYTS) Sri Lanka 2015 Country Report*, World Health Organization, Sri Lanka, 2016, http://www.searo.who.int/tobacco/data/gyts_sri_lanka_2015_report.pdf?ua=1.

[15] Ministry of Health and Nutrition, *Global Youth Tobacco Survey (GYTS)*, Sri Lanka Factsheet, Sri Lanka, 2011.

[16] D. N. Sinha, K. M. Palipudi, C. K. Jones et al., "Levels and trends of smokeless tobacco use among youth in countries of the World Health Organization South-East Asia Region," *Indian Journal of Cancer*, vol. 51, pp. S50–S53, 2014.

[17] I. K. Liyanage, K. Wickramasinghe, H. E. Ratnayake et al., "Use of Illicit Substances Among Schoolchildren in Colombo District, Sri Lanka," *Substance Abuse*, vol. 34, no. 2, pp. 137–142, 2013.

[18] United Nations Office on Drugs and Crime, *World drug report 2014*, United Nations Office on Drugs and Crime, Vienna, Austria, 2014.

[19] M. Holmila and K. Raitasalo, "Gender differences in drinking: why do they still exist?" *Addiction*, vol. 100, no. 12, pp. 1763–1769, 2005.

[20] E. P. Shulman, K. P. Harden, J. M. Chein, and L. Steinberg, "Sex differences in the developmental trajectories of impulse control and sensation-seeking from early adolescence to early adulthood," *Journal of Youth and Adolescence*, vol. 44, no. 1, pp. 1–17, 2015.

[21] A. Rogacheva, T. Laatikainen, K. Patja, M. Paavola, K. Tossavainen, and E. Vartiainen, "Smoking and related factors of the social environment among adolescents in the Republic of Karelia," *European Journal of Public Health*, vol. 18, no. 6, pp. 630–636, 2008.

[22] J. S. Brook, R. E. Adams, E. B. Balka, and E. Johnson, "Early adolescent marijuana use: risks for the transition to young adulthood," *Psychological Medicine*, vol. 32, no. 1, Article ID S0033291701004809, pp. 79–91, 2002.

[23] J. W. Miller, T. S. Naimi, R. D. Brewer, and S. E. Jones, "Binge drinking and associated health risk behaviors among high school students," *Pediatrics*, vol. 119, no. 1, pp. 76–85, 2007.

[24] L. B. Snyder, F. F. Milici, M. Slater, H. Sun, and Y. Strizhakova, "Effects of Alcohol Advertising Exposure on Drinking Among Youth," *Archives of Pediatrics & Adolescent Medicine*, vol. 160, no. 1, pp. 18–24, 2006.

[25] Y.-H. Liu, J.-Y. Teng, Z.-X. Zheng et al., "Emodin regulates glucose uptake by activating sirtl in 3T3-L1 adipocytes," *Journal of Nanjing University of Chinese Medicine*, vol. 30, no. 6, pp. 546–549, 2014.

[26] A. Y. Loke and Y. P. I. Wong, "Smoking among young children in Hong Kong: influence of parental smoking," *Journal of Advanced Nursing*, vol. 66, no. 12, pp. 2659–2670, 2010.

[27] T. M. Kelly, J. R. Cornelius, and D. B. Clark, "Psychiatric disorders and attempted suicide among adolescents with substance use disorders," *Drug and Alcohol Dependence*, vol. 73, no. 1, pp. 87–97, 2004.

24

Determinants of Food Taboos in the Pregnant Women of the Awabel District, East Gojjam Zone, Amhara Regional State in Ethiopia

Wollelaw Getnet,[1] Wubie Aycheh,[2] and Taddele Tessema ⓘ[2]

[1]Amhara Regional Health Bureau, Debre Markos Referral Hospital, East Gojjam Zone, Debre Markos, Ethiopia
[2]Department of Public Health, College of Health Science, Debre Markos University, Debre Markos, Ethiopia

Correspondence should be addressed to Taddele Tessema; mekutaddele@gmail.com

Academic Editor: Jennifer L. Freeman

Background. Food taboos have great effect on pregnant women through prohibited essential food and/or drinks. It is transferred from generation to generation and has negative effect on pregnant mothers' health. *Objective.* To assess magnitude of food taboo and associated factors among pregnant women attending antenatal care at public health institutions in Awabel district, Northwest Ethiopia, 2016. *Methods.* Institutional based cross-sectional study was conducted. Three hundred seven pregnant women were selected for the study. All governmental health institutions in the district were included for the study. Data were entered in to Epi-Data version 3.1 and exported to SPSS version 20 for analysis. Multiple logistic regression analysis was conducted to identify independent predictors of food taboo. *Results.* Twenty-seven percent of pregnant mother encountered food taboos. Avoided food items by pregnant mothers were linseed, coffee, tea, cabbage, porridge, wheat bread, banana, pimento, groundnut, salty diet, nug, sugarcane, pumpkin, and coca drinks. Reasons mentioned for avoidance of this food items were plastered on the fetal head, making fatty baby which is difficult for delivery, fear of abortion, and fetal abnormality. Age of the mother AOR= 2.97 (1.71-5.16), income AOR= 0.28 (0.11-0.72), and previous antenatal care AOR= 2.33 (1.89-5.47) were significantly associated with food taboo. *Conclusion.* Our study revealed that considerable proportion of food taboo exists during pregnancy in the study area. This can be improved by strengthening the nutrition counseling components of antenatal care follow-up.

1. Introduction

Food taboo is abstaining people from food and/or beverage consuming due to religious and cultural reasons [1]. It can be permanent or temporal. Permanent food taboos are avoiding food and/or drinks throughout their life, while some foods are avoided for certain periods of time. These restrictions often apply to women and are related to the reproduction cycle (during pregnancy, birth, and lactation periods) [2].

Pregnant women have faced dietary deficiency due to food taboo. Some pregnant women, who live in rural area, are obliged to have food taboo that restrain calorie and specific nutrients [3]. Although in the real scenario pregnancy requires more calorie, some food items are considered to be good or bad by the community during pregnancy [4]. Food taboos among pregnant women are varying from culture to culture and community to community especially in rural settings. Pregnant women who were practicing food taboos had significance on lower body weight and unhealthier babies [5, 6].

Food taboos have influence on pregnancy even though they need about 300 extra calories per day, especially during the later pregnancy period. When a baby grows quickly, additional calories should come from nutritious foods, so they can contribute to baby's growth and development [7]. The major problem of food taboos is preventing pregnant women from accessing a well-balanced diet, resulting in high prevalence of low birth weight and harm to mother and baby.

Seven percent of disability particularly sight loss and limb malformation is believed to be caused by broken food taboo [8].

Food taboos have an effect on nutritional status of children and women in Ethiopia. The health sector is better to increase its effort to enhance good nutritional practice through health education, treatment of extremely malnourished children, and provision of micronutrients to mother and children. Government's Health Sector Development Plan IV (HSDP IV) (2010/11-2014/15) continues to improve the nutritional status of pregnant mother and children through the following programmers: Enhanced Outreach Strategy (EOS) with Targeted Supplementary Food (TSF) and Transitioning of EOS into the Health Extension Program (HEP), Health Facility Nutrition Service, Community Based Nutrition (CBN), and Micronutrient Intervention and Essential Nutrition Actions [9].

Any country in the world has food taboo due to different factors like culture, norm, and religion. The food taboo is also differing from place to place and time to time. Each religion has its own food taboo [10]. Food taboos during pregnancy are influenced by different factors like dietary counseling, whether attending antenatal care (ANC) clinic or not, younger age, less educational status, and multiparous and pregnant women. Culture and belief also influence maternal eating pattern during pregnancy [11]. Food taboos on pregnant women usually lead to having low nutritional status and put them at high risk of maternal death. For instance, the mean height of Ethiopian women is 156 cm, which shows severe past malnutrition and puts them at high risk during delivery [5].

Study conducted in Ghana has focused on dietary habit of pregnant women but has not addressed the intake of specific nutrient; especially micronutrient had effect on pregnancy and resulted in complication or not [1]. Consistent evidence supported the fact that Ethiopian women dietary status and habits during pregnancy and nutrient intake were assessed [5]; however, prohibition of food during pregnancy in the study area was not addressed. Maintaining well nutritional status of pregnant women and keeping their health are important by assessing the gap about food taboo. This will give scientific evidence for policy maker and programmers to design possible strategy, to address the problem, furthermore, for the health care workers to intervene based on the finding of the study.

2. Method and Materials

2.1. Study Area, Setting, and Period. The study was conducted in Awabel district, East Gojjam Zone, Amhara Region, Ethiopia. Awabel district is 40 km from Debre Markos in the Southeast and 259 km from Addis Ababa in the Northwest and 306 km from Bahir Dar in the Southwest. The district has 5 urban and 15 rural kebeles, six health centers, and one district hospital. It has 137,000 total population. The study was conducted from April 15 to May 17, 2016.

2.2. Study Design and Population. Institutional based cross-sectional study was conducted among women attending ANC follow-up from all governmental heath institutions in the district.

2.3. Sample Size and Sampling Technique. The sample size determination was used with the assumption of confidence level =95%, critical value Z=1.96 (from significance level α=5%), and degree of precision=0.05, by taking 49.8% proportion from Shashmene district study about food taboo [5]. Then the sample size was calculated using the formula for single population proportion.

$n_0 = (S_{0/2})^2. \ P \ (1-p)/W^2 = (1.96)^2. \ (0.498). \ (0.502)/(0.05)^2 = 384$, where n_0 is sample size calculated as follows. Since the target population in the study area was less than 10,000 (i.e., 1250), we use the formula $n = n_0/1 + n_0/N$, where N is the number of pregnant women:

=384/ (1 + 384/1250) =293.

Then we can take/add 5% for nonresponse rate 293*5/100=14.

So, total sample size was 307.

2.4. Sampling Procedure. Based on the previous ANC follow-up number, the sample was allocated for each health institution. So from each of the six health centers we should expect to collect 37 samples and from the primary hospital 82 samples. Sequential sampling technique was used to select study participants. According to the sample size in each health institution samples were taken.

2.5. Data Collection Methods. An interview administered pretested Amharic language questionnaire prepared in English was used. To avoid information contamination, pretest was done on 5% women attending ANC follow-up on the near health center and its finding was used to modify the tool. Data collectors were briefed about the purpose of the study and data were collected after a verbal informed consent obtained from participants. Data collection process was facilitated by seven midwifery professional data collector and two BSc midwives.

2.6. Data Quality Assurance. Data quality was assured through careful design of the questionnaire. Data collector and supervisors were trained one day about the purpose of the study, the questionnaire in detail, the data collection procedure, the data collection setting, and the rights of study participants. Pretest was done prior to the actual data collection.

2.7. Data Processing and Analysis. Data were checked for completeness and consistency and entered in to Epi-Data version 3.1 and then exported to SPSS version 20 for analysis. Descriptive analysis was carried out to determine the magnitude of food taboo. Bivariate logistic regression analysis which was performed for each independent variable with the outcome of interest at $p < 0.05$ was considered statistically significant. Finally multiple logistic regression analysis was conducted to determine independent predictors of food taboo.

TABLE 1: Sociodemographic characteristics of ANC follow-up women in Awabel district, Northwest Ethiopia, April 15-May 17, 2016 (n=307).

Variables		Frequency	Percentage
Age group	15-19 years	49	16.3
	20-24 years	134	44.7
	25-29 years	93	31.0
	≥30 years	24	8.0
Religion	Orthodox	261	87.0
	Muslim	39	13.0
Ethinicity	Amhara	273	91.0
	Oromo	27	9.0
Educationl Status	Cannot read and write	141	47.0
	Can read and write	68	22.7
	Primary school	15	5.0
	secondary school	33	11.0
	College diploma and above	43	14.3
Occupation mother	Farmer	170	56.7
	Government employee	46	15.3
	Merchant	55	18.3
	Housewife	29	9.7
Marital status	Married	289	96.3
	Unmarried	11	3.7
Number of deliver	Primi	161	53.7
	Two times	80	26.7
	Three times	40	13.3
	=/> 4 times	19	6.3
Income	<650birr	140	46.7
	651-1000birr	64	21.3
	1001-1500birr	44	14.7
	≥1500birr	52	17.3
Educational status of husband	Cannot read &write	147	49.0
	Can read and write	87	29.0
	Complete primary and secondary school	26	8.6
	College diploma & above	40	13.4
Previous ANC attendance	Yes	224	74.7
	No	76	25.3
Residence	Rural	239	79.7
	Urban	61	20.3

2.8. Ethical Consideration. The study was conducted after securing approval of proposal by Debre Markos University, Medicine and Health Sciences College Ethical Review Committee. Written permission was obtained from Awabel Administrative Health Office for Selected Health Centers. All the study participants were informed about the purpose of the study and finally verbal consent was obtained before interview. The study participants have the right to refuse participation or terminate their involvement at any point when the interview was secured.

3. Results

3.1. Sociodemographic Characteristics. Among 307 respondents, data were collected from 300 pregnant women; this made the response rate 97.7%.

About 87% of the respondents were orthodox Christian and 91% were from Amhara ethnicity. Around 50% of the pregnant women were illiterate and 79.4% of the pregnant women lived in rural areas (Table 1).

3.2. Food Taboos during Pregnancy. Twenty-seven percent of respondent avoid three or more food/drink items during pregnancy. Twelve food and/or drink items were prohibited by the study participants.

3.2.1. Fruits and Vegetables. Certain fruit and vegetables were taboo during pregnancy such as banana 107 (35.7%), pimento 96 (32%), cabbage 73 (24.3%), and sugarcane 133 (44.3%). Pregnant women believed that the reason for the taboo is that when they consumed banana, something is attached to the head of the fetus, pimento burns the fetus, cabbage disturbs the fetus, and sugarcane increases the seminal fluids (Figure 1).

3.2.2. Cereals and Salty Diet. The result of this study indicated that cereals were taboos like linseed (16.3%), pumpkin (42.7%), nug (32.3%), wheat (28.3%), groundnut (13.7%), and salty diets (11.7%). The study participants avoid pumpkin and ground nut because they assumed that these foods increase

TABLE 2: Determinants of food taboo in public health institution in Awabel district, Northwest Ethiopia, April 15-May 17, 2016 (n=307).

Variables		Having food taboo		COR(95%CI)	AOR (95%CI)	P-Value
		Yes	No			
Age of the mother	15-19 years	11	38	1.00	1.00	
	20-24 years	40	94	0.68(0.316,0.464)	2.971(1.711,5.159)	0.001
	25-29 years	28	65	0.672(0.301,0.502)	3.358(1.638,6.886)	0.001
	≥30 years	2	22	3.18(1.646,15.70)	12.716(2.429,66.58)	0.003
Income of the mother	<650biir	21	119	1.00	1.00	
	650-1000birr	22	42	0.337(0.168,0.674)	0.290(0.132,0.638)	0.002
	1001-1500birr	16	28	0.309(0.143,0.667)	0.281(0.111,0.715)	0.008
	≥1500 birr	22	30	0.241(0.117,0.494)	0.330(0.117,0.929)	0.036
Previous ANC attendants	Yes	63	18	1.00	1.00	
	No	161	58	1.22(1.89,5.408)	2.33(1.257,4.336)	0.007

Note: COR: crude odds ratio; AOR: adjusted odds ratio; CI: confidence interval.

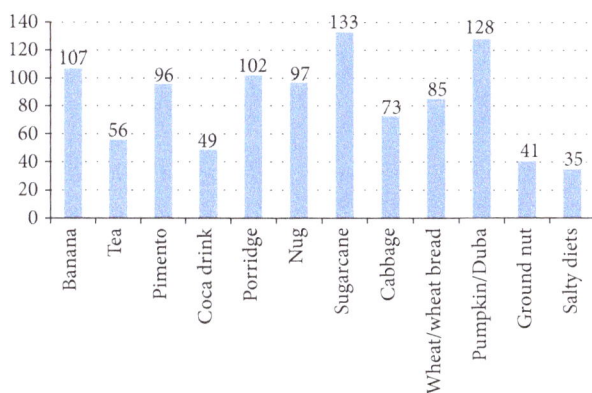

Y-axis Number of pregnant women involved in food taboo

X-axis List of food items

FIGURE 1: Food taboo in ANC attendants in each food items/drinks in Awabel district, Northwest, Ethiopia, April 15-May 17, 2016.

the weight of the fetus, making it difficult to deliver, linseed causes loss strength of the fetus, and nug changes the color of the fetus and makes it black.

3.2.3. Drinks. Drinks like coffee (19%), tea (18.7%), coca (16.3%), and porridge (34%) were restricted due to burning the fetus and causing abnormality and coca drink causes abortion.

These foods were restricted by the following reasons: banana (believing that something is attached to the head), pimento (burning the fetus), cabbage (disturbing the fetus), and sugarcane (increasing the fluids during delivery); coffee and tea were restricted due to burning the fetus and causing abnormality; coca drink causes abortion; pumpkin and ground nut increase the weight of the fetus making it difficult to deliver. Most of pregnant women avoid foods due to plaster on the fetal head, making fatty baby, difficult for delivery, fear of abortion, and fetal abnormality.

3.3. Determinants of Food Taboos in the Pregnant Women. Pregnant women whose age is 20-24 years were 2.97 times

more likely to develop food taboo compared with the age between 15 and 19 years (AOR=2.97, 95% CI: 1.71-5.16); pregnant women who earned 650-1000 birr are 56% less likely to have food taboo compared to pregnant women who have <650-birr monthly income (AOR =0.29, 95% CI: 0.13-0.64); and pregnant women who never have ANC attendance in the health institution were 2.33 times more likely to develop food taboo as compared with pregnant women who have ANC attendance (AOR= 2.3, 95% CI: 1.26-4.34) (Table 2).

4. Discussion

The finding of this study revealed that 27% of study participants had food taboo which is less than the proportion of food taboo in different studies done, in Shashmene district (49.8%) [4].

More than three-fourths (82.1%) of participants in North Costal Paradesh and nearly half (48%) of participants in Surendranagar had food taboo which are higher than our findings [5, 6].

The possible difference may be because of study time, study area, and increase in the knowledge of the mother in the time of the study. In this study, some fruits were avoided even though they are important in the period of pregnancy. Based on this study, banana has not been eaten by 107(35.7%) of pregnant women which is not comparable with the study conducted in Hydya Zone (8.6%). This discrepancy may be due to the study area, culture, and time difference [12].

Ground nut in this study was 13.7% which is in line with the study done in Shashmene (13.6%) [4]. Age of the mother in bivariate regression analysis was significantly associated with food taboos; as age of the mother is increased, adoption of the food taboo is increased. Pregnant women whose age is 20-24 years were 6.8 times more likely to develop food taboos compared with age between 15 and 19 years (COR=8.6, 95% CI: 0.32-0.46)

In multivariate regression analysis, age of the mother was significantly associated with food taboo. As the age of the mother is increased, adoption of the food taboo is increased. Pregnant women whose age is 20-24 years were 2.97 times more likely to develop food taboos compared with the age between 15 and 19 years (AOR=2.97, 95% CI: 1.71-5.16). This study is almost similar to the study in Shashmene [4]. The possible explanation may be that younger women more likely accept modern education and older women have indigenous knowledge.

Previous ANC attendance of study participant is significantly associated with food taboo. Pregnant women who have never had ANC attendance in the health institution were 2.33 times more likely to develop food taboo as compared with pregnant women who have had ANC attendance. This result is comparable with the study conducted in Shashmene [4]. This may be due to the knowledge gained from formal education and experienced health education. In this study, income was significantly associated with food taboo. Pregnant women who earned 650-1000 birr were 56% less likely to have food taboo compared to pregnant women who have <650-birr monthly income, which is in line with the study done in Wondo Genet [12], Bangladesh [13], and Ogan state of Nigeria [14]. As income increases, the avoidance of food taboos decreases.

5. Conclusion

There were low proportion of food taboos in the study area and were obligated to avoid specific food items due to cultural and traditional view. Women, who were of old age, had low income, and had not had previous ANC attendance, were more practicing food taboos.

The food and drink items, which were avoided during pregnancy, were linseed, cabbage, banana, sugarcane, pumpkin/duba, nug, tea, coffee, porridge, coca drink, groundnut, pimento, and salty diets. Reasons which avoid food were plastered on the fetal head, fatty baby, fear of abortion, and fetal abnormality. Age of the mother, income, and previous ANC attendance had significant association with food taboos.

Based on the finding, the following recommendations were forwarded:

(I) Midwives had better work more for creating awareness about food taboos. Women, who had food taboos, assess the reasons and provide health education about the use of appropriate nutrition.

(II) Governmental, nongovernmental organization and various public associations had been better actively involved in eliminating harmful beliefs.

(III) Health education program had better taken cognizance of the popular beliefs regarding food taboos during pregnancy and used innovative means to minimize their negative and maximize their positive nutritional effects.

(IV) The health professionals, who work in Awabel District Health Institutions, had better created awareness for pregnant women who have ANC follow-up to minimize food taboos.

Authors' Contributions

Wollelaw Getnet, Wubie Aycheh, and Taddele Tessema were participated in proposal writing, analyzing the data, and drafting the paper. Taddele Tessema prepared the manuscript for publication. All authors revised subsequent drafts of the paper.

Acknowledgments

The authors' deep gratitude goes to Debre Markos University, College of Medicine and Health Sciences, for proper review and approval of this paper. The authors would also like to extend their gratitude to Awabel district health workers, data collectors, and supervisors for valuable contribution for the success of this study.

References

[1] "Harmful traditional practices affecting the health of women and children," *Factsheet No 23*, vol. 10, 1997.

[2] O. Esther, *Relation of dietary and socio economic characteristics of mothers to child growth [Master thesis]*, 2008.

[3] P. Rajkumar and M. A. Vedapriya, "Taboos and misconceptions about food during pregnancy among rural population of pondichery," *Calicut Medical Journal*, vol. 8, no. 2, p. 1, 2010.

[4] N. Biza Zepro, "Food Taboos and Misconceptions Among Pregnant Women of Shashemene District, Ethiopia, 2012," *Science Journal of Public Health*, vol. 3, no. 3, p. 410, 2015.

[5] A. Parmar and G. H. Khanpara, "A study on taboos and misconceptions associated with pregnancy among rural women of Surendranagar district," *Healthline*, vol. 2, p. 40, 2013.

[6] Lakshmi, "Food preference and taboos during ANC among the tribal women," *Journal of community nutrition and health*, vol. 2, no. 2, p. 33, 2013.

[7] K. A. Samson, "Common food taboos and beliefs during pregnancy in Yilokrobo district, Ghana," *Science Journal of Public Health*, vol. 2, no. 3, p. 41, 2014.

[8] J. DelmaPaofa, N. Kaugla, T. Catherina et al., "Food taboos and traditional customs among pregnant women in Papua New Guinea: Missed opportunity for education in antenatal clinics," *Research Journal reproductive health*, vol. 8, no. 1, p. 6, 2013.

[9] Central Statistical Agency, *Ethiopia Mini Demographic and Health Survey*, vol. 56, Addis Ababa, Ethiopia, 2014.

[10] J. T. Liu, "Taboos in Food Practices during Pre and Post-natal: A Comparative Study between Tribal and Non- Tribal Women in Odisha," *Journal of reproductive health*, vol. 2, no. 3, pp. 141–152, 2015.

[11] O. A. Oni and J. Tukur, "Identifying pregnant women who would adhere to food taboos in a rural community: a community-based study.," *African Journal of Reproductive Health*, vol. 16, no. 3, pp. 68–76, 2012.

[12] D. Kuche, P. Singh, and D. Moges, "Dietary Practices And Associated Factors among Pregnant Women in Wondo Genet District, Southern Ethiopia: A Cross-Sectional Study," *Journal*

of Pharmaceutical & Scientific Innovation, vol. 4, no. 5, pp. 270–275, 2015.

[13] H. B, "Nutritional Status of Pregnant Women in Selected Rural and Urban Area of Bangladesh," *Journal of Nutrition & Food Sciences*, vol. 03, no. 04, 2013.

[14] O. S. Oluwafolahan, A. B. Catherine, and A. J. Olubukunola, "Dietary habits of pregnant women in Ogun-East Senatorial Zone, Ogun State, Nigeria: A comparative study," *International Journal of Nutrition and Metabolism*, vol. 6, no. 4, pp. 42–49, 2014.

25

Skilled Birth Attendance among Women in Tharaka-Nithi County, Kenya

Eliphas Gitonga

School of Public Health, Kenyatta University, Nairobi, Kenya

Correspondence should be addressed to Eliphas Gitonga; eliphasg@gmail.com

Academic Editor: Julio Diaz

Background. The burden of maternal mortality is concentrated in sub-Saharan Africa with an estimation of 500 000 deaths annually. In 2012, about forty million births occurred without a skilled attendant in developing countries. Skilled birth attendance improves maternal and newborn survival. The aim of this study therefore was to establish the level of skilled birth attendance and the associated factors. *Methods.* A cross-sectional survey was carried out using structured questionnaires as tools of data collection. Systematic sampling was used to select the respondents from the facilities that were stratified. The dependent variable was skilled birth attendance. Descriptive statistics were used to generate proportions and percentages while chi-square and Fisher's exact tests were used to draw inferences. Association was significant if $P < 0.05$. *Results.* The level of utilisation of skilled birth attendance was 77%. Skilled birth attendance was noted to be associated with age, level of education, average family income, parity, distance to the health facility, timing of initiation of antenatal care, level of facility attended during pregnancy, and birth preparedness status. *Conclusion.* The level of skilled birth attendance among women in Tharaka-Nithi County, Kenya, despite being higher than in some counties, requires improvement.

1. Introduction

Maternal mortality in Kenya is 362 per 100 000 live births. This is high according to the World Health Organisation that rates figures above 300 deaths per 100 000 live births as high. Skilled birth attendance (SBA) is one of the proven interventions that can reduce maternal mortality [1]. A skilled attendant is an accredited health professional such as a midwife, doctor, or nurse who has been educated and trained to proficiency in the skills needed to manage normal (uncomplicated) pregnancies, childbirth, and the immediate postnatal period and in the identification and management/referral of complications in women and newborns [2]. Countries like Malaysia, Sri Lanka, Thailand, and Egypt reduced at times by half the maternal mortality ratio within ten years by increasing the level of skilled birth attendance. This illustrates the impact of skilled birth attendance [3].

Maternal health is part of the social pillar in Kenya Vision 2030. It is planned that, for Kenya to achieve the vision of middle income economy by 2030, all efforts should be made to reduce maternal mortality. Skilled birth attendance

(SBA) is one of the key strategies that were adopted. It has been identified by the Kenyan government as one of the high impact interventions to reduce maternal deaths. Several initiatives including training and recruitment are underway to increase the number of skilled birth attendants. This is being coupled by improvement of infrastructure in the health facilities [1]. Tharaka-Nithi is one of the 47 counties in Kenya. According to the Kenya Health and Demographic Survey 2014/15, it is one of the middle performers in uptake of skilled birth attendance at 77%. Kiambu County is the highest at 93% while Wajir County is the lowest at 18% [4]. The main aim of this study was to establish the level and the associated factors of skilled birth attendance among women in Tharaka-Nithi County, Kenya.

2. Methods

2.1. Study Design and Target Population. This was a cross-sectional study targeting women who had delivered within a year during the study period.

2.2. Setting. The study was done in Tharaka-Nithi County, Kenya. It has four subcounties: Maara, Chuka/Igamba-ngo'mbe, Tharaka North, and Tharaka South. The county falls in the former eastern province. The county has a total population of 365,330 and a surface area of 2639 km^2. It has only sixty-one kilometres of bitumen (tarmac) road [5]. Tharaka South subcounty was the site of study and has only 7 km of tarmac road. The study was done among women within a catchment area of Nkondi, Lukenya, and Kamwathu dispensaries, Kibung'a, Tunyai, and Chiakariga health centres, Marimanti Level Four Hospital, and St. Orsola Matiri hospitals.

2.3. Variables. The independent variables were age, level of education, distance to the health facility, type of facility attended for antenatal care (level 2: dispensary; level 3: health centre; level 4: hospitals), family income, gravida, parity, uptake of focused antenatal care, timing of booking of antenatal care, and status of birth preparedness. The dependent variable was skilled birth attendance for the previous pregnancy. It is defined for the use in this study as a delivery that occurs in the health facility with necessary equipment and is attended by an approved health worker according to the World Health Organisation (WHO). It was dichotomised as "skilled birth attendance" and "nonskilled birth attendance."

2.4. Sampling, Data Collection, and Data Analysis. Stratified sampling was used to select the health facilities on the basis of ensuring that all the levels of the facilities were represented. The strata included the dispensaries, health centres, and hospitals. They all offer maternal and child health services. Systematic sampling was used to select the respondents. The sample size was 345 respondents determined using Kothari's (2004) formula. Semistructured questionnaires were the instruments for data collection. A pilot study was done at Nkarini mobile clinic to assess the reliability of the tools. Test-retest method was used to achieve validity. Administration was done by trained research assistants under the supervision of the principal investigator. Data was entered in Stata version 11 for analysis. Descriptive statistics, mainly percentages, were initially used after which inferences statistics were applied. Chi-square and Fisher's exact tests were the two statistical tests that were used to draw inferences (associations between the dependent and independent variables).

2.5. Ethical and Logistical Considerations. Ethical approval was sought from Kenyatta University Ethics and Review Committee. A research permit was obtained from the National Commission for Science Technology (NACOSTI-Kenya) and Innovation. Permission was granted by the heads of health facilities and informed consent was obtained from the respondents. Confidentiality was assured and maintained in the entire data collection period.

3. Results

3.1. Skilled Birth Attendance. The objective of this analysis was to establish the proportion of respondents whose deliveries occurred under skilled birth attendance. Skilled birth

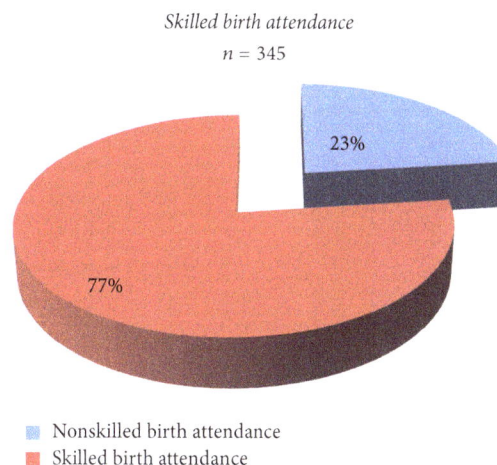

FIGURE 1: Skilled birth attendance.

attendance was deemed to have occurred if the delivery was attended in a health facility with requisite equipment and an approved health worker as prescribed by the World Health Organisation (WHO). Majority (77%) of the three hundred and forty-five women had skilled birth attendance in their most recent delivery. A birth was deemed recent if it occurred within one year of the study. Because of recall bias, births that occurred beyond a year were excluded. A small proportion (23%) delivered either at home, on the way to a health facility, or in a health facility without a skilled birth attendant. Figure 1 shows the proportion of women who had skilled birth attendance.

3.2. Demographic and Institutional Factors Associated with Skilled Birth Attendance. The analysis in this section was to establish the association between demographic/institutional factors that are associated with skilled birth attendance (SBA). Age in years, level of education, family income, and facility attended during antenatal care were found to be associated with SBA. The proportion of women delivering under SBA was the highest among women aged 20–24 years (90%) followed by those aged 25–29 years (80%). It was the lowest among women aged 40–44 years (50%). The proportion of women delivering under SBA increased with the increase in the level of education. This comparative increase was also noted with the increase in the level of income. There was a significant association between the distance to the health facility and skilled birth attendance ($P < 0.001$). Women who attended their antenatal care in a hospital had a higher proportion of delivering under SBA compared to those who used dispensaries for their pregnancy care. Table 1 shows the demographic and institutional factors associated with skilled birth attendance.

3.3. Pregnancy Related Factors Associated with Skilled Birth Attendance. The analysis in this section was done to establish the association between pregnancy related factors that are associated with SBA. The increase in the number of pregnancies (gravida) and deliveries (parity) decreases the proportion of women delivering under SBA. Attendance of

TABLE 1: Demographic and institutional factors associated with skilled birth attendance.

Variable	Group	Nonskilled birth attendance	Skilled birth attendance	Statistical values
Age in years ($N = 345$)	Below 20	9 (28%)	23 (72%)	$\chi^2(5) = 31.32$ $P \leq 0.001$
	20–24	10 (10%)	94 (90%)	
	25–29	16 (20%)	65 (80%)	
	30–34	13 (23%)	44 (77%)	
	35–39	20 (43%)	27 (57%)	
	40–44	12 (50%)	12 (50%)	
Level of education ($N = 345$)	No formal education	11 (58%)	8 (42%)	$\chi^2(2) = 17.05$ $P \leq 0.001$
	Primary education	60 (23%)	196 (77%)	
	Secondary education and above	9 (13%)	61 (87%)	
Family monthly income (Kshs) ($N = 345$)	Below 1000	44 (32%)	93 (68%)	$\chi^2(2) = 13.76$ $P \leq 0.001$
	1000–5000	32 (20%)	124 (79%)	
	Above 5000	4 (8%)	48 (92%)	
Distance to health facility ($N = 345$)	More than 5 km	54 (18%)	238 (82%)	$\chi^2(1) = 23.53$ $P \leq 0.001$
	Within 5 km	26 (49%)	27 (51%)	
Facility attended during ANC ($N = 327$)	Dispensary	15 (21%)	56 (79%)	$\chi^2(2) = 11.66$ $P = 0.003$
	Health centre	26 (31%)	59 (69%)	
	Hospital	22 (13%)	149 (87%)	

TABLE 2: Pregnancy related factors associated with skilled birth attendance.

Variable	Group	Nonskilled birth attendance	Skilled birth attendance	Statistical values
Gravida ($n = 345$)	1-2	32 (17%)	159 (83%)	$\chi^2(2) = 31.72$ $P \leq 0.001$
	3-4	15 (17%)	72 (83%)	
	5+	33 (49%)	34 (51%)	
Parity ($n = 345$)	1-2	33 (17%)	163 (83%)	$\chi^2(2) = 27.19$ $P \leq 0.001$
	3-4	17 (20%)	70 (80%)	
	5+	30 (48%)	32 (52%)	
Attendance of focused antenatal care ($n = 345$)	No	56 (34%)	110 (66%)	$\chi^2(1) = 19.98$ $P \leq 0.001$
	Yes	24 (13%)	155 (87%)	
Trimester of ANC booking ($n = 327$)	3rd	26 (36%)	47 (64%)	$\chi^2(2) = 16.17$ $P \leq 0.001$
	2nd	31 (14%)	184 (86%)	
	1st	6 (15%)	33 (85%)	
Birth preparedness ($n = 345$)	Unprepared	73 (27%)	202 (73%)	$\chi^2(2) = 8.58$ $P = 0.003$
	Prepared	7 (10%)	63 (90%)	

four or more antenatal visits in a targeted manner (focused antenatal care) resulted in a higher proportion of women delivering under SBA (87%). Booking of antenatal clinics in the first and second trimester resulted in a higher proportion of women delivering under SBA compared to booking in the third trimester. Birth preparedness encompassed planning for place of delivery, means of transport, skilled birth attendance, funds for the process, and caretaker of the family during the delivery time. Birth preparedness was associated with SBA (90%) compared to nonpreparedness. Table 2 shows the pregnancy related factors associated with skilled birth attendance.

4. Discussion

The main aim of the study was to establish the uptake of skilled birth attendance and the factors associated with it. The proportion of skilled birth attendance was average among the study respondents. The uptake of skilled birth attendance at Tharaka South subcounty is similar to that in Tharaka-Nithi County at 77%. This means that more than 20% still deliver at home despite the risks to the mother and to the baby. The level of skilled birth attendance was higher than the national proportion that is at 62% [1]. It is still higher than the national proportion of rural women that is at 50%. The national figure is lowered by marginalised and hardship counties like Wajir (18%) and Tana River (32%) but also boosted by counties like Mombasa at 82% and Kiambu at 93% [4]. This finding is also higher than that found in Makueni County, Kenya [6], which was found to be at 44%. In a follow-up study in 2012 in Makueni County, it was found to be at 37% [7]. The difference may be explained by the difference in approaches of study. A study in West Pokot, Kenya, found the uptake to be much lower at 33%. West Pokot County has fewer health facilities and long distances to cover to access care which may explain the lower levels of uptake. The general socioeconomic status is low in the county coupled by poor transport/communication infrastructure. Women in these environments opt for home deliveries because of the logistical and economic limitations [8].

Skilled birth attendance is associated with age, level of education, type of employment, average family income, level of facility attended during antenatal care (dispensary, health centre, or hospital), timing of initiation of antenatal care, distance to the health facility, birth preparedness status, and parity.

An increase in age is also associated with an increase in parity. Women with advanced age may have had negative experiences in their previous hospital visits for delivery and thereby chose home deliveries. In studies in Ghana, it was found that women aged 15–19 years were more likely to deliver under skilled birth attendance compared to those aged 40–45 years [9]. Education influences decision-making. It also improves the ability to assess risks of home deliveries. Educated women are also able to synthesise the information given in health facilities or accessed in media platforms. This concurs with the findings of the Ministry of health, Kenya, where only a quarter of women without education were attended by skilled birth attendants during birth while more than 85% delivered under SBA [1]. Education has been noted in previous studies as a positive predicator of birth preparedness [10], health facility delivery [11], and focused antenatal care [12]. In South Ethiopia, education was noted to influence both skilled birth attendance and birth preparedness. Women with a higher level of education were noted to more likely prepare for birth and deliver under SBA [13].

Average family income is linked to economic status. The economic status is associated with skilled birth attendance. Birth is accompanied with costs (hospital charges, transport fees, and supplies for the baby). The ability to meet these costs influences the decision on skilled birth attendance. This agrees with findings in West Pokot County, Kenya [8]. Women in Ghana in a higher wealth index had greater autonomy in decision-making on reproductive health and more likely delivered under skilled birth attendance [9].

Distance to the health facility has implications on cost and time spent to the health facility. It by extension influences the decision to deliver in a health facility or not. Some women at times deliver on the way to the health facility due to long distances. A study in West Pokot, Kenya, found concurring results [8]. An analysis of Kenya Demographic and Health Survey 2008-2009 indicated that physical access to health facilities through distance and/or lack of transport

and economic considerations are important barriers to SBA. Access to appropriate transport for mothers in labour and improving the experiences and outcomes for mothers using health facilities at childbirth augmented by health education may increase the uptake of health facility delivery in Kenya [14]. In a related study in Makueni County, Kenya, the type of transport used to the place of delivery was associated with the place of delivery. Access to a vehicle for transport at the onset of labour was associated with a 24-fold increase in utilisation of a healthcare facility for delivery compared to other modes of transportation. The two logistical barriers to skilled birth attendance were availability and cost of transportation. For women to deliver in the presence of a skilled birth attendant, they may need support with transport and cost of services [15].

Parity (number of births) and the number of pregnancies were found to be associated with skilled birth attendance. This may be associated with previous experiences. Women who have had negative experiences and outcomes following health facility deliveries at times choose to deliver at home. There is also a category of women who have had no complications following home deliveries. This group may perceive home deliveries to be safer, though it may just be by chance. Delivery is associated with unseen complications that may not be managed at home when they set in. An occurrence, for example, of disseminated intravascular coagulation is a big risk to life that traditional birth attendants or other assistants at home may not manage because of requisite skills and facilities. This may lead to maternal death. This is consistent with other studies that have found that an increase in pregnancies and births decreases the chances of health facility deliveries [13]. Maternal mortality has been found to be higher among women with high parity [16].

Focused antenatal care, which is the attendance of at least targeted visits, was found to be associated with skilled birth attendance. The targeted visits increase the contact time of the women and the health workers for effective counselling and prompt intervention of any complications. Targeted visits place emphasis on skilled birth attendance especially during booking and the fourth visit. This is consistent with findings in a study in Ethiopia [13]. This finding also concurs with multicountry analysis on the association of antenatal care and skilled birth attendance. It was found especially in Kenya and Tanzania that the amount and quality of antenatal care have an influence on the uptake of skilled birth attendance. Quality of care and uptake of at least four antenatal visits have a positive effect on SBA [16].

Booking antenatal care early (first trimester) was noted in this study to be associated with skilled birth attendance. Early booking gives provision for more time to achieve a variety of objectives of antenatal care. This includes counselling on birth preparedness and significance of skilled birth attendance. Uptake of focused antenatal care is also feasible because of the time remaining before birth.

Birth preparedness was also noted to be associated with skilled birth attendance. The various aspects of birth preparedness could be associated with skilled birth attendance. For instance, saving money for delivery expenses and arranging for transport are expected to enable one to reach the health facility. Identifying a skilled birth attendant early enough can also ensure that one is attended by one during delivery. Birth preparedness is one of the community strategies to reduce the two delays in accessing healthcare. When a woman is prepared for birth, she is likely to make swift decisions in seeking and reaching care. The finding in this study relates to those published on determinants of health facility delivery in Eastern Kenya where birth preparedness was found to be one of the key predictors [11]. A study in South Ethiopia on the association of birth preparedness and skilled birth attendance indicated similar findings where the probability of skilled birth attendance was increased by birth preparedness [13]. Birth preparedness uses a participatory approach where the health worker discusses with the women early enough their birth plans. It also involves the family and the community especially in the resource mobilisation part. Some resources are communal like means of transport. This involvement could be part of what results in better outcomes contrary to approaches that were unidirectional.

5. Conclusion

This study has shown that the level of skilled birth attendance is high (77%). Skilled birth attendance is associated with age, level of education, average family income, parity, distance to the health facility, timing of initiation of antenatal care, level of facility attended during pregnancy, and birth preparedness status.

Additional Points

The national and county governments in collaboration with health stakeholders should initiate measures to sensitise and increase the uptake of skilled birth attendance among rural women.

References

[1] Ministry of Health, "Kenya Reproductive, Maternal, Newborn, Child And Adolescent Health (Rmncah) Investment Framework," 2016, Nairobi, MOH.

[2] WHO, "Making pregnancy safer," WHO, Geneva.

[3] U. Högberg, "The World Health Report 2005: "Make every mother and child count"—Including Africans," *Scandinavian Journal of Public Health*, vol. 33, no. 6, pp. 409–411, 2005.

[4] KNBS, *Kenya Health and Demographic Survey 2014*, KNBS, Nairobi, Kenya, 2015.

[5] "Commission for revenue allocation," 2011, Kenya County facts, CRA.

[6] A. Gitimu, C. Herr, H. Oruko et al., "Determinants of use of skilled birth attendant at delivery in Makueni, Kenya: A cross sectional study," *BMC Pregnancy and Childbirth*, vol. 15, no. 1, article no. 9, 2015.

[7] H. Kimani, C. Farquhar, and P. Wanzala, "Determinants of delivery by skilled birth attendants among pregnant women in Makueni county, Kenya," *Public Health Research*, vol. 5, no. 1, pp. 1–6, 2015.

[8] J. O. Ogolla, "Factors associated with home delivery in west pokot county of Kenya," *Advances in Public Health*, vol. 2015, Article ID 493184, pp. 1–6, 2015.

[9] E. K. Ameyaw, A. Tanle, K. Kissah-Korsah, and J. Amo-Adjei, "Women's health decision-making autonomy and skilled birth attendance in Ghana," *International Journal of Reproductive Medicine*, vol. 2016, Article ID 6569514, 9 pages, 2016.

[10] E. Gitonga, M. Keraka, and P. Mwaniki, "Birth preparedness among women in Tharaka Nithi County, Kenya," *African Journal of Midwifery and Women's Health*, vol. 9, no. 4, pp. 153–157, 2015.

[11] E. Gitonga and M. Felarmine, "Determinants of health facility delivery among women in Tharaka Nithi County," *The Pan African Medical Journal*, vol. 2, supplement 2, p. 9, 2016.

[12] E. Gitonga, "Determinants of focused antenatal care uptake among women in tharaka nithi county, Kenya," *Advances in Public Health*, vol. 2017, Article ID 3685401, pp. 1–4, 2017.

[13] Y. Lakew, F. Tessema, and C. Hailu, "Birth preparedness and its association with skilled birth attendance and postpartum checkups among mothers in Gibe Wereda, Hadiya Zone, South Ethiopia," *Journal of Environmental and Public Health*, vol. 2016, Article ID 6458283, pp. 1–11, 2016.

[14] J. Kitui, S. Lewis, and G. Davey, "Factors influencing place of delivery for women in Kenya: an analysis of the Kenya demographic and health survey, 2008/2009," *BMC Pregnancy and Childbirth*, vol. 13, article 40, 2013.

[15] J. Bongaarts, "WHO, UNICEF, UNFPA, World Bank Group, and United Nations Population Division Trends in Maternal Mortality: 1990 to 2015 Geneva: World Health Organization, 2015," *Population and Development Review*, vol. 42, no. 4, pp. 726–726, 2016.

[16] Adjiwanou Vissého. and LeGrand Thomas, "Does antenatal care matter in the use of skilled birth attendance in rural Africa? a multi-country analysis," *Social Science Medicine*, vol. 86, pp. 26–34, 2013.

Permissions

List of Contributors

Fabiola V. Moshi and Stephen M. Kibusi
School of Nursing and Public Health,The University of Dodoma, Dodoma, Tanzania

Flora Fabian
School of Medicine and Dentistry, The University of Dodoma, Dodoma, Tanzania

Addisu Tesfaw
Gendewoyin Health center, Gonchasiso EneseWoreda, North West Ethiopia, Ethiopia

Dube Jara
Department of Public Health, College of Health Sciences, Debre Markos University, Debre Markos, Ethiopia

Habtamu Temesgen
Department of Human Nutrition and Food Science, College of Health Sciences, Debre Markos University, Debre Markos, Ethiopia

Eliphas Gitonga
School of PublicHealth, Kenyatta University,Nairobi, Kenya

Tenaw Gualu and Abebe Dilie
Department of Nursing, College of Health Sciences, Debre Markos University, Debre Markos, Ethiopia

Elizabeth AKu Baku
School of Nursing and Midwifery, University of Health and Allied Sciences, Ho, Volta Region, Ghana

Isaac Agbemafle
Department of Family and Community Health, School of Public Health, University of Health and Allied Sciences, Ho,Volta Region, Ghana

Agnes Millicent Kotoh
Department of Population, Family and Reproductive Health, School of Public Health, University of Ghana, Legon,Greater Accra Region, Accra, Ghana

Richard M. K. Adanu
Office of the Dean, School of Public Health, University of Ghana, Legon, Greater Accra Region, Accra, Ghana

Neko M. Castleberry
Research Department, American College of Obstetricians and Gynecologists (ACOG), 409 12th Street SW, Washington, DC 20024, USA

Katherine M. Jones and Laura H. Taouk
Research Department, American College of Obstetricians and Gynecologists (ACOG), 409 12th Street SW, Washington, DC 20024, USA
Department of Psychology, American University, 4400 Massachusetts Avenue NW, Washington, DC 20016, USA

Michele M. Carter
Department of Psychology, American University, 4400 Massachusetts Avenue NW, Washington, DC 20016, USA

Jay Schulkin
Department of Obstetrics and Gynecology, University of Washington School of Medicine, Seattle, WA 98195, USA

Yohannes Mehretie Adinew and Shimelash Bitew Workie
College of Health Sciences and Medicine, Wolaita Sodo University, Wolaita Sodo, Ethiopia

Senafikish Amsalu Feleke and Zelalem Birhanu Mengesha
Department of Reproductive Health, Institute of Public Health, University of Gondar, Gondar, Ethiopia

John C. Ssempebwa and GeofreyMusinguzi
Department of Disease Control and Environmental Health, School of Public Health, College of Health Sciences, Makerere University, Kampala, Uganda

Simon Peter Sebina Kibira
Department of Community Health and Behavioural Sciences, School of Public Health, College of Health Sciences, Makerere University, Kampala, Uganda

Matilda Kweyamba
Cornerstone Surgery, Kampala, Uganda
School of Public Health, Makerere University College of Health Sciences, Kampala, Uganda

Esther Buregyeya and Aggrey David Mukose
School of Public Health, Makerere University College of Health Sciences, Kampala, Uganda

Joy Kusiima
FETP Fellowship Program, Uganda Cancer Institute, Kampala, Uganda

Vianney Kweyamba
Department of Surgery, Naguru Regional Referral Hospital, Kampala, Uganda

Menberu Molla
Save the Children International,West Amhara, Bahir Dar, Ethiopia

Tadese Ejigu
School of Public Health (SPH), College of Medicine and Health Sciences, Bahir Dar University, Bahir Dar, Ethiopia

Girma Nega
School of Food and Chemical Engineering, Department of Applied Nutrition, Bahir Dar University, Bahir Dar, Ethiopia

Mamo Nigatu, Tsegaye Tewelde Gebrehiwot and Desta Hiko Gemeda
Department of Epidemiology, Institute of Health, Jimma University, Jimma, Ethiopia

Eric Badu
Centre for Disability and Rehabilitation Studies, Kwame Nkrumah University of Science and Technology, Kumasi, Ghana
The University of Newcastle, Callaghan, NSW, Australia

Peter Agyei-Baffour
Department of Health Policy, Management and Economics/School of Public Health, Kwame Nkrumah University of Science and Technology (KNUST), Kumasi, Ghana
Isaac Ofori Acheampong St. John of God Nursing Training College, Ministry of Health, Sefwi Asafo, Western Region, Ghana

Maxwell Preprah Opoku
University of Tasmania, Hobart, TAS, Australia

Kwasi Addai-Donkor
Ghana Health Service, Kwame Nkrumah University of Science and Technology, Kumasi, Ghana

Freda Intiful, Claudia Osei, Rebecca Steele-Dadzie, Ruth Nyarko and Matilda Asante
School of Biomedical and Allied Health Sciences, Department of Nutrition and Dietetics, University of Ghana, Accra, Ghana

Mengesha Boko Geta
Kebado Primary Hospital, Hawassa, Ethiopia

Walelegn Worku Yallew
Institute of Public Health, College of Medicine and Health Sciences, University of Gondar, Gondar, Ethiopia

Yetnayet Abebe Weldsilase, Tolossa Wakayo and Mulusew Gerbaba
Jimma University, Institute of Health Sciences, Department of Population and Family Health, Ethiopia

Melaku Haile Likka
Jimma University, Institute of Health Sciences, Department of Health Economics, Management and Policy, Ethiopia

R. Constance Wiener
Department of Dental Practice and Rural Health, School of Dentistry, 104A Health Sciences Addition, West Virginia University, Morgantown,WV 26506-9448, USA

Nilanjana Dwibedi and Usha Sambamoorthi
Department of Pharmaceutical Systems and Policy,West Virginia University School of Pharmacy, Robert C. Byrd Health Sciences Center [North], Morgantown,WV 26506-9510, USA

Chan Shen
Departments of Health Services Research and Biostatistics, University of Texas MD Anderson Cancer Center, 1400 Pressler St., Houston, TX 77030, USA

Patricia A. Findley
Rutgers University, School of SocialWork, 536 George Street, New Brunswick, NJ 08901, USA

Kasu Tola, Haftom Abebe and Yemane Gebremariam
Mekelle University College of Health Sciences School of Public Health, Mekelle, Ethiopia

Birhanu Jikamo
Hawassa University College of Medicine and Health Sciences School of Public and Environmental Health, Hawassa, Ethiopia

Mekdes Mekonnen, Tsigereda Behailu and Negash Wakgari
School of Nursing and Midwifery, College of Medicine and Health Sciences, Hawassa University, Hawassa, Ethiopia

Gertrude Nancy Annan
Nursing and Midwifery Training College, Kumasi, Ghana

Yvonne Asiedu
SDA Midwifery Training College, Asamang, Ghana

Kwamena Sekyi Dickson
Department of Population and Health, College of Humanities and Legal Studies, University of Cape Coast, Cape Coast, Ghana

Hubert Amu
Department of Population and Behavioural Sciences, School of Public Health, University of Health and Allied Sciences, Hohoe, Ghana

Svetla Gadzhanova and Elizabeth Roughead
Quality Use of Medicines and Pharmacy Research Centre, University of South Australia, Australia

Demis Berhan and Hanna Gulema
Addis Continental Institute of Public Health, Addis Ababa, Ethiopia

Sameera Senanayake and Ayesha Lokubalasooriya
Family Health Bureau, Ministry of Health, Sri Lanka

Shanthi Gunawardena
Non-Communicable Diseases Unit, Ministry of Health, Sri Lanka

Mahesh Kumbukage and Champika Wickramasnghe
Ministry of Health, Sri Lanka

Nalika Gunawardena
World Health Organization, Sri Lanka

Renuka Peiris
Ministry of Education, Sri Lanka

Wollelaw Getnet
Amhara Regional Health Bureau, Debre Markos Referral Hospital, East Gojjam Zone, Debre Markos, Ethiopia

Wubie Aycheh and Taddele Tessema
Department of Public Health, College of Health Science, Debre Markos University, Debre Markos, Ethiopia

Eliphas Gitonga
School of PublicHealth, Kenyatta University,Nairobi, Kenya

Index